TUBERCULOSIS
An Interdisciplinary Perspective

TUBERCULOSIS
An Interdisciplinary Perspective

Edited by

John D H Porter
London School of Hygiene and Tropical Medicine, UK

John M Grange
Imperial College School of Medicine, National Heart and Lung Institute, UK

Imperial College Press

Published by

Imperial College Press
57 Shelton Street
Covent Garden
London WC2H 9HE

Distributed by

World Scientific Publishing Co. Pte. Ltd.

P O Box 128, Farrer Road, Singapore 912805

USA office: Suite 1B, 1060 Main Street, River Edge, NJ 07661

UK office: 57 Shelton Street, Covent Garden, London WC2H 9HE

Library of Congress Cataloging-in-Publication Data
Tuberculosis : an interdisciplinary perspective / editors, John D. H.
  Porter, John M. Grange.
      p.   cm.
  Includes bibliographical references.
  ISBN 1-86094-143-5
    1. Tuberculosis.   2. Tuberculosis -- Government policy.
  3. Tuberculosis -- Epidemiology.   I. Porter, John D. H.   II. Grange,
  John M.
  RA644.T7T726   1999
  362.1'96995--dc21   98-43593
                                                                CIP

British Library Cataloguing-in-Publication Data
A catalogue record for this book is available from the British Library.

First published 1999
Reprinted 1999

Printed in Singapore.

PREFACE

Tuberculosis presents the global health care community with a paradox — the development of modern short course chemotherapy is one of the greatest triumphs of 'evidence-based' medical science as it is not only one of the most effective, but also one of the most cost-effective of all known therapies. Yet, far from being conquered or even controlled, tuberculosis is currently the most prevalent infectious cause of human suffering and mortality and, in 1993, the World Health Organization took the unprecedented step of declaring it a 'Global Emergency'. For the sake of the millions who suffer and die from this preventable and curable affliction each year, it is essential that we look carefully at the reason for the paradox and seek novel ways of addressing this major public health problem, even if this means challenging the very axioms and structures on which current health care practices are based.

The principal theme of this book is evident in its title 'Tuberculosis — An Interdisciplinary Perspective'. A wide range of disciplines is represented, including clinical medicine, social science, epidemiology, health policy, economics, nursing, education, ethics and history. By bringing together different academic disciplines to address a health issue such as tuberculosis, we are provided with an opportunity to study and understand different perspectives and approaches and, thereby, through a different vision, to approach the global issues of disease control in perhaps more creative and effective ways.

Interdisciplinary collaboration is, however, not the only theme in this book. As we read each of the chapters, we were struck by the other major themes that emerged: poverty, vulnerability, health care structures, globalisation, transcultural issues and the uneasy relation between quantitative and qualitative research methodology. It is apparent that perspectives on health are changing and that there is an increasing awareness that an overarching and all-embracing concept of health can help to link people working in different disciplines and even in different sectors. There is, within the field of public health, the increasing realisation that it is not sufficient merely to prevent disease, but that we need to be involved in the active creation of health and 'healthy communities'.

A feature of this book is the interaction and cross-over of the disciplines that occur in each of the chapters. Although a person may, for example, be labelled as an epidemiologist, their writing indicates that they resort to other disciplines such as history and the qualitative methods of the social sciences to construct their arguments. Each chapter stands alone and there is thus an inevitable overlap. Nevertheless, the contexts are quite different, as are the processes that are described. They amply demonstrate the *complexity* of ideas expressed in the field of public health — a complexity which, though fascinating, often makes arguments difficult to understand. This complexity should, however, be seen positively and as an incentive to developing novel ways of working together. For this purpose, each of us needs to develop a clarity of vision and engage in 'healthy' debate in order to resolve any conflict that might ensue.

One possible area of conflict is between those who espouse the reductionist 'evidence-based' approach and those who advocate a more 'holistic' viewpoint. But there need be no conflict. Implicit throughout this book is the fundamental importance of modern short course therapy, and the vast amount of effort devoted to its development by many distinguished scientists over the last half century is in no way denigrated. Likewise, recent developments in immunology and molecular biology are to be welcomed as the likely key to much more effective preventive, diagnostic and therapeutic approaches. We do, however, agree with Sir Douglas Black (1998) that 'evidence-based' biomedicine is but one facet of the whole complex structure of modern medicine and not without its limitations in addressing major public health challenges. We also acknowledge the dangers of 'scientism', defined by Leggett (1997) as "an approach to medical practice that regards the scientific understanding of the disease as the only relevant issue, whilst ignoring any other factors". This belief system — and it is surely no more than a belief system — is firmly entrenched in many sectors of academic medicine and may prove to be a very powerful barrier to interdisciplinary communication and collaboration.

One of the represented disciplines, ethics, is a focus for the development of concepts, ideas and reasoning. Interestingly, the changes and shifts witnessed in health care and in public health are also occurring in the discipline of ethics. Over the last decade, in the field of bioethics for example, there has been an eclipse of 'foundationalist' projects aimed at the development of a moral theory capable of providing the framework for the deduction of principles and rules that could then be applied to particular cases. There has, in fact, been a shift away from the search for the foundations of morality towards a greater reliance upon the coherence of practical moral reasoning and common sense. According to Rawls, moral reasoning is based on the linkages between "a rich tapestry of principles, intuitions and norms" that together constitute a relatively stable, coherent, wide reflective equilibrium (Turner, 1998). Indeed, Murphy (1995) has remarked that "Bioethics seems to be shifting from the image of a layer cake, with theories supporting principles that justify rules which lead to particular conclusions in specific cases, towards the image of the web, where the web consists of a rich, 'thick' body of maxims, rules and norms that are a matter of shared public reason". The various strands of this web are mutually strengthening, with no one aspect providing a 'foundation' for the other components.

This book provides us with a web of complexity — a mosaic — around the subject of tuberculosis. All of those who have contributed have provided us with a "rich tapestry of principles, intuitions and

norms" that can facilitate the development of a structure for tuberculosis control that is part of the overall public health goal of 'creating
health' and 'healthy communities'. Rhetoric, however, is not enough.
To create this process we need to engage in debate and, possibly, conflict, with a clear understanding of who we are and of the power vested
in our roles as health professionals and how this power can be used
to a positive or negative effect. We are living in a time of complexity
and change — the expression 'paradigm shift' is often heard today —
and, far from being led to despair, we are provided with an opportunity
to challenge axioms and dogmas and to create novel approaches to the
control of tuberculosis to the betterment of the health of communities
worldwide.

We hope you enjoy reading this book. We feel that it is an important
contribution to the subject of tuberculosis and we hope that it will also
be of use to people working in many different disciplines of health care.

John Porter and John Grange
August 1998

References

Black D. 1998. The limitations of evidence. *J. R. Coll. Phys. Lond.* **32**, 23–26.
Leggett JM. 1997. Medical scientism: good practice or fatal error? *J. R. Soc. Med.*
90, 97–101.
Turner L. 1998. An anthropological exploration of contemporary bioethics: The va-
rieties of common sense. *J. Med. Ethics.* **24**, 127–133.
Murphy N. 1995. Postmodern non-relativism: Imre Lakatos, Theor Meyerling and
Alasdair MacIntyre. *Philosoph. Forum* **27**, 37–53.

CONTENTS

AUTHORS

Fazle H. Abed
Executive Director, BRAC, 75 Mohakhali, Dhaka 1212, Bangladesh.

Ruairí Brugha
Department of Public Health Policy, London School of Hygiene and Tropical Medicine, Keppel Street, London WC1E 7HT, United Kingdom.

A. M. R. Chowdhury
Director, Research and Evaluation Division, BRAC, 75 Mohakhali, Dhaka 1212, Bangladesh.

Sadia Chowdhury
Director, Health and Population Division, BRAC, 75 Mohakhali, Dhaka 1212, Bangladesh.

Freda Festenstein
Imperial College School of Medicine, National Heart and Lung Institute, Dovehouse, London SW3 6LY, United Kingdom.

Susan Foster
Department of Public Health Policy, London School of Hygiene and Tropical Medicine, Keppel Street, London WC1E 7HT, United Kingdom. [Present address: Department of International Health, Boston University School of Public Health, 715 Albany Street, Boston MA 02118, USA.]

Virginia Gleissberg
Shrewsbury Centre, Shrewsbury Road, London E7 8QP, United Kingdom.

John M. Grange
Imperial College School of Medicine, National Heart and Lung Institute, Dovehouse Street, London SW3 6LY, United Kingdom.

Patricia Hudelson
Task Force on Gender Sensitive Interventions, Special Programme for Research and Training in Tropical Diseases (TDR), World Health Organization, Avenue Appia 20, CH-1211 Geneva 27, Switzerland.

Klaus Jochem
International Division, Nuffield Institute for Health, 71-75 Clarendon Road, Leeds LS2 9PL, United Kingdom

Peter Mwaba
Department of Medicine, University of Zambia School of Medicine, University Teaching Hospital, Lusaka, Zambia.

Ravi Narayan
Community Health Cell, No. 367, Srinivasa Nilaya, Jakkasandra, 1 Main, 1 Block, Koramangali, Bangalore – 560 034, India.

Thelma Narayan
Community Health Cell, No. 367, Srinivasa Nilaya, Jakkasandra, 1 Main, 1 Block, Koramangali, Bangalore – 560 034, India.

David Nyheim
FEWER — Forum on Early Warning and Early Response, FEWER, 1 Glyn Street, London SE11 5HT, United Kingdom.

Jessica A. Ogden
Department of Public Health Policy, London School of Hygiene and Tropical Medicine, Keppel Street, London WC1E 7HT, United Kingdom.

John Porter
Departments of Infectious and Tropical Diseases and Public Health Policy, London School of Hygiene and Tropical Medicine, Keppel Street, London WC1E 7HT, United Kingdom.

Paul Pronyk
Health Systems Development Unit, Northern Province of South Africa, Department of Community Health, University of Witwatersrand, Johannesburg, South Africa.

Sheela Rangan
Foundation for Research in Community Health, 84 QA R.G. Thadani Marg, Worli, Bombay 400018, India.

M. Angélica Salomão
Chief of the Division of Endemic Diseases, Ministry of Health, CP 264, Maputo, Mozambique.

Carolyn Stephens
Department of Public Health Policy, London School of Hygiene and Tropical Medicine, Keppel Street, London WC1E 7HT, United Kingdom.

Elizabeth Tayler
Global Tuberculosis Programme, World Health Organization, CH-1211 Geneva 27, Switzerland. Present address: Department for International Development, 94 Victoria St., London SW1E 5JL, UK

Mukund Uplekar
Foundation for Research in Community Health, 84 QA R.G. Thadani Marg, Worli, Bombay 400018, India.

Andrew Ustianowski
Centre For Infectious Diseases, University College London Medical School, Windeyer Building, 46 Cleveland Street, London W1P 6DB, United Kingdom.

J. Patrick Vaughan
Department of Public Health Policy, London School of Hygiene and Tropical Medicine, Keppel Street, London WC1E 7HT, United Kingdom.

John Walley
International Division, Nuffield Institute for Health, 71–75 Clarendon Road, Leeds LS2 9PL, United Kingdom.

Gill Walt
Department of Public Health Policy, London School of Hygiene and Tropical Medicine, Keppel Street, London WC1E 7HT, United Kingdom.

Alimuddin Zumla
Centre For Infectious Diseases, Royal Free and University College Medical School, Windeyer Building, 46 Cleveland Street, London W1P 6DB, United Kingdom.

Anthony Zwi
Department of Public Health Policy, London School of Hygiene and Tropical Medicine, Keppel Street, London WC1E 7HT, United Kingdom.

Acknowledgments

We wish to express our heartfelt thanks to all the authors for finding the time in their very busy professional lives to prepare their contributions. We hope that our readers are as impressed as we are with the quality of their writing and of the contents, as well as with their obvious dedication to, and enthusiasm for, their respective disciplines, and their openness to concepts from other disciplines.

Since 1995, the Department for International Development (DFID) of the United Kingdom has supported a 'Tuberculosis Research Programme' which links the London School of Hygiene and Tropical Medicine (LSHTM) and the Nuffield Institute for Health, Leeds. Much of the creation and development of this book has come from work within this programme and also from the previous DFID AIDS Research programme at the LSHTM (1990–1995), which supported the development of work in Africa on the interaction between tuberculosis and HIV infection. We would like to thank DFID for its support and continued interest in interdisciplinary research work on tuberculosis.

Finally, we would like to thank Andrea Darlow and Helen Pennel for the book cover and we gratefully acknowledge the friendliness, helpfulness, encouragement and patience of Geetha Nair and Joy Marie Tan at Imperial College Press.

PART I

INTRODUCTION TO TUBERCULOSIS AND ITS CONTROL

CHAPTER 1

THE GLOBAL BURDEN OF TUBERCULOSIS

John M. Grange

Introduction

Tuberculosis has long ranked among the most feared and dreaded of all of the many afflictions of the human race and names for the disease such as John Bunyan's 'Captain of all of these Men of Death' truly reflect its unenviable reputation in days gone by. Tragically, though, the disease is still so prevalent that, in 1993, 111 years after the causative organism was identified and half a century after the introduction of effective therapy, the World Health Organization (WHO) deemed it necessary to take the unprecedented step of declaring it a Global Emergency (World Health Organization, 1994a).

Although being among the most widespread and prevalent of the chronic diseases that plague mankind, the precise impact of tuberculosis on human health worldwide can only be estimated indirectly. Even in some developed nations, notification and record-keeping are far from being optimal (Sheldon *et al.*, 1992), while in many regions where the burden of tuberculosis is high disease surveillance is rudimentary. Surveys of the prevalence of the disease based on case-finding and bacteriological surveys are notoriously unreliable as they are critically dependent on the quality of medical services and diagnostic facilities. In 1994, 3.3 million cases of tuberculosis worldwide were notified whereas, as outlined below, the estimated total number of cases was between two and three times higher.

A major problem faced by epidemiologists is the complex 'timetable' of human tuberculosis. Infection by the tubercle bacillus induces certain immunological changes, notably a conversion to dermal reactivity to tuberculin. From the results of tuberculin testing surveys, it has been estimated that about one third of the human population has been infected by the tubercle bacillus: approximately 2,000 million people (Kochi, 1991; Raviglione *et al.*, 1995; Raviglione and Luelmo, 1996; Raviglione and Nunn, 1997). It is assumed, though never formally proven, that all infected persons who convert to tuberculin positivity develop the so-called primary complex, consisting of a small lesion at the site of bacillary implantation (usually the lung) and enlarged regional lymph nodes. Dissemination of bacilli to other organs may occur via the lymphatic system or blood stream. In most cases, though, the primary complex remains undetected and the infected person never experiences the clinical features of tuberculosis.

There is indirect evidence that, in infected persons who do not succumb to primary tuberculosis, the disease enters a latent state and that bacilli remain within the tissues in a poorly understood 'persister' form (Grange, 1992). These quiescent foci of infection can potentially reactivate at any time during the remainder of the infected person's life. For many years it was dogmatically asserted that, once infected, a person was protected against exogenous reinfection so that all tuberculosis developing later in life was due to endogenous reactivation. There is now, however, considerable evidence — some of it provided by the application of highly discriminative DNA 'fingerprinting' techniques — that exogenous reinfection does indeed occur in both immunosuppressed and non-immunosuppressed persons (Dwyer *et al.*, 1993; Small *et al.*, 1994; Marchal, 1997).

Not all those infected by the tubercle bacillus develop overt disease. Indeed, only a minority do so. The ratio of infection to development of overt tuberculosis is termed the *disease ratio*. As a general rule, about 5% of those infected develop so-called primary tuberculosis within five years of infection and a further 5% subsequently develop post-primary disease, giving a total of 10% (Raviglione and Nunn, 1997). The actual risk of developing tuberculosis after infection varies throughout life, but on average the annual risk is about 0.2%.

The disease ratio shows some regional variation and, as discussed below, it is much higher in the presence of certain predisposing factors, notably human immunodeficiency virus (HIV) infection. In addition, neonates and infants are more likely to develop overt tuberculosis following infection. There have been many attempts to link susceptibility to tuberculosis to race and ethnicity, but numerous confounding factors such as differing socio-economical and environmental conditions render such analyses very difficult. Although this issue awaits clarification, it appears that genetic factors play only a minor role in determining susceptibility to this disease.

Overt primary tuberculosis is the result of either local complications of the primary complex or of non-pulmonary lesions resulting from blood-borne dissemination to other organs. In both cases, the bacilli are unable to escape from the lesions so that the patients are usually not infectious.

Post-primary disease, by contrast, usually involves the lung, irrespective of the site of the initial infection, and the gross tissue destruction characteristic of this form of the disease causes the formation of well-oxygenated cavities that favour the growth of bacilli and facilitate their access to the sputum. Thus, patients with post-primary lesions are often infectious and are said to have 'open' tuberculosis. There is a close relationship between 'smear positivity', i.e. the presence of enough acid-fast bacilli in the sputum (at least 5,000 bacilli per ml) for them to be detected microscopically, and infectivity (Rouillon *et al.*, 1976). The relative infectivity of smear-positive and negative-patients is shown in Table 1. Sputum microscopy therefore plays a key role in disease control by providing a rapid, robust, sensitive and specific means of detecting infectious patients in a community.

As infection by the tubercle bacillus leads to conversion to tuberculin positivity, skin testing surveys are used to determine the *annual infection rate*, or *annual risk of infection*, in a community (Enarson and Rouillon, 1998). Ideally, representative groups from the population

J. M. Grange

Table 1. Prevalence of infection by the tubercle bacillus according to closeness of contact. Data from a study in the Netherlands. Data from Rouillon *et al.* (1976).

Microscopical status of source case sputum	% subjects infected among contacts of source case		
	At home (n = 858)	Near relative or friend (n = 4207)	Colleague at work (n = 3931)
Smear positive	20.2	3.7	0.3
Smear negative	1.1	0.2	0.0

should be tested at yearly intervals in order to determine the number of persons who actually convert from negative to positive in a given year. This approach is, however, usually impractical and indirect estimates of the annual infection rate are arrived at by testing a group of similar age range, such as military recruits, or even a population of mixed ages, provided the average age is known. Owing to serious methodological problems, such estimates must be interpreted with caution (Rieder, 1995).

The Global Burden of Tuberculosis

As the annual risk of a tuberculin-positive person developing active tuberculosis is about 0.2%, data on the annual infection rate from many countries can be used, subject to the methodological problems discussed above, to calculate the total number of new cases of tuberculosis developing from the infected pool each year. According to the WHO, the numbers of new cases in 1990 and 1995 were 7.5 million and 8.8 million respectively and the numbers are predicted to rise to 10.2 million by the year 2000, a 37% increase from the 1990 estimate (Dolin *et al.* 1994; Raviglione and Nunn, 1977). Some authorities, such as Enarson and Rouillon (1998), regard the WHO figures for incidence and deaths as an overestimate. Using modified methods, the WHO estimate for 1997 was

Table 2.   The global toll of tuberculosis in 1997. Adapted from the World Health
Organization (1998).

Region	Persons infected	Incidence (New cases)	Prevalence	Deaths
Africa	293,000,000	1,650,000	3,586,000	,770,000
Americas	237,000,000	448,000	988,000	160,000
Eastern Mediterranean	161,000,000	427,000	1,035,000	173,000
Europe	205,000,000	342,000	710,000	118,000
South-East Asia	704,000,000	2,800,000	6,553,000	1,095,000
Western Pacific	610,000,000	1,583,000	3,429,000	591,000
Total	2,210,000,000	7,250,000	16,301,000	2,907,000

slightly lower, at 7.3 million (World Health Organization, 1998). The
geographical distribution of the patients in 1997 is shown in Table 2.

Being a very chronic disease with a clinical course often lasting well
over a year, except in the case of the minority of patients who have
access to good diagnostic facilities and adequately-supervised therapy,
the number of people with active tuberculosis at a given time (the *point
prevalence*) is about double the annual incidence of new cases and may
therefore be as high as 16 million (World Health Organization, 1998).
Roughly half of these patients have open or infectious pulmonary tuberculosis and may transmit the infection to others. If the average number
of persons infected by one infectious patient (the *contagion parameter*)
and the annual rate of infection are known, the number of infectious
cases in a community may be calculated. In practice, the contagion
parameter is not easily estimated and, depending on the region and
socio-economic factors such as overcrowding, may vary from two to 20.

In most countries of the world, tuberculosis ranks high among the
major causes of illness and death, as shown in Table 3 which lists the
ten leading causes of mortality worldwide. Infectious diseases are, collectively, the commonest cause of mortality in the world today, accounting
for around one third of all deaths. Infectious diseases are relatively well
controlled in the industrialised nations, but 'lifestyle plagues' such as

Table 3. The leading causes of mortality worldwide. Data from World Health Organization, Annual Report, 1997.

Disease	Number of deaths annually (millions)
Coronary heart disease	7.2
Cancer (all types)	6.3
Cerebrovascular (stroke)	4.6
Acute lower respiratory tract infection	3.9
Tuberculosis	3.0
Chronic obstructive pulmonary disease	2.9
Diarrhoea (including dysentery)	2.5
Malaria	2.1
HIV/AIDS	1.5
Hepatitis B	1.2

cancer, heart disease, stroke and chronic lung disease, resulting largely from smoking, poor diet and stress, are an increasing cause of morbidity and mortality. The WHO has predicted that the developing world will experience an increase in such conditions in addition to their burden of infectious disease. Tuberculosis is estimated to be responsible for between 2.2 and three million deaths annually, including at least 100,000 children in whom — after malaria, acute respiratory and gastrointestinal disease — it is a leading cause of mortality. Amongst infectious agents, tuberculosis is the single most important cause of adult death, killing more people than AIDS, malaria and other tropical diseases together, and is the cause of 7% of all adult deaths and 26% of *preventable* adult deaths. The impact of tuberculosis can also be assessed by calculating the number of years of healthy life that are lost. This is expressed as disability-adjusted life years (DALY). Of all DALYs lost as a result of disease worldwide, tuberculosis accounts for 7% among women, and 8.4% among men, in those aged between 15 to 49 years (Raviglione and Luelmo, 1997).

The Resurgence of Tuberculosis

Tuberculosis is a resurgent disease in most regions of the world. Until the 1980s, the incidence of the disease remained steady or showed a slight decline in the developing nations, but since that time increases have been reported in many nations as a result of the HIV/AIDS pandemic. There has also been an absolute increase in prevalence as a result of the rapid increase in the population size.

There has also been an increase in the incidence of the disease in developed nations since the mid 1980s, but this must be seen in the perspective of a very low incidence compared with that of the developing nations. Nevertheless, the apparent return of a disease regarded by many as being almost extinct caused considerable consternation and fear among the medical profession and the general public, particularly in the USA as a result of a number of widely-publicised outbreaks in New York City (see below). This resurgence has been attributed to a combination of the HIV/AIDS pandemic, increasing inner city deprivation, the arrival of immigrants and refugees from countries with a high incidence of tuberculosis, a dismantling of surveillance and contact-tracing services, and a loss of diagnostic awareness and clinical skills (Reichman, 1991).

As a result of these and other factors, it is likely that the overall prevalence of tuberculosis will increase for the foreseeable future unless there are radical changes in the global effort to control this disease. The WHO has calculated that, in the absence of such changes, there will be 90 million new cases of tuberculosis and 30 million deaths in the final decade of the millennium and that the annual mortality could rise to four million by the year 2004.

Although not as common a cause of death as cardiovascular disease and cancer, tuberculosis differs from the former in that a highly effective treatment is available and that, by detecting infectious cases and rendering them non-infectious by such treatment, transmission could be prevented and the global burden of this disease thereby considerably reduced. Furthermore, as many patients with tuberculosis are young, and as therapy usually enables them to return to an active and economically-productive life, often with no residual morbidity or disability, tuberculosis ranks among the most cost effective of all diseases to treat (Murray *et al.*, 1990). Indeed, it has been estimated that each year of life saved by effective anti-tuberculosis chemotherapy costs 90 US cents (about 60 UK pence).

The Impact of Control Measures

Effective therapy has, unfortunately, been the exception rather than the rule due to poor supervision of the patients. Although it might be argued that inefficient treatment services are better than none at all, poor therapy may actually be counterproductive for two reasons. First, repeated relapses of the disease prolongs the period of infectivity and facilitates spread of infection and, secondly, it favours the generation of drug- and multidrug-resistance.

In view of encouraging experiences in several countries, notably China (China Tuberculosis Control Collaboration, 1996) and Bangladesh (Chowdhury *et al.*, 1997) the WHO (World Health Organization, 1997a) has stressed that all anti-tuberculosis therapy should be administered under direct observation within the DOTS (Directly Observed Therapy, Short Course) strategy (Chapter 5). Owing to a number of restrictive factors, notably underfunding, only 10% of all cases of tuberculosis receive such therapy (World Health Organization, 1997a). The coverage of DOTS is summarised by the WHO region in Table 4, although within each of these regions the country-to-country variation in coverage varies enormously from almost total coverage to none at all.

Somewhat surprisingly, although a high percentage of patients in the Netherlands, Portugal, Slovenia and the Czech Republic receive DOTS, this strategy does not appear to be used to a significant extent in the European region, including most member states of the European Union. Coker and Miller (1997) have stated that DOTS cannot be implemented effectively in Britain owing to a national shortage of clinical nurse specialists and an unwillingness or inability of district nurses to take on this service.

Table 4. Number and percentage of cases of tuberculosis patients receiving directly observed therapy, short course (DOTS). Data from the World Health Organization.

Region	Total cases (reported and estimated)	Patients receiving DOTS Number	Percentage
Africa	1,285,300	301,113	23
Americas	488,900	67,035	14
Eastern Mediterranean	536,400	55,829	10
Europe	428,200	12,352	3
South-East Asia	3,057,500	46,798	2
Western Pacific	1,636,700	232,813	14
Total	7,433,000	715,940	9.6

Natural Trends in the Epidemiology of Tuberculosis

An understanding of the natural behaviour of tuberculosis in the community is essential for the design and evaluation of control programmes. Tuberculosis has afflicted the human population since the dawn of recorded history and characteristic bone lesions have been found in Egyptian mummies and in skeletons of pre-Columbian Indians in South America (Clark *et al.*, 1987). From the limited historical evidence, it appears that the disease occurred sporadically until populations aggregated in towns and cities, with associated overcrowding and urban squalor. In many industrialised countries, tuberculosis was very common during the middle decades of the 19th century, after which it declined at an annual rate of 1–2%. At the peak of such epidemics, many young people were affected but as the incidence declined, the average age of patients increased. In developing countries, where the prevalence of tuberculosis is high, many more young people have the disease. In 1990, 77% of patients with tuberculosis in the developing world were under 50 years of age, compared to only 20% in most industrialised countries.

These observations have led to the frequently expressed notion that tuberculosis naturally occurs in waves, thereby implying the development of some form of herd immunity. There is, in fact, little evidence that such herd immunity develops and it is more likely that the decline is largely brought about by improvements in socio-economic factors, such as better working conditions and less overcrowding, which reduce the contagion parameter. If this is the case, there is no guarantee that the high incidence of tuberculosis seen in many of the poorer countries will decline significantly unless socio-economic conditions improve or unless more effective health measures are adopted — itself an important aspect of socio-economic development.

Likewise, hopes that the incidence of tuberculosis would continue to fall in developed nations until it eventually disappeared have not been realised. For the reasons outlined above, many developed countries have experienced an upsurge in the incidence of the disease since the 1980s. Effective chemotherapy was introduced in the developed countries at a time when the incidence of tuberculosis was rapidly declining and this appears to have led to over-optimistic expectations that 'scientific' interventions alone would lead to the elimination of tuberculosis. This, in turn, has led to an underestimation of the impact of changing socio-economic conditions on the natural history of the disease. In the centenary year of the discovery of the tubercle bacillus by Robert Koch, Waaler (1982) wrote that "without Koch's discovery, the socio-economic character of tuberculosis would have been clearer, and a demand for redistribution of the wealth of the community would have become a much more important issue".

The Impact of Poverty on Tuberculosis

Poverty, malnutrition and overcrowding have long been recognised as being among the principal predisposing factors for tuberculosis. As discussed above, improved socio-economic conditions contributed more to the dramatic decline in the prevalence of this disease in the industrialised countries from the late 19th century to the present time than medical interventions.

There is a clear association between socio-economic factors and the incidence of tuberculosis in England and Wales where, between 1980 and 1992, the incidence showed a 35% increase among the poorest 10% of the population, a 13% increase among the next poorest 20%, but no increase among the remaining, relatively more affluent, 70% (Bhatti *et al.*, 1995). In the city of Liverpool, the incidence of tuberculosis was significantly related to the Townsend and Jarman deprivation indices (Spence *et al.*, 1993), while in various districts of London the notification rate increased by 12% for each 1% rise in the numbers of persons living under overcrowded conditions, irrespective of their ethnic origin (Mangtani *et al.*, 1995). In the major cities of the UK and other industrialised countries there is a particularly high incidence of tuberculosis among single homeless people, among whom there is also a high incidence of alcoholism. This group of patients is notoriously difficult to treat as they have little confidence or trust in health workers and often abscond (Moore-Gillon, 1998; Citron, 1997).

In the USA, the recent epidemics of tuberculosis have principally affected the socio-economically underprivileged. In New York City, the incidence of tuberculosis, AIDS and death from all causes is much higher among those who receive welfare support and abuse drugs, alcohol or both (Friedman *et al.*, 1996). During an eight year study commencing in 1984, of 858 such persons aged between 18 and 64 years, 47 (5.5%) developed tuberculosis and 84 (9.8%) developed AIDS. A fifth of this population were dead by the end of the study period and infectious disease, principally tuberculosis, AIDS and pneumonia was the cause of 57% of these deaths. The annual incidence of tuberculosis in this group was almost 15 times that in the general population of New York City, and 70 times higher than the rate for the entire USA. Also, at an incidence of 744 per 100,000 of the population, it was very much higher than that encountered in most parts of the developing world. The high prevalence of tuberculosis in this disadvantaged population may be associated with a high prevalence of AIDS, which was ten times higher than in the general population.

The Impact of the HIV/AIDS Pandemic on Tuberculosis

Infection by HIV is now by far the most important of the factors predisposing to the development of overt tuberculosis in those infected by the tubercle bacillus. For this reason, Chretien (1990) referred to the combination of these pathogens as 'The Cursed Duet'.

The HIV pandemic is having three major effects on the behaviour of tuberculosis. It markedly increases the chance of an infected person developing overt disease, it leads to a considerable reduction in the time interval between infection and the manifestation of such disease and it modifies the clinical features of the disease, notably in the more profoundly immunosuppressed. A fourth, indirect and delayed effect is the increased transmission of the infection in the general population as a result of the greater numbers of source cases (Lienhardt and Rodrigues, 1997).

As described above, people infected by the tubercle bacillus have about a 10% chance of developing overt tuberculosis at some period later in their lives. If infected when young, this risk is spread over several decades. If, on the other hand, the infected person is also HIV positive, the chance of developing active tuberculosis is increased to 50% over what is often a considerably shortened life span. The *annual* risk of developing active tuberculosis in HIV-positive persons is between 8 and 10%, which is over 40 times greater than the risk in HIV-negative persons (Dolin *et al.*, 1994; Antonucci *et al.*, 1995). Put another way, a co-infected person has roughly the same chance of developing tuberculosis in a single year as a person infected only by *M. tuberculosis* has in their entire lifetime.

HIV-related tuberculosis may be the result of either primary infection of a previously uninfected person, endogenous reactivation of latent disease or an exogenous reinfection. The proportion of these three possibilities depends on the prevalence of infectious tuberculosis patients in a given community. In high prevalence regions where most at-risk people have been infected by the tubercle bacillus before they become HIV positive, the incidence of reactivation disease in such communities is relatively high. In regions where tuberculosis is an uncommon disease, and the risk of infection is therefore lower, it is more likely that tuberculosis will be due to primary infection occurring after HIV sero-conversion (Leitch *et al.*, 1995). The precise effect of HIV positivity on the risk of developing overt tuberculosis after primary infection is not known but observations on mini-epidemics among HIV-positive persons strongly indicate that the risk is very high (Communicable Disease Report, 1995).

The considerable shortening of the interval between infection and the development of overt tuberculosis has been demonstrated by a number of examples, confirmed by DNA fingerprinting or other bacteriological examinations, of clusters of HIV positive people developing extensive disease within a few months of exposure in a hospital to patients with open tuberculosis (Bouvet *et al.*, 1993; Kent *et al.*, 1994).

The impact of the HIV/AIDS pandemic on tuberculosis has been devastating. In 1994, it was estimated that 5.4 million people were infected with both HIV and *M. tuberculosis*: the global distribution of this dually infected population is shown in Table 5. By 1996 the number had risen to over six million (World Health Organization, 1996). Given that approximately 8% of dually infected people develop overt tuberculosis each year, it may be calculated that HIV was responsible for over half a million *additional* cases of tuberculosis in 1996. The number of additional cases in 1997 may have been much higher, possibly well over one million; as in December of that year it was estimated that the total number of HIV-positive people worldwide was 30.6 million and could rise to 40 million by the year 2000 (UNAIDS/WHO, 1997).

Owing to the global distribution of HIV infection, Africa is the continent most affected by HIV-related tuberculosis. In 1995, it was estimated that about 8% of cases of tuberculosis worldwide, and at least 20% of those in Africa, were HIV related. By the year 2000, 14% of all

J. M. Grange

Table 5. Estimated distribution of HIV-infected adults alive in mid 1994 and those also infected with *M. tuberculosis*. Data from the World Health Organization.

Region	Total HIV positive	Dually infected
Sub-Saharan Africa	8,000,000	3,760,000
North Africa/Middle East	100,000	23,000
Western Europe	450,000	49,000
Eastern Europe/Central Asia	50,000	9,000
Latin America/Caribbean	1,500,000	450,000
North America	800,000	80,000
East Asia/Pacific	50,000	20,000
South/South-East Asia	$> 2,500,000$	$> 1,150,000$
Australia	$> 20,000$	$> 4,000$
Total	c.13,500,000	c.5,600,000

cases of tuberculosis could be HIV related, accounting for 1.4 million cases worldwide and 600,000 cases in Africa alone (Dolin *et al.*, 1994).

In 1996, about 70% of all co-infected persons lived in sub-Saharan Africa and, as a result, many countries in that region are experiencing considerable increases in the prevalence of tuberculosis. The estimated one million cases in the region in 1990 is expected to double by the year 2000, and in ten studied countries there was a close relationship between the number of excess cases, based on pre-1985 trends, and the percentage of patients who were HIV positive (Cantwell and Binkin, 1997). In Tanzania, for example, patients with tuberculosis are between 5.4 and 7.1 times more likely to be HIV positive than the general population (Chum *et al.*, 1996). An association between tuberculosis and HIV positivity is also seen in children in Africa (Chintu and Zumla, 1997). In Lusaka, Zambia, 37% of children admitted to hospital with tuberculosis in 1990 were HIV positive, compared to 11% of those with other conditions. This increased to 56% in 1991 and 68.9% by 1992 (Luo *et al.*, 1994).

Although the burden of co-infection currently falls principally on Africa, the situation in Asia is very worrying as this is a region where two-thirds of all the people infected by *M. tuberculosis* live and where HIV infection is spreading more rapidly than anywhere else in the world. In South India, the incidence of HIV seropositivity in patients with pulmonary tuberculosis rose from 0.77% in 1991 to 3.4% in 1993 (Solomon *et al.*, 1995).

The future epidemiological behaviour of HIV-related tuberculosis will depend on the annual infection rate, particularly in the age group principally at risk from HIV, and the prevalence of HIV infection. Future trends in Africa have been predicted for four different scenarios (Schulzer *et al.*, 1992), as summarised in Table 6. In the worst-case scenario, which is certainly within the bounds of possibility, tuberculosis would affect up to one in 50 of the general population and one in 25 of the population particularly at risk annually.

Table 6. Estimated incidence rates (per 100,000) of tuberculosis in sub-Saharan Africa in the year 2000. Data from Schulzer *et al.* (1992).

Scenario:*	Smear-positive cases				Total cases			
	1	2	3	4	1	2	3	4
15–49 years	142	272	681	1,769	300	573	1,540	4,218
Percentage increase since 1980	59.5	52	280	888	67.5	60	330	1,078
Adjusted for total population	77	150	325	792	162	312	727	1,875
Percentage increase since 1980	40	36	195	620	47	42	230	752

*Scenario 1: 1% risk of tuberculosis infection in 1980, 45% tuberculosis infection prevalence and a 1989 HIV prevalence of 2%.
Scenario 2: 2%, 60%, 2%
Scenario 3: 2%, 60%, 10%
Scenario 4: 2%, 60%, 20%

The nature, presentation and clinical course of tuberculosis in HIV-positive patients differs from that in non-immunosuppressed patients (Festenstein and Grange, 1991). Although the disease in HIV-positive patients with relatively high CD4+ T cell counts may not differ substantially from that occurring in HIV-negative patients, atypical forms are frequently encountered in the more profoundly immunosuppressed.

In particular, the pulmonary cavitation characteristic of post-primary tuberculosis is unusual in those with CD4+ counts of less than $50/mm^3$. Instead, radiology often reveals rather nondescript spreading opacities (Daley, 1995). Disseminated disease is common and may manifest as asymmetrical lymphadenopathy or multi-organ involvement. The sputum of patients with HIV-related tuberculosis who do not show cavity formation is often negative on microscopy although the relationship between sputum negativity and non-infectiousness in HIV-positive patients may not be as straightforward as in those who are HIV negative. For practical purposes, it appears that the infectivity of the two groups of patients is similar (Nunn *et al.*, 1994). Assumptions of infectivity, or the lack of it, based on microscopy could have very serious consequences for other patients and health care workers, particularly in regions where many HIV-positive patients have multidrug-resistant tuberculosis.

Although tuberculosis in HIV positive patients responds bacteriologically to standard short course chemotherapy, provided that the bacilli are susceptible to the drugs, there is a high mortality rate both during and after treatment. Such patients are four times more likely to die than HIV-negative patients within a year of diagnosis, with many deaths occurring early during the course of chemotherapy. Although the details are far from clear, tuberculosis appears to accelerate the progression of HIV infection to the full picture of AIDS. Indeed, tuberculosis in any form is now an AIDS-defining condition in HIV-positive persons (Centers for Disease Control, 1993). This acceleration has been attributed to various forms of immunological synergy and it has been shown that the viral load, determined by detection of RNA copies of the HIV genome, may increase 160-fold when overt tuberculosis develops (Goletti *et al.*, 1996). The consequent foreshortening of life, despite adequate anti-tuberculosis chemotherapy, is a serious cause for concern and emphasises the need for more intensive research into ways of preventing the development of overt tuberculosis in co-infected persons.

The Growing Menace of Drug-Resistant Tuberculosis

The problem of treatment failure due to the emergence of drug resistance became apparent soon after the introduction of anti-tuberculosis chemotherapy and led to the universal advocation of multidrug regimens. Unfortunately, sub-optimal use of the available drugs has led to the widespread emergence of strains resistant to one or more of the first-line anti-tuberculosis drugs and, in some cases, to many of the second-line drugs as well. After the resurgence of tuberculosis caused by the HIV/AIDS pandemic, the world is now faced with the 'third epidemic' of drug- and multidrug-resistant disease (Neville *et al.*, 1994).

There are two forms of drug resistance — acquired and primary (or initial). Acquired resistance occurs as a result of sub-optimal drug regimens which permit the selective growth of drug-resistant mutants. Primary resistance is the result of infection by a tubercle bacillus already resistant to one or more drugs. These two forms of resistance have different epidemiological significances. A high incidence of acquired resistance indicates that drug regimens or supervision of therapy are at fault while the occurrence of primary resistance indicates that control of transmission of disease in the community is inadequate. Sequential selections of mutants results in the development of resistance to several drugs. Multidrug resistance (MDR) is defined by the WHO as resistance to the principal first-line drugs, isoniazid and rifampicin, with or without resistance to other drugs (Kochi *et al.*, 1993).

There are many reasons, almost all avoidable, for the development of drug resistance. These include intermittent drug supplies, unavailability of combination preparations, poorly-formulated combination preparations, use of time-expired drugs, inappropriate prescribing, poor supervision of therapy and unregulated over-the-counter sale of drugs. In respect to the latter, cough mixtures containing isoniazid are readily available without prescription in some countries. A common iatrogenic cause of drug resistance is the addition of a single drug to a failing regimen in the absence of bacteriological control. It is usually assumed that drug resistance does not develop if the patient receives combination preparations of drugs, but Mitchison (1998) has described cases, and explanations, of multidrug resistance arising in patients who take such preparations irregularly and intermittently.

The determination of drug resistance is not easy as it requires laboratories able to isolate the tubercle bacillus and to perform the somewhat lengthy test procedures with good quality control (Vareldzis *et al.*, 1994; Collins *et al.*, 1997). Even in the best equipped centres, errors are not uncommon and may only become apparent if laboratory reports and clinical data are considered together (Nitta *et al.*, 1996). In addition, there are a variety of methods for drug susceptibility testing and there has been a lack of standardisation. For these reasons, information on the incidence of drug resistance worldwide is poorly documented. While the majority of clinical isolates in industrialised countries such as the USA and the UK are subjected to drug susceptibility testing by reliable procedures, surveys in many countries have been based on the testing of small and probably unrepresentative samples. This is evident from a comprehensive review of the world literature of drug resistance surveys carried out between 1985 and 1994 inclusive (Cohn *et al.*, 1997). In view of these problems, the WHO, in cooperation with the International Union Against Tuberculosis and Lung Disease, has established an extensive project on the global surveillance of drug resistance. This has involved the preparation of guidelines for standardised surveillance techniques and the establishment of a network of supra-national reference laboratories to coordinate surveillance and to provide technical aid (World Health Organization, 1994b, 1997b; Drobniewski *et al.*, 1997).

Estimates of the magnitude of the future problem of drug resistance and the cost of managing it are rendered very difficult by the lack of firm epidemiological data on the present incidence. Thus, an analysis of the available data gives a very broad range of possible scenarios. In sub-Saharan Africa, for example, the incidence of multidrug resistance per 100,000 of the population in the year 2000 could range from 2.3 to 32 (Carpels *et al.*, 1995). The latter figure, which is not improbable, implies that there could be as many as 250,000 cases in this region in the year 2000.

Multidrug resistance is not restricted to the developing nations only. A number of well-documented epidemics have occurred in New York City and other parts of the USA (Morse, 1994). Although the blame was laid on the HIV/AIDS pandemic, as over 40% of tuberculosis patients in New York City were HIV positive, this pandemic merely served to accelerate the spread of drug resistance generated by other factors. Thus, the incidence of drug-resistant tuberculosis had been rising in the USA before the occurrence of the HIV-related epidemics: the incidence of initial isoniazid resistance increased from less than 2% in 1968 to 9% in 1991, and rifampicin resistance increased from less than 1% in the period 1982–1986 to 4% in 1991. Almost a fifth of cases of tuberculosis in New York City were caused by multidrug-resistant bacilli in 1991, and 5% of patients were infected with bacilli resistant to six or seven drugs. Fortunately, the problem is a relatively localised one: more than 60% of all cases of multidrug-resistant tuberculosis occurring in the USA in 1994 were reported from New York City.

The cost of treating patients with multidrug-resistant tuberculosis in the USA is very high, sometimes exceeding $250,000, compared to $2,000 for treating a patient with the drug-susceptible disease. Even with very well-supervised therapy and good supportive care, the mortality is high. In some reports up to 45% of HIV-negative, and 85% of HIV-positive, patients die within two years of diagnosis. The prognosis for the patients, most of whom are HIV positive, with disease due to bacilli resistant to six or seven drugs is much worse: about half die within one month of diagnosis. On the other hand, early diagnosis of multidrug-resistant tuberculosis and treatment with at least two drugs to which the organism is susceptible has been reported to prolong life and improve the cure rate, even in severely immunosuppressed HIV-positive persons (Turett *et al.*, 1995).

As mentioned above, HIV infection is not *per se* a predisposing factor for the generation of multidrug resistance. The association between such resistance and HIV positivity, as has occurred in New York (Gordin *et al.*, 1996) and Ethiopia (Mitike, 1997), is probably coincidental. If multidrug-resistant tuberculosis enters a community in which many

HIV-positive persons are crowded together, e.g. in hospitals, prisons or common lodging facilities, then an epidemic of overt multidrug-resistant disease can rapidly develop. No such association is found in other countries such as South Africa (Anastasis et al., 1997) and Burkina Faso (Ledru et al., 1996).

The prevalence of drug resistance often varies considerably in different communities within a country. The example of the USA has been discussed above. Ethnic minority communities, originating in countries where drug resistance is common, often have higher levels of drug resistance than the indigenous populations. An example from South-East England is shown in Table 7 (Grange and Yates, 1993).

Table 7.   Prevalence of tuberculosis due to drug-resistant strains of M. tuberculosis in South-East England, 1984–1991. Data from Grange and Yates (1993).

Type of resistance	Ethnic origin of patients		
	European ($n = 4594$)	Indian subcontinent ($n = 4099$)	Others ($n = 625$)
1. Drug			
Isoniazid	60	119	16
Streptomycin	30	72	21
Pyrazinamide	15	12	2
Rifampicin	3	5	1
Ethambutol	1	–	–
2. Drugs			
Isoniazid + Streptomycin	16	83	22
Isoniazid + Rifampicin	4	4	4
Others	1	7	–
3. Drugs	1	28	1
4. Drugs	1	14	5
5. Drugs	1	3	1
6. Drugs	–	1	–
Total (percent) resistant	133 (2.9)	348 (8.5)	73* (11.7)

*35 African, 31 from the Far East and 7 others.

There is evidence that the incidence of drug-resistant tuberculosis in a community can be reduced by rigorous application of disease control measures. Thus, the incidence of initial single drug resistance declined from over 30% in 1980 to 15% in 1990 in South Korea and from 15% in 1981 to 6.3% in 1985 in Algeria (Vareldzis *et al.*, 1994). The impact of control measures on the incidence of multidrug resistance remains to be determined.

Bovine Tuberculosis and Implications for Human Health

It is generally forgotten nowadays that one of the most effective control measures ever undertaken for any bacterial disease was the virtual eradication of cattle tuberculosis in most developed countries (Moda *et al.*, 1996). Indeed, human tuberculosis caused by *M. bovis* (the bovine tubercle bacillus) in countries where such control measures have been applied successfully is extremely rare. In South-East England, *M. bovis* is responsible for less than 1% of all bacteriologically-confirmed cases of tuberculosis. Almost all patients were born before 1960, the year in which the bovine tuberculosis eradication programme was completed, and developed the disease as a result of late endogenous reactivation (Grange and Yates, 1994). The situation in the USA and most other European countries is very similar. There have been a few reports of human-to-cattle transmission of tuberculosis caused by *M. bovis* in Europe and there is limited and anecdotal evidence for human-to-human transmission but, as a general rule, this disease poses a minor and diminishing health problem in the developed world. Of more concern is the infection of cattle from wildlife reservoirs such as the badger in the UK and Ireland and the opossum in New Zealand (O'Reilly and Daborn, 1995). There have, however, been a few reports of the occurrence of tuberculosis due to *M. bovis* in younger HIV-infected persons, including a small but explosive epidemic of cases due to exposure to a source case in a hospital (Bouvet *et al.*, 1993).

Data on the incidence of cattle tuberculosis in countries in which little or no attempt to control the disease has been made are limited, although the disease is known to exist in 94 of 136 tropical countries

(Cosivi *et al.*, 1995). Information on the impact of such a disease on human health is even more limited, principally because few laboratories isolate tubercle bacilli and even fewer have the facilities or incentive to distinguish between the human and bovine types. Human tuberculosis due to *M. bovis* certainly occurs in the developing world, but few detailed epidemiological studies have been conducted (Cosivi *et al.*, 1998). There is a theoretical possibility that a high incidence of HIV infection could render communities more susceptible to the development of this form of tuberculosis after exposure to infectious cattle and that it might increase the risk of human-to-human transmission (Daborn *et al.*, 1996). Thus, further epidemiological studies on this form of tuberculosis in humans and a consideration of the cost effectiveness of programmes to eradicate it from cattle are required.

Comparison of the Problems of Tuberculosis Control Facing Industrialised and Developing Countries

The burden of tuberculosis is principally borne by developing nations where 95% of all cases of this disease and 98% of deaths due to it, occur.

Developing countries are faced with an enormous burden of disease of which tuberculosis, though one of the most prevalent, is nevertheless just one of many issues competing for very limited financial resources. In Uganda, for example, US$2.50 is spent annually per head of the population on health whereas US$30 is spent on paying interest on loans from the wealthier nations. In many countries, patients must pay for treatment and meet other expenses, such as travel to the health centre. Although the costs are small by Western standards, they may be very burdensome to poor people (Bevan, 1997). Successful tuberculosis control programmes based on subsidised directly observed therapy have been conducted in China and Bangladesh and a further one is in progress in India, but all are dependent on loans from the World Bank, thereby adding to the burden of international debt.

In industrialised countries, by contrast, tuberculosis has become an uncommon disease. Even though many such countries have experienced small increases in incidence since the mid 1980s, the number of cases remains very low relative to the developing world. The demographical characteristics of tuberculosis in industrialised countries have changed considerably during the course of the 20th century. As the incidence of the disease in the indigenous population has fallen, tuberculosis has become relatively more prevalent in certain minority groups, notably immigrant populations and refugee populations. As discussed in detail in Chapter 13, the management of the disease in these populations poses a considerable challenge to established medical practice, particularly with respect to effective communication. As a general principle, the impact of HIV-related tuberculosis has not been as evident as in developing nations as the majority of patients are not in the age group at risk of becoming infected with HIV, although important exceptions occur. The particular association between tuberculosis, socio-economic deprivation and HIV-related tuberculosis in New York City has been described above.

A further problem facing industrialised nations is generated by the very fact that tuberculosis is an uncommon disease. As discussed in a classic paper by Reichman (1991) entitled 'The U-shaped Curve of Concern', loss of interest in, and diagnostic awareness of, a disease that is both uncommon and declining in incidence is more or less inevitable. This leads to delays between the onset of symptoms and commencement of therapy (Pirkis *et al.*, 1996), a loss of clinical experience among physicians, a dismantling of dedicated treatment facilities and a reduction in screening and surveillance measures, thereby enabling the incidence of tuberculosis to rise unobserved until, as has happened in the USA, a serious outbreak jolts the medical profession out of complacency and into a state of concern. These problems are not easily resolved, especially as so many other medical problems clamour for the time of physicians in an increasingly complex and stressful environment in which financial constraint is a regrettable but unavoidable reality.

Conclusions

"If preventable, why not prevented?" This question was posed by King Edward VII when visiting a tuberculosis sanatorium several decades before the discovery of anti-tuberculosis drugs. It is a question that should rightly challenge the conscience of the world community today. Tuberculosis is among the most effective and cost effective of all diseases to treat yet it has been declared a global emergency. Clearly something is radically wrong with either the available therapy, the way in which it is administered or, more likely, the extent of interest, care, compassion and altruism shown by the wealthier nations — in which a mere 5% of cases of tuberculosis and 2% of deaths due to it occur — to those where the greatest burden of the disease falls. It is tempting for those in the industrialised countries to say 'tuberculosis is not our problem', but if potentially untreatable multidrug resistant forms of the disease continue to spread, and if HIV-related tuberculosis devastates the economies of the developing world, the global community will learn too late that it is everyone's problem. The WHO has stated that if it received funding equivalent to the cost of one jet fighter annually for ten years, the incidence of tuberculosis worldwide could be halved.

Obviously, the fight against tuberculosis would be greatly aided by the introduction of novel control measures, such as highly-effective vaccines and immunotherapeutic agents and improved diagnostic tests. However, we cannot wait for these innovations: there is a huge burden of unnecessary suffering to be addressed now, and this will take a much greater effort than we, as a global community, appear to be willing to make. It is worth bearing in mind the words of Dr. Arata Kochi, Manager of the World Health Organization Global Tuberculosis Programme: "The growing tuberculosis epidemic is no longer an emergency only for those who care about health, but for those who care about justice", and also the words of King Solomon (Proverbs 12:28): "Along the way of justice there is life."

References

Anastasis, D., Pillai, G., Rambiritch, V. and Abdool Karim, S. S. (1997) A retrospective study of human immunodeficiency virus infection and drug-resistant tuberculosis in Durban, South Africa. *Tubercle. Lung Dis.* 1, 220–224.

Antonucci, G., Girardi, E., Raviglioni, H. C. and Ippolito, G. (1995) Risk factors for tuberculosis in HIV-infected persons. A prospective cohort study. *J. Am. Med. Assoc.* **274**, 143–148.

Bevan, E. (1997) Tuberculosis treatment is expensive for patients in developing countries. *Br. Med. J.* **315**, 187–188.

Bhatti, N., Law, M. R., Morris, J. K., Halliday, R. and Moore-Gillon, J. (1995) Increasing incidence of tuberculosis in England and Wales: A study of the likely causes. *Br. Med. J.* **310**, 967–969.

Bouvet, E., *et al.* (1993) A nosocomial outbreak of multidrug-resistant *Mycobacterium bovis* among HIV-infected patients. A case-control study. *AIDS* **7**, 1453–1460.

Cantwell, M. F. and Binkin, N. J. (1997) Impact of HIV on tuberculosis in sub-Saharan Africa: A regional perspective. *Tubercle. Lung Dis.* 1, 205–214.

Carpels, G., *et al.* (1995) Drug resistant tuberculosis in sub-Saharan Africa: An estimation of incidence and cost for the year 2000. *Tubercle. Lung Dis.* **76**, 480–486.

Centers for Disease Control. (1993) The 1993 revised classification system for HIV infection and expanded surveillance case definition for AIDS among adolescents and adults. *Morb. Mort. Wkly. Rep.* **41–17**, 1–19.

China Tuberculosis Control Collaboration. (1996) Results of directly observed short-course chemotherapy in 112,842 Chinese patients with smear-positive tuberculosis. *Lancet* **347**, 358–362.

Chintu, C. and Zumla, A. (1997) Pediatric Tuberculosis and the HIV Epidemic. In: Zumla, A., Johnson, M., Miller, R. F., eds. *AIDS and Respiratory Medicine*. London: Chapman and Hall, pp. 153–163.

Chowdhury, A. M. R., Chowdhury, S., Islam, M. N., Islam, A. and Vaughan, J. P. (1997) Control of tuberculosis by community health workers in Bangladesh. *Lancet* **350**, 169–172.

Chretien, J. (1990) Tuberculosis and HIV. The cursed duet. *Bull. Int. Union Tuberc. Lung Dis.* **65**(1), 25–28.

Chum, H. J., O'Brien, R. J., Chonde, T. M., Graf, P. and Rieder, H. L. (1996) An epidemiological study of tuberculosis and HIV infection in Tanzania, 1991–1993. *AIDS* **10**, 299–309.

Citron, K. M. (1997) *Coming Out of the Shadow*. London: Crisis — Working for Homeless People.

Clark, G., Kelley, M., Grange, J. M. and Hill, C. (1987) A re-evaluation of the evolution of mycobacterial disease in human populations. *Curr. Anthropol.* **28**, 45–62.

Cohn, D. L., Bustreo, F. and Raviglione, M. C. (1997) Drug resistant tuberculosis: Review of the worldwide situation and the WHO/IUATLD global surveillance project. *Clin. Infect. Dis.* **24** (Suppl. 1), S121–S130.

Coker, R. and Miller, R. (1997) HIV associated tuberculosis. *Br. Med. J.* **314**, 1847.

Collins, C. H., Grange, J. M. and Yates, M. D. (1997) *Tuberculosis Bacteriology. Organization and Practice.* 2nd edn. Oxford: Butterworth-Heinemann.

Communicable Disease Report. (1995) Outbreak of hospital acquired multidrug resistant tuberculosis. *CDR Weekly* **5**(34), 161.

Cosivi, O., Meslin, F. X., Daborn, C. J. and Grange, J. M. (1995) Epidemiology of *Mycobacterium bovis* infection in animals and humans, with particular reference to Africa. *OIE. Sci. Tech. Rev.* **14**, 733–746.

Cosivi, O., *et al.* (1998) Zoonotic tuberculosis due to *Mycobacterium bovis* in developing countries. *Emerg. Infect. Dis.* **4**, 59–70.

Daborn, C. J., Grange, J. M. and Kazwala, R. R. (1996) The bovine tuberculosis cycle — an African perspective. *J. Appl. Bacteriol.* **81** (Symposium Supplement), 27S–32S.

Daley, C. L. (1995) The typically 'atypical' radiographic presentation of tuberculosis in advanced HIV disease. *Tubercle. Lung Dis.* **76**, 475–476.

Dolin, P. J., Raviglione, M. C. and Kochi, A. (1994) Global tuberculosis incidence and mortality during 1990–2000. *Bull. Wld. Hlth. Org.* **72**, 213–220.

Drobniewski, F., Pablos-Méndez, A. and Raviglione, M. C. (1997) Epidemiology of tuberculosis in the world. *Semin. Resp. Crit. Care. Med.* **18**, 419–429.

Dwyer, B., *et al.* (1993) DNA restriction fragment analysis to define an extended cluster of tuberculosis in homeless men and their associates. *J. Infect. Dis.* **167**, 490–494.

Enarson, D. A. and Rouillon, A. (1998) The Epidemiological Basis of Tuberculosis Control. In Davies, P. D. O., ed. *Clinical Tuberculosis*, 2nd edition. London: Chapman and Hall. pp. 36–52.

Festenstein, F. and Grange, J. M. (1991) Tuberculosis and the acquired immune deficiency syndrome. *J. Appl. Bacteriol.* **71**, 19–30.

Friedman, L. N., Williams, M. T., Singh, T. P. and Frieden, T. R. (1996) Tuberculosis, AIDS, and death among substance abusers on welfare in New York City. *New Engl. J. Med.* **334**, 828–833.

Goletti, D., *et al.* (1996) Effect of *Mycobacterium tuberculosis* on HIV replication. Role of immune activation. *J. Immunol.* **157**, 1271–1278.

Gordin, F. M., *et al.* (1996) The impact of human immunodeficiency virus infection on drug resistant tuberculosis. *Am. J. Resp. Crit. Care. Med.* **154**, 1478–1483.

Grange, J. M. (1992) The mystery of the mycobacterial persistor. *Tubercle. Lung Dis.* **73**, 249–251.

Grange, J. M. and Yates, M. D. (1993) Re-emergence of tuberculosis. *Br. Med. J.* **306**, 931–932.

Grange, J. M. and Yates, M. D. (1994) Zoonotic aspects of *Mycobacterium bovis* infection. *Vet. Microbiol.* **40**, 137–151.

Kent, R. J., Uttley, A. H., Stoker, N. G., Miller, R. and Pozniak, A. L. (1994) Transmission of tuberculosis in British centre for patients infected with HIV. *Br. Med. J.* **309**, 639–640.

Kochi, A. (1991) The global tuberculosis situation and the new control strategy of the World Health Organization. *Tubercle.* **72**, 1–6.

Kochi, A., Vareldzis, B. and Styblo, K. (1993) Multidrug-resistant tuberculosis and its control. *Res. Microbiol.* **144**, 104–110.

Ledru, S., et al. (1996) Impact of short-course therapy on tuberculosis drug resistance in South-West Burkina Faso. *Tubercle. Lung Dis.* **77**, 429–436.

Leitch, A. G., et al. (1995) Why disease due to *Mycobacterium tuberculosis* is less common than expected in HIV-positive patients in Edinburgh. *Resp. Med.* **89**, 495–497.

Lienhardt, C. and Rodriguez, L. C. (1997) Estimation of the impact of the human immunodeficiency virus infection on tuberculosis: Tuberculosis risks revisited? *Tubercle. Lung Dis.* **1**, 196–204.

Luo, C., et al. (1994) Human immunodeficiency virus type-1 infection in Zambian children with tuberculosis: Changing seroprevalence and evaluation of a thiacetazone-free regimen. *Tubercle. Lung Dis.* **75**, 110–115.

Mangtani, P., Jolly, D. J., Watson, J. M. and Rodrigues, L. C. (1995) Socioeconomic depravation and notification rate for tuberculosis in London 1982–91. *Br. Med. J.* **310**, 963–966.

Marchal, G. (1997) Recently transmitted tuberculosis is more frequent than reactivation of latent infections. *Tubercle. Lung Dis.* **1**, 192.

Mitchison, D. A. (1998) How drug resistance emerges as a result of poor compliance during short course chemotherapy for tuberculosis. *Int. J. Tuberc. Lung Dis.* **2**, 10–15.

Mitike, G., Kebede, D. and Yenneneh, H. (1997) HIV infection and antituberculosis drug resistance among pulmonary tuberculosis patients in Harar Tuberculosis Centre, Ethiopia. *East Afr. Med. J.* **74**(3), 154–157.

Moda, G., Daborn, C. J., Grange, J. M. and Cosivi, O. (1996) The zoonotic importance of *Mycobacterium bovis*. *Tubercle. Lung Dis.* **77**, 103–108.

Moore-Gillon, J. (1998) Tuberculosis and poverty in the developed world. In: Davies, P. D. O, ed. *Clinical Tuberculosis*, 2nd edition. London: Chapman and Hall. pp. 383–393.

Morse, D. L. (1994) Multidrug resistance. The New York experience. In: Porter, J. D. H, McAdam, K. P. W. J., eds. *Tuberculosis: Back to the Future*. Chichester: John Wiley, pp. 225–230.

Murray, C. J., Styblo, K. and Rouillon, A. (1990) Tuberculosis in developing countries: Burden, intervention and cost. *Bull. Int. Union Tuberc. Lung Dis.* **65**(1), 6–24.

Neville, K., et al. (1994) The third epidemic — multidrug-resistant tuberculosis. *Chest* **105**, 45–48.

Nitta, A. T., Davidson, P. T., De Koning, M. L. and Kilman, R. J. (1996) Misdiagnosis of multidrug tuberculosis possibly due to laboratory-related errors. *J. Am. Med. Assoc.* **276**, 1980–1983.

Nunn, P., *et al.* (1994) The effect of human immunodeficiency virus type-1 on the infectiousness of tuberculosis. *Tubercle. Lung Dis.* **75**, 25–32.

O'Reilly, L. M. and Daborn C. J. (1995) The epidemiology of *Mycobacterium bovis* infection in animals and man: A review. *Tubercle. Lung Dis.* **76** (Supplement): 1–46.

Pirkis, J. E., *et al.* (1996) Time to initiation of anti-tuberculosis treatment. *Tubercle. Lung Dis.* **77**, 401–406.

Raviglione, M. C., Snider, D. E. and Kochi, A. (1995) Global epidemiology of tuberculosis. Morbidity and mortality of a worldwide epidemic. *J. Am. Med. Assoc.* **273**, 220–226.

Raviglione, M. C. and Luelmo, F. (1996) Update on the global epidemiology of tuberculosis. *Curr. Iss. Publ. Hlth.* **2**, 192–197.

Raviglione, M. C. and Nunn, P. (1997) Epidemiology of Tuberculosis. In: Zumla, A., Johnson, M. A., Miller, R. F., eds. *AIDS and Respiratory Medicine*. London: Chapman and Hall, pp. 117–141.

Reichman, L. B. (1991) The U-shaped curve of concern. *Am. Rev. Resp. Dis.* **144**, 741–742.

Rieder, H. L. (1995) Methodological issues in the estimation of the tuberculosis problem from tuberculin surveys. *Tubercle. Lung Dis.* **76**, 114–121.

Rouillon, A., Perdrizet, S. and Parrot, R. (1976) Transmission of tubercle bacilli: The effects of chemotherapy. *Tubercle.* **57**, 275–799.

Schulzer, M., Fitzgerald, J. M., Enarson, D. A. and Grzybowski, S. (1992) An estimate of the future size of the tuberculosis problem in sub-Saharan Africa resulting from HIV infection. *Tubercle. Lung Dis.* **73**, 52–58.

Sheldon, C. D., King, K., Cock, H., Wilkinson, P. and Barnes N. C. (1992) Notification of tuberculosis: How many cases are never reported? *Thorax* **47**, 1015–1018.

Small, P. M., *et al.* (1994) The epidemiology of tuberculosis in San Francisco — A population-based study using conventional and molecular methods. *N. Engl. J. Med.* **330**, 1703–1709.

Solomon, S., Anuradha, S. and Rajasekaran, S. (1995) Trend of HIV infection in patients with pulmonary tuberculosis in South India. *Tubercle. Lung Dis.* **76**, 17–19.

Spence, D. P. S., Hotchkiss, J., Williams, C. S. D. and Davies, P. D. O. (1993) Tuberculosis and poverty. *Br. Med. J.* **307**, 759–761.

Turett, G. S., *et al.* (1995) Improved outcomes for patients with multi-drug resistant tuberculosis. *Clin. Infect. Dis.* **21**, 1238–1244.

UNAIDS/WHO. (1997) Fact sheet: *Report on the Global HIV/AIDS Epidemic, December 1997*. Geneva: World Health Organization. November 26th 1997.

Vareldzis, B. P., *et al.* (1994) Drug resistant tuberculosis: Laboratory issues. World Health Organization recommendations. *Tubercle. Lung Dis.* **75**, 1–7.

Waaler, H. T. (1982) Tuberculosis and socio-ecconomic development. *Bull. Int. Union Tuberc.* **57**, 202–205.

World Health Organization. (1994a) *TB — A Global Emergency.* Geneva: World Health Organization (WHO/TB/94.177).

World Health Organization. (1994b) *Guidelines for Surveillance of Drug Resistance in Tuberculosis.* Geneva: World Health Organization (WHO/TB/94.178).

World Health Organization. (1996) *Tuberculosis in the Era of HIV. A Deadly Partnership.* Geneva: World Health Organization (WHO/TB/96.204).

World Health Organization. (1997a) *Global Tuberculosis Control. WHO Report 1997.* Geneva: World Health Organization Global Tuberculosis Programme (WHO/TB/97.225).

World Health Organization. (1997b) *Anti-Tuberculosis Drug Resistance in the World. The WHO/IUATLD Project on Anti-Tuberculosis Drug Resistance Surveillance.* Geneva: World Health Organization Global Tuberculosis Programme.

World Health Organization. (1998) *The World Health Report 1998.* Geneva: World Health Organization.

CHAPTER 2

DETERMINANTS OF THE TUBERCULOSIS BURDEN IN POPULATIONS

Klaus Jochem and John Walley

Introduction — The Population Biology of Tuberculosis

In this chapter we review the dynamics of tuberculosis in populations and the risk factors for infection and disease in individuals.

There have, in the last two decades, been considerable conceptual advances in understanding the associations between infectious agents and host populations (Anderson and May, 1992). In terms of the population biology of an infectious agent, the most fundamental distinction is between those organisms that replicate within the host, such as most viruses and bacteria as well as many protozoa and fungi (classified as microparasites), and those parasites, including most helminths and arthropods that do not reproduce within the definitive host (classified as macroparasites). This classification of infectious agents into micro- and macroparasites is conceptual rather than taxonomic and is based on the observed similarities and differences in the interactions between various agents, the environment and their hosts.

For microparasites such as *Mycobacterium tuberculosis* (*M. tuberculosis*), the interaction with the host population can be described by a compartment model comprising, in its simplest form, three basic classes of individuals: susceptible, infected or immune (Fig. 1). Further compartments may distinguish between individuals who are infected but not

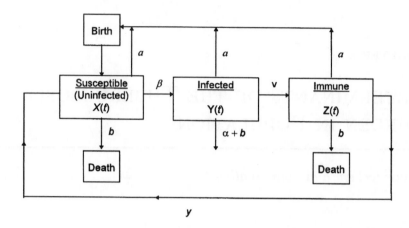

Fig. 1. Basic model for the interactions between microparasites and host populations. Schematic representation of the flow of hosts between susceptible $(X(t))$, infected $(Y(t))$ and immune $(Z(t))$ classes, which records the dynamic interaction between a directly transmitted microparasite and its host population. In this diagram hosts reproduce at a per capita rate, a, and die at a per capita rate, b. The infected hosts experience an additional death rate, α, induced by microparasitic infection. The average durations of stay in the infected and immune classes are denoted by $1/v$ and $1/y$, respectively. The transmission coefficient, which determines the rate at which new infections arise as a consequence of mixing between the susceptible and infected individuals, is defined by β. Source: Anderson and May (1992).

yet diseased and those who are diseased but not infectious. Immunity, following subclinical infection, overt disease, or a medical intervention such as BCG vaccination, may be limited in degree or duration.

Three important observations may be made about the population biology of microparasites such as *M. tuberculosis*. First, when an organism is in a state of equilibrium with its host population, each infection will on average produce one secondary infection. Where tuberculosis is endemic, it has been estimated that each untreated case of infectious tuberculosis will be responsible for 20 to 28 new infections and between 6 and 10% of these infections or re-infections will result in active disease, including one case of infectious tuberculosis, thereby maintaining the equilibrium (Sutherland and Fayers, 1975; Styblo, 1991; Murray *et al.*, 1990).

Secondly, that a state of equilibrium between the host population and organism will persist only if the rate at which susceptible individuals appear (either by birth, immigration, or lowered immunity) is balanced by the rate at which they are infected and develop disease capable of transmission. If, for instance, the infection rate of susceptibles decreases, then the organism will be unable in the long term to maintain itself in the population. In the case of tuberculosis, where transmission generally follows prolonged exposure in closed environments, a change in social organisation can have an impact on the infection rate. It is thought that reduced crowding, a smaller average family size, and better ventilation in households and workplaces, as well as the isolation of infectious cases in sanatoria, are some of the factors accounting for the decline of tuberculosis in industrialised countries during the century before the introduction of chemotherapy. The possibility of tuberculosis elimination through a reduction in transmission sufficient to alter the equilibrium in favour of the host was postulated 30 years ago by Frost (1937) when he wrote: "However, for the eventual eradication of tuberculosis, it is not necessary that transmission be immediately and completely prevented. It is necessary only that the rate of transmission be held permanently below the level at which a given number of infection spreading (i.e. open) cases succeed in establishing an equivalent number to carry on the succession".

The third observation is that the interaction between the host population and the organism will change if the average susceptibility of the host population to infection and disease changes. The degree to which changes in host susceptibility contributed to the dramatic decline in tuberculosis mortality and morbidity observed in industrialised countries before the introduction of chemotherapy has been a subject of speculation. In addition to the social factors contributing to reduced exposure to sources of infection, a higher level of innate immunity secondary to improved nutrition may have lowered both the susceptibility to infection and the susceptibility to active disease among those infected.

Others (Grigg, 1958) have argued that, since immunity has a genetic basis, the fall in tuberculosis mortality and morbidity observed in

Europe and North America in the century before chemotherapy represents the expected course of an epidemic which had selected a human population that survives because of an inherited resistance to tuberculosis. On theoretical grounds, Grigg postulated that the time course of tuberculosis death, disease and infection rates in a population would follow three epidemic curves staggered in time, each with a rapid rise and a slow decline that peaked successively at intervals spaced over several centuries. Tuberculosis mortality peaks first, reflecting the preferential elimination of those at highest susceptibility to the fatal disease; disease incidence, representing changes in the morbidity pattern in a population with an increasing average resistance to the development of active disease, reaches its peak later; and the prevalence of infection, reflecting the trends in transmission as the number of infectious cases falls, declines last.

The notion of epidemic waves of tuberculosis is supported by the incomplete data on trends in tuberculosis mortality and morbidity in Europe. Death rates in England probably neared their peak towards the end of the 18th century following rapid urbanisation during the industrial revolution, with annual deaths in excess of 500 per 100,000 population (Grigg, 1958; Dubos and Dubos, 1952). Mortality rates in England began to decline in the middle of 19th century (Wolff, 1926, quoted in Styblo, 1991) and had fallen to about 200 per 100,000 at the turn of the century and to about 50 per 100,000 by 1950. Although the introduction of effective chemotherapy in the 1950s hastened the decline in tuberculosis incidence and mortality, 90% of the decline had occurred in the century before the availability of curative drugs (Dubos and Dubos, 1952; Lowell et al., 1969).

Grigg concluded that the high death rates recorded in the first half of the 19th century would have been associated with an infection prevalence of close to 100% in the adult population. Infection prevalence remained high throughout the 19th century, though the annual risk of infection (ARI), or the probability that an individual will be infected (or reinfected) with M. tuberculosis in a given year, was declining. A recent extrapolation of transmission trends in England inferred from the association between fatal meningitis in children under five and the ARI observed in the Netherlands and Sweden in this century (Styblo *et al.*, 1969; Sjögren and Sutherland, 1975) suggests that the ARI was in the order of 19% in 1880, 12.7% in 1901 and only 1.9% by 1949 (Vynny-cky and Fine, 1997a). The population prevalence of infection remained high well into this century, despite the rapid decrease in the ARI. In the Netherlands in 1945, the estimated prevalence of infection was 57% and a similar value for England can be presumed (Styblo, 1991).

Changes in host immunity over time is one reason for a change in the risk of infection or disease. The second is changes in the organism. In general, variability in transmission rates observed in outbreaks have been largely attributed to the characteristics of the setting or infectious-ness of the source case. Variations in the virulence of strains of *M. tuberculosis* has been shown in animal models (Sultan *et al.*, 1960) but is difficult to document as an independent factor in human transmission. In a recent outbreak in the American states of Tennessee and Kentucky, in which unusually high rates of transmission were documented, it was possible to identify the infecting strain by genetic markers and com-pare its virulence in mice with other well-characterised strains, demon-strating that the high infectivity was associated with an accelerated replication of the organism in mice (Valway *et al.*, 1998). Because of aggressive contact tracing and the application of preventive treatment in those identified as infected by tuberculin skin testing, it is not clear whether the strain is characterised by a higher rate of disease in those infected. The term virulence is usually applied to the capacity of an organism to cause death or serious morbidity, and in the simplest mod-els of host–parasite interaction is assumed to be directly proportional to its rate of proliferation in the host (Levin, 1996). The relationship between infectivity (the ability to colonise a host), pathogenicity (the ability to cause clinical disease) and virulence (the ability to cause se-rious disease or death) may, however, be more complex and vary over time, since both the population of hosts and of a particular micropar-asite will exhibit genetic diversity which is constantly evolving (World Health Organization, 1997). The selective pressure on *M. tuberculosis* by anti-tuberculosis agents is an additional complicating factor, since the selective advantage of drug resistance to one or more specific drugs may alter infectivity, pathogenicity or virulence.

Until recently, evidence of genetic variability in human susceptibility to tuberculosis has been inconclusive. Several decades ago, Lurie (1964) demonstrated that rabbits could be bred with differential susceptibility to tuberculosis and subsequent genetic studies identified a single dominant gene in mice, originally named *Bcg*, which regulated natural resistance to the BCG strain of *M. bovis* (Gros *et al.*, 1981; Skamene, 1994) and other intracellular organisms (Skamene *et al.*, 1982). A candidate gene was eventually isolated and designated the natural-resistance-associated macrophage protein 1 gene, or Nramp1 (Vidal *et al.*, 1993). Soon after this, the human homologue, designated NRAMP1, was cloned and mapped (Cellier *et al.*, 1994). A recent case-control study comparing the frequency of several polymorphisms in the NRAMP1 gene in West Africans with smear-positive tuberculosis and ethnically-matched healthy controls showed that individuals heterozygous for two independent alleles were significantly associated with susceptibility to tuberculosis (Bellamy *et al.*, 1998). These findings are the first direct confirmation of an association between variation in a single gene and susceptibility to tuberculosis, and support earlier indirect evidence of racial variation in the susceptibility to tuberculosis and data from studies on twins suggesting the inheritance of susceptibility (Stead *et al.*, 1990; Comstock, 1978).

High rates of tuberculosis in populations previously unexposed, and therefore with a higher average susceptibility, were recorded in Inuit populations in Canada, Greenland and the USA (Fellows, 1934; Johnson, 1973; Stein *et al.*, 1968). Annual death rates in the order of 1% were recorded between 1920 and 1950. Among North American prairie Indians, following their forced relocation to reserves, tuberculosis mortality rose from 1% per annum in 1881 to 9% per annum in 1886, declining to 1% by 1900 (Ferguson, 1955). A similar situation was recorded among Sudanese recruits to the Egyptian army at the turn of the century, where previously unexposed young men from a presumably susceptible population developed rapidly fatal disease (Cummins, 1920). More recently, an emerging epidemic of tuberculosis has been reported among the Yanomami Indians of Brazil, who had been isolated from contact with European immigrants to South America until the mid-1960s (Sousa *et al.*, 1997). Out of 625 individuals examined, 6.4% were found to have active tuberculosis with fewer than half showing a positive skin test response to tuberculin. Observational studies on the immune responses of the Yanomami showed a diminished cell-mediated immunity and increased antibody production compared to Brazilians of European descent, suggesting that tuberculosis has exerted a profound selective pressure on human immune responses, a hypothesis predicted by the historical epidemiology of tuberculosis.

The questions of individual susceptibility to tuberculosis infection and disease and the evolutionary biology of *M. tuberculosis* in human populations have no clear answers. Virulence factors of the agent and the host mechanisms by which immunity is mediated are poorly understood. The variable latency between infection and disease, the variable immunity conferred by prior infection and disease, genetic factors of susceptibility and the role of exposure to other mycobacteria (including BCG) in modulating the immune response are all aspects of the complex pathogenesis of tuberculosis and the unstable association between *M. tuberculosis* and the human host. What is clear, however, is that individual susceptibility is dramatically increased by co-infection with HIV, itself a microparasite in evolution, and that the epidemiology of tuberculosis in a population will be altered in relation to the prevalence of HIV infection. The following section moves away from the broad perspective of population biology and takes up more familiar epidemiological indices.

Risk of Infection and Risk of Disease

The major environmental determinants of infection risk are the intensity and duration of exposure to droplets containing *M. tuberculosis* aerosolised by pulmonary tuberculosis patients during forced exhalation, such as coughing or sneezing (Loudon and Spohn, 1969). For the purpose of epidemiological modelling, patients have been categorised as infectious or non-infectious based on whether acid-fast bacilli (AFB) can be detected by direct microscopic examination of a smear made from a sputum specimen (Styblo, 1991; Murray *et al.*, 1990). When the bacillary concentration in the sputum exceeds 10^5 per ml, AFB are easily detectable but when the concentration falls to 10^4 per ml, the likelihood of detecting an AFB in 100 high-power fields is only 50%. Below 5000 bacilli per ml it is unlikely that AFB will be detected by smear examination (Hobby *et al.*, 1973; Yeager *et al.*, 1967). Thus, though the number of bacilli in sputum is a continuum, the microscopic smear status is dichotomous, though technical factors not relating to the concentration of bacilli in the sputum are also important in determining the yield of smear examination in different settings (Toman, 1979). Despite the relatively poor sensitivity of smear microscopy in detecting all cases of pulmonary tuberculosis, there is generally a good correlation between smear positivity and infectiousness. Numerous studies on the risk of infection in household contacts have confirmed that the incidence of infection is highest for contacts of smear positive cases, intermediate for contacts of smear negative culture positive cases and lowest for contacts of smear negative culture negative cases (Shaw and Wynn-Williams, 1954; Van Zwanenberg, 1960; Grzybowski *et al.*, 1975; Rouillon *et al.*, 1976; Rose *et al.*, 1979; Menzies, 1997). Notwithstanding the general association between smear positivity and infectiousness, variation in infectivity between patients with similar clinical characteristics was demonstrated under experimental conditions by exposing guinea pigs to air from rooms of hospitalised tuberculosis patients (Sultan, 1960), suggesting that certain strains of *M. tuberculosis* may be more likely to cause disease in susceptible hosts, a hypothesis that is best able to explain the outbreaks in Tennessee and Kentucky described above (Valway, 1998).

High-risk settings for tuberculosis transmission include those where undiagnosed tuberculosis cases are likely and where close contact is probable, e.g. health care institutions, correctional facilities, poorly-ventilated and crowded work environments, slum dwellings and temporary shelters for the homeless, migrant workers, and displaced populations. Some of these settings are commonly associated with other risk factors that may depress general immunity and predispose an individual to tuberculosis infection and disease. These include malnutrition, intercurrent illness, alcohol abuse and psychological stress.

Tubercle bacilli reaching the pulmonary alveolus through inhalation cause a non-specific inflammatory response which may result in a primary lesion in the lung and adjacent lymph nodes. In newborn or young children, and less frequently in adolescents and adults, infection may progress to life-threatening forms of tuberculosis, but in most infected individuals (who are members of populations with a long historical association with tuberculosis) a cell-mediated immune response rapidly ensues, resulting in the elimination of infection or in foci of tubercle bacilli surrounded by inflammatory cells. The likelihood of progressing from primary infection to clinical disease and the delay between infection and disease varies with the age at infection. In children under the age of four years, disease may develop in up to 60% within the first year of infection and among unvaccinated adolescents enrolled in the British Medical Research Council vaccine trials, 80% of tuberculin converters who developed clinical disease during ten years of follow up did so within two years of infection; overall, 8% of tuberculin converters developed clinical tuberculosis within 15 years (Styblo, 1991; Sutherland, 1968, 1976). The lifetime risk of active disease will vary according to the age at first infection and the likelihood of re-infection. A commonly-quoted figure for the lifetime risk of active tuberculosis in newly infected children and young adults is 10%, with half that risk occurring within the first five years of infection (Sutherland, 1976). For the purposes of modelling, Murray *et al.* (1990) assumed that 6–10% of people with primary infection will eventually develop clinical disease, a figure that does not take into account disease due to re-infection.

In developing countries today, where the annual risk of infection varies from 0.5 to 2.5% (Cauthen *et al.*, 1988; Murray *et al.*, 1990) the risk of multiple infections is high. The contribution of re-infection to tuberculosis incidence is difficult to assess. The dramatic decline in tuberculosis incidence among the Inuit population in Alaska, Canada and Greenland that followed the decline in the ARI in the second half of this century was observed in all age groups, including older people who were previously infected, suggesting that where infection rates are high, re-infection contributes significantly to tuberculosis morbidity. Recent studies using molecular techniques to differentiate strains of *M. tuberculosis* have demonstrated that re-infection can occur in outbreak situations and is common in endemic countries (Daley *et al.*, 1992; Edlin *et al.*, 1992; Nolan *et al.*, 1991; Small *et al.*, 1994; Wilkinson *et al.*, 1997; Gilks *et al.*, 1997). In persons not infected with HIV, the risk of active disease is lower after re-infection than following primary infection. Tuberculin skin test studies carried out on students in nursing and medicine in the pre-antibiotic era in Europe and North America, when the annual risk of work-related tuberculosis exposure was between 50 and 80%, have shown that the risk of disease over a two- to four-year period was lower among those initially tuberculin positive, with an average protective effectiveness of 80% (Heimbeck, 1938; Daniels, 1944; Badger and Ayvazian, 1949; Karns, 1961; Menzies, 1997). A similar value of 79% for the protection conferred by remote primary infection was calculated from age-specific rates of infection prevalence and disease incidence in the Netherlands (Sutherland, 1976). [Vynnycky and Fine (1997b), using an age-dependent model of the dynamics of tuberculosis infection and disease in England and Wales since 1990, have confirmed the contribution of reinfection to tuberculosis morbidity, but estimated that prior infection confers less than 50% protection against disease subsequent to reinfection.] In summary, infection that does not progress to disease within the first three months, while associated with a decreasing risk of reactivation over time, confers protection against disease from re-infection, but this protection is variable in degree and duration.

An increased risk of disease following infection is associated with certain medical conditions such as diabetes, malignancy, haemophilia, renal failure, gastrectomy and jejuno-ileal bypass, but these have little public health significance because of their low prevalence in the general population (Rieder, 1995). Miners with silicosis are at an increased risk of developing tuberculosis (Snider, 1978; Cowie *et al.*, 1989; Sherson and Lander, 1990; Hong Kong Chest Service/Tuberculosis Research Centre Madras/British Medical Research Council, 1991) and an association has also been reported with potters whose occupational exposure to silica dust is high (Cole, 1989). The impact of general malnutrition and micro-nutrient deficiencies on the incidence of tuberculosis is hard to assess and cannot be directly studied (Chan *et al.*, 1996). A lack of vitamin D can impair the action of macrophages in killing intracellular *M. tuberculosis* and has been linked to the incidence of tuberculosis in the UK among South Asian immigrants (Davies, 1985; Rook, 1988). Given the widespread prevalence of malnutrition in some tuberculosis-endemic countries such as India where 360 million consume less than 80% of minimum energy requirements and more than half the children under five are undernourished (United Nations, 1997; UNICEF, 1996), it may be an important population attributable risk factor (Chandra, 1996). Gender-related differences in risk have also been observed and are discussed in Chapter 14, but in recent years by far the most important risk factor has been HIV infection and, as described in Chapters 1 and 12, this has had a major impact on the global burden of tuberculosis.

Conclusions

Before the advent of molecular biology applied both to micro-organisms and host responses, a great deal had been learned about the transmission of tuberculosis as well as the risk factors and time course of disease following infection.

The epidemiological associations between tuberculosis infection and disease were based on assumptions of a relative stability between the organism and the human host. Recent advances in the genetic fingerprinting of *M. tuberculosis* have revealed a heterogeneity of strain diversity worldwide, and have modified our view of the dynamics of tuberculosis transmission, the relative contribution of new infection, reactivation and re-infection, and the impact of chemotherapy on the selection of *M. tuberculosis* strains. Advances in immunology have improved our understanding of the host response, the genetic basis of human susceptibility and the mechanism of protection from BCG and other mycobacteria. It has been the HIV pandemic, however, which has shattered the notion of an apparent stable association between the tubercle bacillus and the human host. In areas of high HIV transmission, the annual tuberculosis incidence has increased more rapidly than services can cope with and this has played a major role in shaking off the general complacency towards this disease.

References

Anderson, R. M. and May, R. M. (1992) *Infectious Disease of Humans — Dynamics and Control.* Oxford: Oxford University Press.

Badger, T. and Ayvazian, L. (1949) Tuberculosis in nurses: Clinical observations on its pathogenesis as seen in a fifteen year follow-up of 745 nurses. *Am. Rev. Tuberc.* **60**, 305–331.

Bellamy, R., Ruwende, C., Corrah, T., McAdam, K. P., Whittle, H. C. and Hill, A. L. (1998) Variations in the *NRAMP1* gene and susceptibility to tuberculosis in West Africans. *N. Engl. J. Med.* **338**, 640–644.

Cauthen, G., *et al.* (1988) Annual risk of tuberculosis infection. Geneva: World Health Organization.

Cellier, M., *et al.* (1994) Human natural resistance-associated macrophage protein: cDNA cloning, chromosomal mapping, genomic organization and tissue-specific expression. *J. Exp. Med.* **180**, 1741–1752.

Chan, J., *et al.* (1996) Effects of protein calorie malnutrition on tuberculosis in mice. *Proc. Natl. Acad. Sci. USA* **93**, 14857–14861.

Chandra, R. K. (1996) Nutrition, immunity and infection: From basic knowledge of dietary manipulation of immune responses to practical application of ameliorating suffering and improving survival. *Proc. Natl. Acad. Sci. USA* **93**, 14304–143307.

Cole, R. (1989) Respiratory tuberculosis in the potteries. *Ann. Occu. Hyg.* **33**, 387–395.

Comstock, G. (1978) Tuberculosis in twins: A re-analysis of the Prophit survey. *Am. Rev. Resp. Dis.* **117**, 621–624.

Cowie, R. L., Langton, M. E. and Becklade, M. R. (1989) Pulmonary tuberculosis in South African gold miners. *Am. Rev. Resp. Dis.* **139**, 1086–1089.

Cummins, S. (1920) Tuberculosis in primitive tribes and its bearing on tuberculosis of civilized communities. *Int. J. Publ. Hlth.* **1**, 10–171.

Daley, C. L., *et al.* (1992) An outbreak of tuberculosis with accelerated progression among persons infected with the human immunodeficiency virus: An analysis using restriction-fragment-length polymorphism. *N. Engl. J. Med.* **326**, 2331–2335.

Daniels, M. (1944) Primary tuberculosis infection in nurses: Manifestations and prognosis. *Lancet*, 165–170.

Davies, P. D. O. (1985) A possible link between vitamin D deficiency and impaired host defence to Mycobacterium tuberculosis. *Tubercle* **66**, 301–306.

Dubos, R. and Dubos, J. (1952) *The White Plague: Tuberculosis, Man and Society.* Boston: Little and Brown.

Edlin, B., *et al.* (1992) An outbreak of multidrug-resistant tuberculosis among hospitalized patients with acquired immunodeficiency syndrome. *N. Engl. J. Med.* **326**, 1514–1521.

Fellows, D. (1934) Mortality in the native races of the Territory of Alaska, with special reference to tuberculosis. *Publ. Hlth. Rep.* **49**, 289–299.

Ferguson, R. (1955) *Studies in Tuberculosis.* Toronto: University of Toronto Press.

Frost, W. (1937) How much control of tuberculosis? *Am. J. Publ. Hlth.* **27**, 759–766.

Gilks, C., *et al.* (1997) Recent transmission of tuberculosis in a cohort of HIV-1 infected female sex workers in Nairobi, Kenya. *AIDS* **11**, 911–918.

Grigg, E. (1958) The arcana of tuberculosis. *Am. Rev. Tuberc. Pulmonary Dis.* **78**, 151–172.

Gros, P., Skamene, E. and Forget, A. (1981) Genetic control of natural resistance to *Mycobacterium bovis* in mice. *J. Immunol.* **127**, 417–421.

Grzybowski, S., Barnett, G. D. and Styblo, K. (1975) Contacts of cases of active pulmonary tuberculosis. *Bull. Int. Union Tuberc.* **50**, 90–106.

Heimbeck, J. (1938) Incidence of tuberculosis in young adult women, with special reference to employment. *Br. J. Tuberc.* **32**, 154–166.

Hobby, G. L., Holman, A. P., Iseman, M. D. and Jones, J. M. (1973) Enumeration of tubercle bacilli in sputum of patients with pulmonary tuberculosis. *Antimicrob. Agents Chemother.* **4**, 94–104.

Hong Kong Chest Service/Tuberculosis Research Centre/British Medical Research Council. (1991) A controlled clinical comparison of 6 and 8 months of antituberculosis chemotherapy in the treatment of patients with silicotuberculosis in Hong Kong. *Am. Rev. Resp. Dis.* **143**, 262–267.

Johnson, M. (1973) Results of 20 years of tuberculosis control in Alaska. *Hlth. Serv. Rep.* **88**, 247–254.

Karns, J. (1961) Tuberculin sensitivity and tuberculosis in nursing and medical students. *Dis. Chest* **40**, 291–301.

Levin, B. (1996) The evolution and maintenance of virulence in microparasites. *Emerg. Infect. Dis.* **2**, 93–102.

Loudon, R. and Spohn, S. (1969) Cough frequency and infectivity in patients with pulmonary tuberculosis. *Am. Rev. Resp. Dis.* **99**, 109–111.

Lowell, A. *et al.* (1969) *Tuberculosis.* Cambridge MA: Harvard University Press.

Lurie, M. (1964) *Resistance to Tuberculosis: Experimental Studies in Native and Acquired Defensive Mechanisms.* Cambridge MA: Harvard University Press.

Menzies, D. (1997) Issues in the management of contacts of patients with active pulmonary tuberculosis. *Can. J. Publ. Hlth.* **88**, 197–201.

Murray, C. J., Styblo, K. and Rouillon, A. (1990) Tuberculosis in developing countries: Burden, intervention and cost. *Bull. Int. Union Tuberc. Lung Dis.* **65**, 6–24.

Nolan, C. M., Elarth, A. M., Barr, H., Saeed, A. M. and Risser, D. R. (1991) An outbreak of tuberculosis in a shelter for homeless men: A description of its evolution and control. *Am. Rev. Resp. Dis.* **143**, 257–261.

Rieder, H. (1995) Epidemiology of tuberculosis in Europe. *Eur. Resp. J.* **8** (Suppl. 20), S620–S632.

Rook, G. A. W. (1988) The role of vitamin D in tuberculosis. *Am. Rev. Resp. Dis.* **138**, 768–770.

Rose, C. E., Zerbe, G. O., Lantz, S. O. and Bailey, W. C. (1979) Establishing priority during investigation of tuberculosis contacts. *Am. Rev. Resp. Dis.* **119**, 603–609.

Rouillon, A., Perdrizet, S. and Parrot, R. (1976) Transmission of tubercle bacilli: The effects of chemotherapy. *Tubercle* **57**, 275–299.

Shaw, J. and Wynn-Williams, N. (1954) Infectivity of pulmonary tuberculosis in relation to sputum status. *Am. Rev. Tuberc.* **69**, 724–732.

Sherson, D. and Lander, F. (1990) Morbidity of pulmonary tuberculosis among silicotic and nonsilicotic foundary workers in Denmark. *J. Occu. Med.* **32**, 110–113.

Sjögren, I. and Sutherland, I. (1975) The risk of tuberculous infection in Sweden. *Tubercle* **56**, 97–112.

Skamene, E. (1994) The *Bcg* gene story. *Immunobiol.* **191**, 451–460.

Skamene, E., Gros, P., Forget, A., Kongshavn, P. A., St Charles, C. and Taylor, B. A. (1982) Genetic regulation of resistance to intracellular pathogens. *Nature* **297**, 506–509.

Small, P. M., *et al.* (1994) The epidemiology of tuberculosis in San Francisco. *N. Engl. J. Med.* **330**, 1703–1709.

Snider Jr., D. E. (1978) The relationship between tuberculosis and silicosis. *Am. Rev. Resp. Dis.* **118**, 455–460.

Sousa, A. O., *et al.* (1997) An epidemic of tuberculosis with a high rate of tuberculin anergy among a population previously unexposed to tuberculosis, the Yanomami Indians of the Brazilian Amazon. *Proc. Natl. Acad. Sci. USA* **94**, 13227–13232.

Stead, W. W., Senner, J. W., Reddick, W. T. and Lofgren, J. P. (1990) Racial differences in susceptibility to infection by *Mycobacterium tuberculosis*. *N. Engl. J. Med.* **322**, 422.

Stein, K. P., Lange, P. K., Gad, U. and Wilbek, E. (1968) Tuberculosis in Greenland. *Arch. Environ. Health.* **17**, 501–506.

Styblo, K., Meijer, J. and Sutherland, I. (1969) The transmission of tubercle bacilli: Its trend in a human population. Tuberculosis Surveillance Research Unit Report No. 1. *Bull. Int. Union Tuberc.* **42**, 5–104.

Styblo, K. (1991) *Epidemiology of Tuberculosis*. The Hague: Royal Netherlands Tuberculosis Association.

Sultan, L., *et al.* (1960) Tuberculosis disseminators: A study of the variability of aerial infectivity of tuberculous patients. *Am. Rev. Resp. Dis.* **82**, 358–369.

Sutherland, I. (1968) The ten-year incidence of clinical tuberculosis following 'conversion' in 2,550 individuals aged 14 to 19 years. The Hague: Royal Netherlands Tuberculosis Association.

Sutherland, I. and Fayers, P. (1975) The association of the risk of tuberculosis infection with age. *Bull. Int. Union Tuberc.* **50**, 70–81.

Toman, K. (1979) *Tuberculosis Case-Finding and Chemotherapy: Questions and Answers*. Geneva: World Health Organization.

UNICEF. (1996) The progress of nations.

United Nations. (1997) UN system position statement — India.

Valway, S. E., *et al.* (1998) An outbreak involving extensive transmission of a virulent strain of *Mycobacterium tuberculosis*. *N. Engl. J. Med.* **338**, 633–639.

Van Zwanenberg, D. (1960) The influence of the number of bacilli on the development of tuberculosis disease in children. *Am. Rev. Resp. Dis.* **119**, 603–609.

Vidal, S. M., Malo, D., Vogan, K., Skamene, E. and Gros, P. (1993) Natural resistance to infection with intracellular parasites: Isolation of a candidate for *Bcg*. *Cell* **73**, 469–485.

Vynnycky, E. and Fine, P. E. M. (1997a) The annual risk of infection with *Mycobacterium tuberculosis* in England and Wales since 1901. *Int. J. Tuberc. Lung Dis.* **1**, 389–396.

Vynnycky, E. and Fine, P. E. M. (1997b) The natural history of tuberculosis: The implications of age-dependent risks of disease and the role of reinfection. *Epidemiol. Infect.* **119**, 183–201.

Wilkinson, D., Pillay, M., Crump, J., Lombard, C., Davies, G. R. and Sturm, A. W. (1997) Molecular epidemiology and transmission dynamics of *Mycobacterium tuberculosis* in rural Africa. *Trop. Med. Int. Hlth.* **2**, 747–753.

Wolff, G. (1926) *Der Gang der Tuberkulose Sterblichkeit und die Industrialisierung Europas*. Leipzig: Barth.

World Health Organization. (1997) *Anti-Tuberculosis Drug Resistance in the World. Report of the World Health Organization/IUATLD Global Project on Anti-tuberculosis Drug Resistance Surveillance, 1994–1997*. Geneva: World Health Organization Global Tuberculosis Programme.

Yeager Jr., H., Lacey, J., Smith, L. R. and LeMaistre, C. A. (1967) Quantitative studies of mycobacterial populations in sputum and saliva. *Am. Rev. Resp. Dis.* **95**, 998–1004.

CHAPTER 3

A CRITIQUE OF THE GLOBAL EFFORT: DO TUBERCULOSIS CONTROL PROGRAMMES ONLY EXIST ON PAPER? — A PERSPECTIVE FROM A DEVELOPING COUNTRY

M. Angélica Salomão

Is Tuberculosis Actually Dealt with by Countries' Health Authorities as a Public Health Problem?

It is very likely that tuberculosis is as old as mankind itself. But, taking into account Darwin's theory of the survival of the species, the fact that the tubercle bacillus still exists in the 20th century means that the human race and this bacillus have tolerated each other for a long time. Many deaths due to tuberculosis have occurred over the centuries, but neither the human race nor the bacillus have shown sufficient supremacy to win this drawn-out battle (Styblo, 1986). The aim of the World Health Organization Global Programme on Tuberculosis, launched in 1990, is to swing the struggle in favour of the human race by creating worldwide conditions capable of controlling tuberculosis (Kochi, 1991).

In industrially developed countries, tuberculosis, which was a major killer until the first half of the 20th century, has now reached such low levels that certain tuberculosis programmes are orientating themselves towards elimination rather than merely control. Indeed, in 1990, the

49

World Health Organization (WHO) and the European region of the
Union Against Tuberculosis and Lung Disease held a workshop entitled
'The last fight against tuberculosis until elimination' (Report, 1991).

In total contrast to this picture, many developing countries are still
at the point of either deciding how to establish tuberculosis control
programmes or not yet seriously addressing the issue at all. Fortunately,
though, even when facing resource and financial constraints, a number
of developing countries, including my own country — Mozambique —
are already applying tuberculosis control measures and obtaining encouraging results.

Although tuberculosis occurs throughout the world, the burden of
the disease is greatest in the developing word, including sub-Saharan
Africa, and the age groups most affected are the most economically productive ones, as shown in Fig. 1 (Murray *et al.*, 1993; see also Chapter 1).

The situation appears to be gloomy, but the means to combat tuberculosis effectively have been available for several decades. The current
tuberculosis control strategy consists of case finding and treatment,

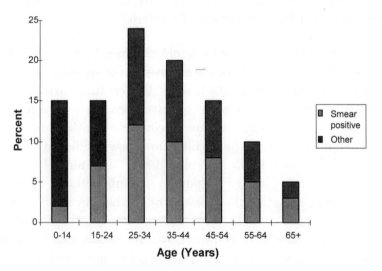

Fig. 1.   Estimated age distribution of cases of tuberculosis in the developing world,
1990.

chemoprophylaxis and BCG vaccination (Rodrigues and Smith, 1990; see also Chapter 6 for a detailed description). The BCG vaccine has been available since the 1920s and tuberculosis drugs since the early 1940s, with the more powerful short course drug regimens being used since the 1970s.

The attitude towards this world-wide public health problem is variable. In some countries there is indifference to the problem, some deal with tuberculosis control as though health care is a *commodity* to be traded like goods, while others are already involved in tuberculosis control activities but have not yet been able to establish partnership links with the beneficiaries of the programmes — the patients with tuberculosis and their communities.

The resources may be available but the community is unaware of, or afraid of approaching, the services. The presence of undiagnosed infectious tuberculosis is the normal state of affairs in many countries, the developing ones in particular (Styblo and Salomão, 1993). The present global situation of tuberculosis shows that only a small group of countries have achieved a partnership link between the health providers and the population. The global emergency of tuberculosis is commonly acknowledged, as is the need for political will as the starting point for practical steps towards control of the disease. A frank and open environment to address the problem is evolving, resulting in health care providers and patients uniting to fight the 'common enemy', *Mycobacterium tuberculosis*. The myth of tuberculosis as an incurable disease has begun to fade away and this should pave the way to the successful application of control measures.

Is Tuberculosis Really Understood as a Burden?

The majority of developing countries — from Africa to Asia and from America to the Pacific rim — show a similar pattern of social structure, with young people constituting a significant part of the population. Resources to meet the basic needs of the population are insufficient, financial resources are meagre and general knowledge concerning tuberculosis is not seen to be disseminated in these communities. Furthermore, the level of socio-economic development is not high and services such as education, primary health care, clean water supplies and sanitation are not widely available.

Children are affected by conditions such as acute respiratory infections, malnutrition and measles while women suffer from malnutrition and problems related to reproductive activity. The general population faces many problems as a direct result of their poor socio-economic status. As these countries are mostly in the tropics, the population also faces the threat of the tropical diseases. Thus, tuberculosis is just one of a large list of public health concerns. Some diseases causing long-term suffering are so common that some societies simply have to accept such suffering and learn to live with it. People may be aware of the various diseases but they cannot dissociate their poor health status from their general outlook on life. Thus, tuberculosis often goes untreated and spreads silently through the community.

Is the Tuberculosis Situation Regarded as a Public Health Problem and are there Any Means to Modify the Present Situation?

The mid-1980s witnessed the launching of economic adjustment programmes worldwide. Developing countries like Mozambique, that have been hit by bad performance of their economies, high external debts and a decrease of exports, were forced to reduce resources allocated to health. In these cases, the reduction in the budget created a gloomy outlook for health programmes in general and primary health care and tuberculosis control in particular, even when services and infrastructure had already been established.

As financial resources declined sharply, social sectors — health and education programmes — were adversely affected. Countries which used to have resources for health, even if only limited ones, could no longer cope with the expenditures. Therefore, tuberculosis programmes suffered as a result of economic reversals.

In the mid-1980s, the International Union Against Tuberculosis and Lung Disease began to give assistance to the establishment of control programmes in certain developing countries where the disease has been a heavy burden on communities. At that time, tuberculosis control was often regarded by governments and donors as a difficult matter. In addition, as there had been no systematic collection of data in many developing countries, there was no information on which to base health care advocacy. The results of a key analysis conducted by Murray and his colleagues in 1990 on the control programmes in Mozambique, Malawi and Tanzania were of great importance for tuberculosis advocacy both nationally and internationally as they firmly established the effectiveness and cost effectiveness of short course chemotherapy under different settings and socio-economic conditions (Murray *et al.*, 1991a). Some of the programmes supported by the International Union Against Tuberculosis and Lung Disease, like those in Mozambique, had been carried out under conditions of political unrest but, nevertheless, as shown in Table 1, the results were good and have therefore been used in advocacy for further programmes (World Health Organization, 1992).

Table 1.   Results of treatment in 41,720 new smear positive patients enrolled on short course chemotherapy in national tuberculosis programmes, 1983–1988.*

Country	Percentage of patients (%)				
	Cured	Sputum Positive	Died	Dropped out	Transferred
Malawi	87	1	7	2	2
Mozambique	78	1	2	11	8
Nicaragua	78	2	3	13	5
Tanzania	77	2	7	10	4
Total	79	2	6	9	4

*Compiled with the help of the International Union Against Tuberculosis and Lung Disease.

The World Health Organization Global Tuberculosis Programme and all the other international groups are working together to attempt to obtain resources and channel them towards the treatment of more tuberculosis patients by providing technical and financial support to countries and programmes. Sadly, however, the overall funding of tuberculosis control is far from adequate. The cost effectiveness of treating tuberculosis is no longer questioned (Murray *et al.*, 1991a; see Chapter 10), but what seems to be missing is the acceptance of the significance of this fact by those responsible for the funding of health care worldwide.

Does the Appearance of HIV/AIDS Affect the Impact of Tuberculosis in the Community?

Over the last 20 to 25 years the emergent HIV/AIDS epidemic has stricken communities throughout the world. The intensity of the impact of this epidemic varies from region to region, but one notable effect is the increase of the number of HIV-related cases of tuberculosis. The actual and predicted impact of HIV on tuberculosis is summarised in

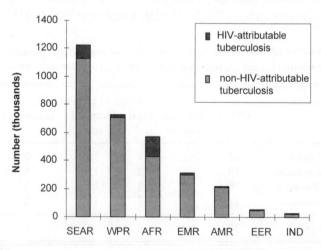

Fig. 2. Estimated deaths due to non-HIV-attributable and to HIV-attributable tuberculosis by World Health Organization regions in 1995 (estimates in thousands).

Chapter 1 and the effect of the HIV pandemic in Africa is described in Chapter 12. Many deaths are occurring (Fig. 2) and more are expected in people co-infected with HIV and the tubercle bacillus.

As HIV infection increases the number of people infected by the tubercle bacillus who develop active tuberculosis, and reduces the length of time between infection and manifestation of disease, the HIV epidemic is leading to an increased incidence of tuberculosis. If treatment is made available, HIV-tuberculosis cases will be cured, but because of the rapid onset and course of the disease, control measures have to be prompt and effective.

What are the Tuberculosis Control Strategies?

As outlined above, the current tuberculosis control measures consist of case finding and treatment, chemoprophylaxis and BCG vaccination. Case-finding is important for the detection of sufferers who need to be put on treatment. Case-finding is pointless if the objective of treating the detected cases is not met (Toman, 1979).

BCG is known to be effective in preventing the severe forms of tuberculosis such as meningitis and miliary disease in children, but not in preventing the disease among adults. The disease in adults is usually infectious. As it is, BCG vaccination programmes do not substantially influence the chain of transmission or decrease the transmission of the disease. Thus, the various national and international BCG vaccination campaigns have done little to reduce the global burden of disease (Styblo and Meijer, 1976).

Chemotherapy, rather than vaccination, is therefore considered to be the key tool for reducing the sources of infection in a community and for making a progressive impact on the magnitude of the disease. If the aim of the fight against tuberculosis for individual patients is to cure and restore them to their previous capabilities, the aim for the community is to reduce the spread of infection and hasten the eradication of the disease (International Union Against Tuberculosis and Lung Disease, 1996; Styblo, 1980).

Is Health Education Important?

Health Education of populations plays a key role in encouraging patients to seek treatment for tuberculosis and adhere to the treatment regimen. Thus, health education involves providing the patients with information to motivate them to be compliant (see also Chapter 21). *Health education is not a way for the health provider to set rules and expect the patient to be obedient. It is a partnership process to improve mutual understanding.* Ignoring this aspect of treatment management has been a major cause of the failure in the control of tuberculosis. Health care providers are often more preoccupied with diagnosing more cases than with the outcome of treatment. What is the use of diagnosis if patients are not prevented from absconding after the initial phase of treatment?

Patients must feel motivated to seek and comply with treatment. This means that they must know what the treatment consists of and for how long it is going to last.

After some days of treatment, patients will feel better (Styblo and Salomão, 1993), but they should not forget that it is important to continue treatment for the entire duration explained to them by the health care provider. Thus, they must realise that the 'cure' that they are experiencing will only be a 'mirage' unless they continue with the prescribed treatment until they are discharged. Only then will the cure be real and sustained.

For patients to understand the basic and simple principles of tuberculosis treatment, they have to be aware of the transmissibility and risk of progression of the disease, the importance of directly observed therapy and the discipline that this demands from them (World Health Organization, 1997).

If properly motivated, patients will be able to comply with the treatment regimen. Motivation is thus a basic condition for the achievement of cure and requires information and support from the health care provider, relatives and friends. A positive environment is also essential. The only way to obtain the patients' support is to make them aware of the need to *collaborate* with the health care provider and know what is expected of them in the treatment process.

Are Health Care Providers Ready to Educate, Motivate and Create Awareness Among Tuberculosis Patients, their Households and their Friends?

Why do health care providers and national control programmes fail to improve results? Patients are left alone with their suffering, social isolation and depression because the services act too technically. If patients can trust the health care provider, they will visit the health facility regularly and their sufferings will be relieved. This is a mandatory condition for successful management of the disease. A mutual confidence has to be established and tailored to each patient — fears and misunderstandings differ from patient to patient and should be considered for each individual (see also Chapter 21).

Health care providers and national control programmes must be prepared to start the 'missionary' role of setting the rules for a successful outcome. The results will always be a failure if:

- The health care provider does not provide support, love and respect and is just concerned with providing drugs without showing any feelings and providing adequate information;
- The health care provider fails to educate patients and communities against taboos necessary to prevent them from absconding and to help them to face segregation and social pressures; or
- The system fails to create positive attitudes and thereby to make the patients understand that success depends firstly on them, secondly on drugs and thirdly on the treating staff.

An example of inappropriate behaviour of health care providers is the use of technical language which the patients fail to understand. Either the staff must learn to use a down-to-earth and accessible language when

approaching the patients, their relatives and friends or the patient will
be lost.

It is not enough merely to establish a national control programme
based on technical considerations. This alone will not achieve the desired results. A national control programme must have faces — that is,
the patients must be treated by humane and compassionate carers and
not merely by competent technicians.

A national programme is, of course, an important element in the control of tuberculosis in a country or region, but it must be able to adapt to
individual situations. A national tuberculosis control programme is the
path along which patients may travel in order to obtain treatment, get
cured and return to a healthy life. *But treatment will not be a miracle.*
It is a process that needs organisation and time (Crofton *et al.*, 1992).

Are National Control Programmes Prepared for this Role?

Good management is mandatory. It is through management of the programme that the agenda to be followed by the 'partners' in tuberculosis
treatment is determined. Additionally, it is good treatment management which will bring results, since procedures in each phase are defined by both partners — the patients and health care providers. This
is why investing in good management of tuberculosis treatment is both
essential for a successful and cost-effective outcome.

Compliance does not come free. It is the result of patience of planning of the strategies for follow up on the part of health care providers
that are essential to attracting and keeping the patient in the network of
treatment. Modern tuberculosis chemotherapy does not even stop with
compliance. The concept of *adherence* is gaining popularity and starting to replace compliance. Adherence is the necessary bond between the
health care providers and their patients that is required for to achieve
cure of the disease. The patient has to be considered as an active element of the process not just an element playing a passive role in a

process directed by the health care provider (Report, 1994). The more recently introduced concept of *concordance* stresses on 'a partnership of equals' in achieving cure (Fox, 1997).

Are We Short of the Means to Fight Tuberculosis?

The experiences of the tuberculosis programmes in developed countries over the last 40 to 50 years, the research conducted during that period to improve treatment results, the positive contributions of the International Union Against Tuberculosis and Lung Disease and the global organisation of tuberculosis control through the Global Tuberculosis Programme of the World Health Organization have provided ample information to health care providers and donors on ways of fighting tuberculosis.

It has already been mentioned that drugs and essential resources for the diagnosis and treatment of tuberculosis are available but control does not depend only on the availability of resources (financial, equipment, drugs and other essential items). Tuberculosis control depends primarily on human beings and their motivation. When political will exists, tuberculosis control is possible, but political will alone is not enough.

The crucial step is the organisation of National Tuberculosis Control Programmes and their management at all levels, paying special attention to organisation at the national level in order to ensure a modern, functional, effective and sustainable programme.

The WHO and the International Union Against Tuberculosis and Lung Disease have persuaded the producers of drugs to lower the prices of anti-tuberculosis drugs, paving the way to allow poorer countries to afford treatment. The prices of anti-tuberculosis drugs and regimens are given respectively, in Tables 3 and 4 of Chapter 10.

It must be stressed that the success of chemotherapy is based on the proven effectiveness of the anti-tuberculosis regimen, either standard or short course, that is used. The former lasts between 12

Table 2. Examples of anti-tuberculosis chemotherapy regimens used in developing countries.

Regimen	Duration
New smear-positive cases	
Standard	
2SH/10TH	12
2SH/10EH	12
2SH/10S$_2$H$_2$	12
Shortcourse	
2SHRZ/6TH	8
2SHRZ/4HR or 2EHRZ/4HR	6
2HRZ/4HR	6
2HRZ/4H$_3$R$_3$	6
New smear-negative cases	
2STH/10TH	12
2SHRZ/6TH	8
Re-treatment	
2SHRZE/1HRZE/3H$_3$R$_3$E$_3$	6
2SHRZE/1HRZE/5TH	8

S = Streptomycin 1 g; H = Isoniazid 300 mg; R = Rifampicin 450/600 mg; E = Ethambutol 25 mg/kg; T = Thiacetazone 150 mg; Z = Pyrazinamide 1,500/2,000 mg. Subscript numbers refer to intermittent therapy, in which drugs are given on a limited number of days (two or three) each week.

to 18 months, and the latter between six to eight months (Murray *et al.*, 1991b) but based on more expensive drugs. Examples of anti-tuberculosis chemotherapy regimens used in developing countries are given in Table 2.

The effectiveness of standard and short course chemotherapy regimens depends on three major factors: the cure rate; the emergence of acquired drug resistance; and the impact of the transmission of the tubercle bacillus in the community (Murray *et al.*, 1991b). It goes without saying that the cure rate is the most important factor.

Do Tuberculosis Control Programmes Only Exist on Paper?

- A National Tuberculosis Control Programme is *not* the Manual of Diagnosis, Treatment and Evaluation.
- A National Tuberculosis Control Programme is *not* a group of health educators or home visitors who know the rules of treatment and offer drugs, with no interest in the numerous problems faced by the patients.
- A National Tuberculosis Control Programme is *not* a system for providing drugs to patients without knowing what the outcome of the treatment is.
- A National Tuberculosis Control Programme is the *ensemble* of rules and behaviours that, at the end of the day, provides guidelines for the management of those suffering from tuberculosis and adequate interventions to reduce the magnitude of the burden of the disease in the community.

People involved in any National Tuberculosis Control Programme must realise that patients are all different and that each one has their own problems and perceptions. What ought to link the programme and the patients is the *partnership* or *concordance* that they build to achieve positive treatment outcomes (Fox, 1997). If this happens, the spill-over effect of stopping disease transmission will bring changes — the outcome of treatment results will improve and the magnitude of the burden of the tuberculosis problem will, in time, show a downward trend.

In a study conducted in Maputo City, Mozambique (Report, 1986), it was shown that cultural beliefs and social factors may prevent people with symptoms suggestive of tuberculosis from approaching health facilities. These beliefs, associated with the uncaring attitudes of health care providers, make the patient feel afraid to visit a health facility (Crofton *et al.*, 1992; Report, 1986).

A high prevalence of tuberculosis in a community is sound evidence of poor living conditions. A tuberculosis patient is usually somebody who has, among other factors, a low socio-economic position, poor standard of housing and a poor nutritional status. Another factor which influences the prevalence of tuberculosis in an area is the level at which health care is provided. If the sources of infection are detected and treated and the living conditions and standards of hygiene are improved, the incidence of the disease may then be lowered. It is, however, important to stress that finding the cases and maintaining them on treatment until they are cured poses the major difficulty. Why is this so?

There are usually two scenarios. The first is that the health authorities do not care about tuberculosis and there are no anti-tuberculosis drugs or specific services to attend to the needs of the patients. The situation therefore remains unchanged. The second scenario is that health authorities organise tuberculosis services and patients seek treatment, but again the situation remains unchanged despite the expectations that good tuberculosis control programmes will reduce the incidence of tuberculosis.

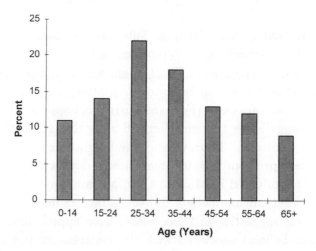

Fig. 3.   Estimated age distribution of deaths due to tuberculosis in the developing world, 1990.

Why does the situation need to be changed?

Taking again into consideration the age distribution of smear-positive cases (Murray *et al.*, 1993) and the socio-economic implications of this fact, there is an urgent need to modify the situation. It does not matter what the actual level of prevalence is. What is important is that health care providers realise that the situation can be progressively changed — and this will also benefit the economy and the quality of life.

Figure 3 shows the estimated age distribution of deaths due to tuberculosis in the developing world in 1990. When this figure is compared with Fig. 1, it is clear that the case fatality rate is high in the young age group, which is the one with the responsibility for improving national wealth and household income.

Why is progress in tuberculosis control disappointing?

Even though patients are detected, tuberculosis control programmes have been established and, with major or minor difficulties, drugs and laboratory supplies are distributed to countries and programmes, the results are not satisfactory throughout the world. This situation raises three key questions:

- Has tuberculosis been regarded as a top high health priority?
- Do we have programmes which are not effective and only exist on paper?
- What ought to be changed in order to implement the resources for detecting and curing cases and for reducing the burden of tuberculosis?

What is the Way Forward?

Tuberculosis control is a *process* which entails organisation, perseverance, finance and motivation. There is no shortage of patients to be treated — and the numbers have increased as a direct result of the HIV pandemic — and more and more money and resources are being channelled to tuberculosis control, even if they are far from adequate.

What seems to be missing is a strong motivation in the people responsible for providing care. Strong motivation has to be merged with capable programme management. In the absence of a permanent, interested, problem-solving and supportive management, the various directives and guidelines for tuberculosis control, however well intended, will lead to nowhere.

Better performance of National Tuberculosis Control Programmes depends on upgrading and educating the peripheral staff who are a sensitive part of the chain of treatment management.

The future of the battle against tuberculosis control depend critically on the effectiveness of establishing a global coalition in order to maintain the political will to defeat this disease, provide adequate supplies of drugs and diagnostic reagents, and prepare strongly-motivated and effective tuberculosis managers.

Acknowledgements

While preparing this chapter I learned that Dr. Karel Styblo had passed away. For all that he has done for my people, my country and my continent, and for the encouragement he had given me, I will always be indebted to him. For his commitment to the fight against tuberculosis and the reduction of human suffering, the world will always be grateful to him and remember him as the advocate for tuberculosis global coalition.

References

Crofton, J., Horne, N. and Miller, F. (1992) Clinical Tuberculosis. London: MacMillan. Chpt. 6, pp. 141–158.
Fox, R. (1997) Are you a commander or a guide? J. R. Soc. Med. 90, 242–243.

International Union Against Tuberculosis and Lung Disease (1996) *Tuberculosis Guide for Low Income Countries*, 4th edition. Paris: International Union Against Tuberculosis and Lung Disease.

Kochi, A. (1991) The global tuberculosis situation and the new control strategy of the World Health Organization. *Tubercle* **72**, 1–6.

Murray, C. J. L., *et al.* (1991a) Cost-effectiveness of chemotherapy for pulmonary tuberculosis in three sub-Saharan countries. *Lancet* **338**, 1305–1308.

Murray, C. J. L., Styblo, K. and Rouillon, A. (1991b) Tuberculosis. In: *Health Sector Priorities Review*, HSPR-24. Washington: The World Bank, pp. 23–38.

Murray, C. J. L., Styblo, K. and Rouillon, A. (1993) Tuberculosis. In: *Disease Control Priorities in Developing Countries*, Oxford University Press, N.Y., **11**, pp. 233–259.

Report. (1986) Direcção Nacional de Acção Social. *Aspectos Sociais Psicológicos, Culturais e Psicopatológicos relacionados com a Tuberculose*. Mozambique: Ministério da Saúde.

Report. (1991) Tuberculosis elimination in the countries of Europe and other industrialized countries. *Eur. Resp. J.* **4**, 1288–1295.

Report. (1994) US Department of Health and Human Services. *Improving Patient Adherence to Tuberculosis Treatment*. Atlanta: CDC. pp. 3–13.

Rodrigues, L. C. and Smith, P. G. (1990) Tuberculosis in developing countries and methods for its control. *Trans. R. Soc. Trop. Med. Hyg.* **84**, 739–744.

Styblo, K. (1980) Recent advances in epidemiological research in tuberculosis. *Selected Papers R. Netherlands Tuberc. Assoc.* **20**, 19–46.

Styblo, K. (1986) Tuberculosis control and surveillance. In: *Recent Advances in Respiratory Medicine*. Edinburgh: Churchill Livingstone. Chpt. 20, pp. 78–86.

Styblo, K. and Meijer, J. (1976) Impact of BCG vaccination programmes in children and young adults on the tuberculosis problem. *Tubercle* **57**, 17–43.

Styblo, K. and Salomão, M. A. (1993) National tuberculosis control programs. In: Reichman, L. B., Hershfield, E. S., eds. *Tuberculosis — A Comprehensive International Approach*. New York: Marcel Dekker Inc. Chpt. 26, pp. 573–600.

Toman, K. (1979) *Tuberculosis. Case Finding and Chemotherapy*. Geneva: World Health Organization. pp. 3–5.

World Health Organization. (1992) *Bull. Wld. Hlth. Org.* **70**, 17–21.

World Health Organization. (1997) *Global Tuberculosis Programme. Report on Tuberculosis Epidemic*. Geneva: World Health Organization.

CHAPTER 4

THE POLITICS OF TUBERCULOSIS: THE ROLE OF PROCESS AND POWER

Gill Walt

Recognising the place of politics in infectious diseases is not new. In 1513, the political scientist, Machiavelli, compared a physician contemplating tuberculosis with politicians looking at public policy:

> 'It happens then as it does to physicians in the treatment of Consumption, which in the commencement is easy to cure and difficult to understand; but when it has neither been discovered in due time nor treated upon a proper principle, it becomes easy to understand and difficult to cure. The same thing happens in state affairs: by foreseeing them at a distance, which is only done by men of talents, the evils which might arise from them are soon cured; but when, from want of foresight, they are suffered to increase to such a height that they are perceptible to everyone, there is no longer any remedy'.[a]

Renewed concern about the resurgence of tuberculosis suggests that 'men of talents' have been found wanting, and many would agree that public health foresight might have kept this problem at more

[a]I owe this quote to Bloom and Murray (1992) who closed their paper with it.

manageable levels. Others might argue that, since tuberculosis is principally a disease of poverty and deprivation, the problem is one for politicians and not for public health specialists. Among this latter group
there are important exceptions, from Virchow's 19th century belief that
a physician's responsibility is to act as 'attorney for the poor' (Porter,
1997), to contemporary observations that politics is not outside the domain of the medical profession, since over the ages, physicians have been
powerful advocates of social reform and change (Grange, 1997).

How can politics help us to understand the re-emergence of a disease
which Selwyn Waksman, who won the Nobel Prize for his research on
streptomycin, described as having been conquered (Ryan, 1992)?

Politics can be defined in many ways: it may be about the exercise of
power or authority, the public allocation of goods and services that are
valued, the negotiation of interests between individuals and groups, and
the resolution of conflict. It is the determination of who gets what, when
and how, where the 'who' is not limited to individuals or groups, but
also to countries or parts of the world. In this chapter a policy analysis
approach is used to explore the different dimensions of politics: by looking at the *context* within which tuberculosis occurs and public policies
have been developed; by looking at the *actors* involved in tuberculosis
control at global, national and local levels; by looking at the *processes* of
policymaking, from policy initiation to implementation; and by looking
at policy outcomes — the *content* of policy. A descriptive framework becomes an explanatory framework as we explore who has wielded power
in order to influence change in the world of infectious diseases, why some
issues regarding infectious disease have made the policy agenda above
others, and how public policies have been negotiated between different
groups and parts of the world.

Some caveats are necessary. Much has been written about tuberculosis, although surprisingly little about the politics of the disease, even
given widespread acceptance of the relationship of tuberculosis with
poverty. It is much easier to impute causality of pathogens to individuals or groups using the methods of laboratory science or standard epidemiology, than to apply the tools of the social sciences such as politics

or sociology. Yet, it is these latter disciplines which are likely to throw light on the multitude of factors that describe the contours of infectious diseases: the ecological or human demographic changes and behaviour, travel and commerce, technology and industry, microbial adaptation, or weaknesses in public health systems (Morse, 1995). Farmer (1996, p. 266) has argued for new, complex models to deepen our understanding of the complexity of factors that promote or retard the emergence or re-emergence of infectious diseases. Furthermore, exploring the politics of tuberculosis from an international perspective provides only one layer of an extremely complex cake.

Context

1940s – 1970s: The promise of control

Scientific politics may be played out between competing scientific ideas, between ideologies, and because scientific discovery brings its own rewards in terms of status and financial gain. A number of political struggles surrounded the science that established the bacterial cause of tuberculosis and then the attempts to find drugs to treat it. Ryan (1992) describes the tension between two schools of thought in the Germany of the late 19th century, where Virchow's scepticism about bacterial causes of disease collided with Koch's announcement of his discovery of the tuberculosis bacterium. Virchow regarded medicine as a social science, and believed that physicians had to be able to understand the social roots of patients' illness, as well as the social conditions needed for their recovery. Koch's work was entirely laboratory based and, according to Ryan, it was on account of Virchow's antipathy to his ideas that the meeting at which Koch reported his finding of the tubercle bacillus was held in the School of Physiology rather than the School of Medicine, over which Virchow presided. Politics, it seems, had other effects on Koch, and rumours abounded about his later refusal to divulge the nature and preparation of the material which became the tuberculin skin test. Some suggest it was due to national and self-interest: to assure a monopoly for the German government and an institute for himself (Bloom and Murray, 1992), others that Koch sold his 'secret' to a drug company for a million marks, to help finance his divorce and remarriage (Porter, 1997).

Dissension also dogged the award of the 1952 Nobel Prize to Waksman. He was challenged by a young researcher, Albert Schatz, who claimed that it was he and not Waksman who had discovered streptomycin (Ryan, 1992). Some scientists also felt that the Nobel Prize that year should have been shared with Jorgen Lehmann, a Swede who discovered PAS (*para*-aminosalicylic acid) around the same time as streptomycin (although he published his findings a little later). Ryan (1992, p. 369) suggests that Lehmann's failure to be awarded the Nobel Prize jointly with Waksman was possibly due to jealousy among his own Swedish colleagues.

The politics involved in early scientific endeavours in looking for chemical cures for tuberculosis is not surprising in view of the impact that the new discoveries made. Once drugs were available, it seemed tuberculosis could be controlled. The anti-tuberculosis drugs of the late 1940s were hailed with enthusiasm by public health specialists who foresaw a potential eradication of the disease, by drug companies which foresaw large returns on their investments, and by patients who had suffered for years. The following two decades were unique in building confidence in the power of drugs to treat and control disease (not only tuberculosis). The addition of rifampicin in 1963 (which facilitated the development of shorter treatment regimes) seemed to offer significant choice in treatment in the face of existing problems associated with some of the older drugs. The era of the 'magic bullet' heralded a change in the assumptions and behaviour of patients and their physicians alike. Optimism was further supported as epidemiological data apparently provided evidence for the impact the new drugs had on morbidity and mortality, especially in industrialised countries. The impact of drugs was only challenged later, as long-term analysis showed that tuberculosis was declining in the industrialised world long before antibiotics were introduced. For example, in 1845, tuberculosis was killing about 500 out of 100,000 Europeans; by 1950 — before streptomycin was used generally — incidence had already fallen to 50 per 100,000 (Porter, 1997, p. 427).

In the white heat of technological advance, attention was on bacteria and their control, and by the 1960s it is probably fair to say that most public health physicians assumed that tuberculosis control and treatment was largely a managerial problem. This was strengthened by the collaboration between the Indian government, the United Kingdom's Medical Research Council (MRC) and World Health Organization (WHO) in India in the late 1950s, which demonstrated that ambulatory care was both feasible and effective and probably less stigmatising than incarcerating patients in sanitoria. It was reinforced by the apparent success of bacille Calmette-Guérin (BCG) vaccination, where, in the best case, children were protected from the disseminated forms of the disease (for example, tuberculous meningitis). It was only in the late 1970s and early 1980s that it was realised that BCG generally failed to control adult pulmonary disease. By this time BCG vaccination was already an accepted strategy for tuberculosis control (Colditz *et al.*, 1996).

The fact that developing countries in the greatest need, with high prevalence rates, were the least able to adopt the new ways of diagnosing and treating tuberculosis, became buried in the complacent belief that drugs and ambulatory care could cure those with disease and BCG vaccination could prevent further cases. Scientific journals reflected the lack of interest and attention of the public health policy and practitioner networks: the number of papers published on tuberculosis dropped to almost zero, until 1990, when they began appearing again. For example, the *Transactions of the Royal Society of Tropical Medicine* published fewer than six papers between 1970 and 1989, but 15 between 1990 and 1993.

1970s – 1990s: The nightmare of resurgence

Complacency was challenged in the 1970s, when tuberculosis began appearing in the industrialised countries among injecting drug users, the growing group of homeless people, and from the early 1980s, among those with HIV/AIDS. The recognition that tuberculosis was re-emerging in industrialised countries grew slowly. Garrett (1994, p. 279) claims that Reichman, then head of tuberculosis control in New York City, was unable to get papers published in scientific journals at the end of the 1970s because they were about a social group of marginal in-terest — 'junkies'. But by the mid-1980s the links between HIV/AIDS and tuberculosis were established and creating concern among public health scientists. In 1987 the Commission on Health Research for De-velopment, an influential group of international health policymakers, started a process of extensive global consultation through workshops and meetings to establish research needs for developing countries. By the time their final report was published in 1990, they had established tuberculosis as 'a neglected disease' (Commission on Health Research for Development, 1990, p. 22), and others were sharing their view. A World Bank review of problems in developing countries concluded that tuberculosis had been overlooked, and began lending for national pro-grammes of tuberculosis control in the early 1990s (Jamison and Mosley, 1992).

Work prepared for the Commission on Health Research and the World Bank to quantify the cost effectiveness of reported successes in tu-berculosis control was undertaken by a small number of interconnected researchers and practitioners in the USA and Europe, drawing on expe-rience such as that of the International Union Against Tuberculosis and Lung Disease which had achieved high cure rates in their East Africa tuberculosis programmes using few resources. Policy diffusion was rapid — especially as data was disseminated about the surge in tuberculosis among AIDS patients — and tuberculosis was back firmly on the health policy agenda by the end of the 1980s. In 1993, the WHO took the unprecedented step of declaring tuberculosis a 'global emergency'.

Regenerated interest in tuberculosis was undoubtedly fuelled by self-interest: although drug-resistant strains had long been diagnosed in de-veloping countries, multidrug resistance was a new and growing problem in industrialised countries, and was extremely expensive to manage. In

New York City almost a fifth of tuberculosis strains were resistant to the two main drugs, rifampicin and isoniazid, and 80% of those with such multidrug-resistant tuberculosis died. The cost of treating a tuberculosis patient in the USA jumped from US$2,000 for ambulatory care to as much as US$250,000 in the case of multidrug resistance (World Health Organization, 1994). Furthermore, the prevalence of tuberculosis amongst immigrants and increased travel among citizens were recognised as having some effect on infection levels (Driver *et al.*, 1994), although their relative contribution to growing incidence and outbreaks of tuberculosis was disputed, especially in relation to immigrants. Bloom and Murray (1992, p. 1059) reported that only 31% of excess cases of tuberculosis could be attributed to foreign-born individuals. Tuberculosis was recognised to be one of several emerging infectious diseases that did not respect national boundaries (Lederburg, quoted in Farmer, 1996). Recognising the externalities — "spillovers of benefits or losses from one individual to another" (World Bank, 1993, p. 55) of tuberculosis control services — legitimised their provision by governments and the provision of subsidies for such programmes, even in an era in which neo-liberal economists were questioning the role of government in health care provision and encouraging growth in the private sector.

The reappearance of tuberculosis (and the increasing incidence of HIV infection and AIDS) on the policy agenda was thus due to a combination of socio-economic and political factors exacerbated in some countries by the structural adjustment policies being promoted by the World Bank and International Monetary Fund (Lurie *et al.*, 1995). As the problem returned to the industrialised world, a small group of international health specialists, with backgrounds in medicine, public health and economics, recognised its serious consequences for international health and began working — through consultations, collecting evidence and calculating costs — to give prominence to a disease whose requiem had been presumptuous. This epistemic community, described by Haas (1992), as networks of professionals with recognised expertise and competence in a particular domain or issue area, was relatively small, authoritative and interconnected; and although individuals had

quite close contacts with the WHO, the organisation was not a major
actor in getting tuberculosis onto the international health policy agenda
until a few years later.

Actors: The Changing Face of Authority

World Health Organization: Diverted from tuberculosis

The WHO's position of leadership and authority in international health
was generally high until the late 1980s. From the 1970s, however, it
entered an era punctuated by dissension, initiated by its promotion of
the primary health care approach. This policy encouraged the exten-
sion and integration of preventive and curative health services especially
in developing countries where, historically, health services tended to be
urban based and hospital orientated. Although the treatment of common diseases such as tuberculosis and the provision of essential drugs
(including anti-tuberculosis drugs) were part of primary health care, focus shifted away from diseases and towards the development of health
systems, focusing on principles of equity, community participation, and
prevention and promotion of health — all issues which had social, economic and political implications. The WHO was drawn more explicitly
than ever before into political discussion and conflict (Walt, 1993).

While primary health care was strongly promoted and supported
within and outside the organisation, it had its opponents. Walsh and
Warren (1979), for example, concluded that while the goals of primary
health care were 'above reproach' they were not feasible because of the
cost and numbers of trained personnel required. Instead, they suggested a selective primary health care approach which would focus on
diseases which were both common and for which there were cost-effective
treatments. By their reckoning (their paper was published before HIV
was discovered or multidrug resistance was generally recognised), tuberculosis was only of 'medium' priority even in developing countries,
because of the difficulties in treating it. It is interesting to note that

Walsh and Warren also suggested that polio was a medium priority disease for developing countries, and yet within a decade the WHO had announced support for a Polio Eradication Programme, and by the 1990s there are signs that this goal may be achieved. There have been considerable debates, however, about some of the ethical and political dilemmas in supporting this programme (Taylor *et al.*, 1997) and claims that it has been unsuccessful in India (Mudur, 1998, p. 1264).

While proponents of primary health care were highly critical of what came to be known as 'selective primary health care' — many international agencies adopted a selective approach — supporting, for example, vertically-organised child immunisation programmes. Within the WHO, however, the policy trajectory through the 1980s continued to support primary health care — even under the Director-Generalship of Dr. Nakajima — through a process of 'Renewal for Health for All' (World Health Organization, 1996). Although diseases were still part of the WHO's programmes, they were in high profile only in those programmes such as the Special Programme on Research and Training in Tropical Diseases (TDR) which had significant extrabudgetary funds (Vaughan *et al.*, 1996). Thus, tuberculosis, which was not included in TDR (probably because of the prevailing view that the problem of tuberculosis was solved, and that it was now the task of national governments to implement proven strategies), was overshadowed by much better resourced programmes. Within the WHO, the Tuberculosis Unit was allowed to stagnate, and by 1989 it had only one member of staff. With few resources, the WHO played little more than a supportive or facilitating role in countries with national tuberculosis programmes. This was not necessarily through lack of interest. Adetokunbo Lucas (Director of TDR from 1976 to 1986) suggests that the WHO was "optimistic that countries would take up the challenge and use the available tools that were of proven efficacy. Developed countries did. Developing countries couldn't." (Lucas A, Personal communication). Thus, it was left to organisations such as the International Union Against Tuberculosis and Lung Disease, which Bloom and Murray (1992, p. 1061) call 'hero of the piece', to act as the 'operational arm' of the WHO, and run successful tuberculosis programmes in a number of countries during this period when tuberculosis hardly figured as a public health issue.

What *is* surprising is that the WHO, an organisation of more than 180 member states, many of which were low income and with high prevalence rates for tuberculosis, reflected so blatantly the public health complacency of its richer member states rather than the priorities of its low-income developing member states. Although, in theory, policy within the WHO is decided by member states at the World Health Assembly meetings every year, policies are being developed and designed by the staff who make up the Secretariat in Geneva, who are advised and assisted by scientists and health professionals all over the world, but probably dominated by those from the industrialised nations. In the 1960s and 1970s this epistemic community perceived tuberculosis as a problem which could be resolved through the proper use of drugs, or conditioned by poverty and, therefore, resolved through development and economic growth. Few of those working in public health saw development and economic growth as being within their domain of concern.

World Bank: Funding for tuberculosis

By the early 1990s, however, other powerful actors were joining forces to put tuberculosis back on the public policy agenda. The World Bank's 1993 Development Report added authority by categorising tuberculosis as a part of an essential clinical services package, and it began lending to countries embarking on revised tuberculosis control programmes. As authority in health policy shifted from the WHO to the World Bank (Mills and Zwi, 1995) so governments from the industrialised world took their cue from the Bank, and tried to stop the spread of the disease. Support grew for a different approach to managing the disease: directly observed therapy using short course chemotherapy. This rapidly became known as DOTS, and was heavily promoted by both the WHO and the World Bank as the preferred policy for treatment of tuberculosis, as the former organisation struggled to re-assert its authority in this field. The Global Tuberculosis Programme staff grew in number to 12 in 1994, through the mobilisation of extra resources (in 1992–1993 the WHO regular budget funds provided less than one-sixth of the tuberculosis budget — the rest came from external sources). The Tuberculosis Unit produced several glossy and accessible publications, which were clear advocacy bids for attention to, and renewed action on, tuberculosis. One used a dramatic table to illustrate the difference between the number of deaths from infectious and parasitic diseases and funding for those diseases. It drew graphic attention to the fact that the number of deaths from tuberculosis was much larger than from AIDS or leprosy (a disease similarly haunted by stigma, dormancy and slow growth) and yet, as shown in Table 1, AIDS and leprosy received, respectively, eleven and four times more funds (World Health Organization, 1994).

Table 1. Deaths per annum of people aged over five years from infectious and parasitic diseases and external aid given for their control. Data from the World Health Organization (1994).

Disease	Deaths	External aid (US$)
Tuberculosis	1,900,000	16,000,000
Malaria	400,000	55,000,000
AIDS	200,000	185,000,000
Parasitic disease	200,000	74,000,000
Leprosy	2,000	77,000,000

The pharmaceutical industry: Concern for profit

The other actors who neglected tuberculosis after the great discoveries of the early 20th century were the pharmaceutical companies. Garrett (1994, p. 440) claims that with the increase in tuberculosis, the global supply of streptomycin (unpatented, cheap and needed overwhelmingly in developing countries) was 'tapped out', and that the United States' Federal Drugs Agency had to convince drug companies to begin making the drug again. The drug was being made in countries such as India, but even domestic manufacturers were not enthusiastic producers of the cheap, non-brand named drugs where there was a market for second- and third-line drugs (Narayan, 1998). By the 1990s one of the acknowledged factors standing in the way of tuberculosis treatment was the market —

> *"commercial competition will not drive development of new anti-tuberculosis drugs as long as 95% of cases are in poor countries."* (Horton, 1995, p. 790).

Even when pharmaceutical companies began to explore the possibilities of testing potentially useful drugs, a complex and multi-actored global market led to conflicts between companies. Reichman (1996, p. 175) describes one such 'entanglement' between an American and a Japanese company. The American company wanted to start clinical trials of sparfloxacin (to which it held mycobacterial development rights) to test its usefulness in tuberculosis. The Japanese company which held the world licence for sparfloxacin argued, however, that if it was specifically tested for, and was found to have advantages for, the treatment tuberculosis, it might preclude the drug being used for other conditions such as chronic bronchitis, pneumonia "or other more prevalent (or profitable) conditions". The licence to the Americans was withdrawn. Others have noted some of the global complexities of drug manufacture and licensing (Reich and Govindaraj, 1998) in relation to other drugs.

Lack of investment in research on anti-tuberculosis strategies was, however, not limited to drugs or to the pharmaceutical sector. Research into vaccines and production decreased to the point that, by 1990, more than half of all vaccine manufacturers had stopped producing vaccines for some immunisable diseases and, although biotechnology was pointing the way to exciting new possibilities for vaccine design, enthusiasm was not strong in the industry (Garrett, 1994, p. 617). Within the publicly-funded research institutes, research on tuberculosis virtually stopped in the early 1950s, when antibiotics came on to the market. As late as 1992 Bloom and Murray (1992, p. 1057) lamented the 'wealth of ignorance' about the 'daunting' tubercle bacillus. This situation changed slowly as the realisation of the implications of the resurgence of tuberculosis spread and many more funds were accessed for both basic and applied research on tuberculosis. For example, in 1995 Glaxo-Wellcome announced a £10 million five-year grant for research into the biology of mycobacteria; governments began to give extrabudgetary support to the WHO and national research institutes; and aid agencies such as USAID announced additional funds of $50 million to fight infectious diseases in 1997 (Brown, 1997).

Technical co-operation specifically for tuberculosis control also increased in the 1990s, sometimes encouraging partnerships between donors and drug manufacturers, or very large tenders of drugs for national programmes. The political consequences were often marked. Fryatt (1995) describes the generous Japanese gift of rifampicin for three to four years to the Nepal tuberculosis control programme which raised a number of questions for managers of programmes, not only because of supply difficulties, erratic prescribing and sustainability, but because the drug could only be given as a single tablet because the Japanese pharmaceutical industry does not make combination therapy drugs. Managers were concerned that this would have a poor impact on treatment and was potentially less attractive to patients. Narayan (1998) points to accusations in the media of high-level illegal transactions over the huge tenders for tuberculosis drugs in the Revised National Strategy on Tuberculosis in India.

Community level actors

The public, patients and health workers

Possibly the most important actors in the tuberculosis story are those at the local level — the patients, their families, and the health professionals with whom they come into contact. At the beginning of the century, as the idea gained currency that the disease could be controlled, many local-level alliances were made between organised medicine and the public in Europe and the USA (Porter, 1997). Mass mobilisation efforts were expended in publicising the disease, educating people (against spitting, for example), and promoting preventive techniques. Local societies appealed to their communities for funding and ran local campaigns. By 1950 the American Lung Association was raising $20 million through its sale of Christmas seals alone. In India, local tuberculosis societies also existed, but by the 1990s had languished into relative inactivity (Narayan, 1998). In some countries, the International Union Against Tuberculosis and Lung Disease was an important player at the local level through its provision of services. However, by the time tuberculosis found its way back onto the health policy agenda, patients were, on the whole, being dealt with by often demotivated, overstretched, under-resourced health care personnel in public health services or in the unregulated and unaudited private sector. There was little community activity, or public, non-governmental advocacy on behalf of tuberculosis patients.

Health services: providing a useless bottle of cough medicine?

Treatment of tuberculosis depends on patients and their families presenting to public health care facilities or to private practitioners, and adhering to drug regimens. But it also depends on health professionals adhering to therapeutic guidelines and monitoring and following up cases. While it is acknowledged that these are singularly difficult goals to achieve, there has been surprisingly little written on the socio-economic, structural, political or cultural barriers to the implementation of tuberculosis programmes from the point of view of patients or health professionals. Where research has focused on social relations, it has been dominated by social scientists looking at families or households, with little attention being given to the societal political-economic factors which also affect social relations. Thus, patient non-compliance is often explained as being due to cultural or personality factors rather than to what Farmer (1997) calls 'structural violence' — the economic, social, ethical and political dimensions that underpin societal relations. One of the best examples of 'structural violence' is that of South Africa during the Apartheid years, where tuberculosis control measures involved the application of exclusionary policies designated to keep the disease out of the social and economic centres of white society, and where legislation was used to ensure this: through public health acts, urban area acts, influx control laws, slum clearance acts, group area acts and 'bantustans' (Packard, 1989, p. 299). Farmer suggests that explanations that rely on culture or personality tend to minimise the role of poverty in influencing behaviour and result in victim-blaming around compliance. Quoting from a number of other studies and experiences, he shows that even where patients believe that their tuberculosis is due to cultural factors such as witchcraft or 'susto' they will adhere to drug regimes at considerable costs to themselves. These factors, plus the tendency of academic researchers to promote their own disciplinary interests, means that inadequate attention has been paid to the political-economy of risk for patients and health workers. "Throughout the world, those least likely to comply are those least able to comply" (Farmer, 1997, p. 353).

It is acknowledged that the structure of the health system influences health seeking behaviour. Some studies have indicated that patients may visit a number of health providers (both private and public) before being diagnosed, delays which are exacerbated by "useless bottles of cough medicine" (Banerji, 1993, p. 79; Narayan, 1998). It is also acknowledged that private practitioners do not necessarily promote agreed therapeutic guidelines and are notorious for poor follow up of patients. Delays in diagnosis have costs to patients and their families, as curtailment or incomplete treatment has for society at large, by increasing the opportunities for development of drug resistance. In one study in Uganda, Saunderson (1995) found that 70% of total costs, from the initial symptoms to cure, were borne by the patient. He pointed out that considerable savings to the individual would be made by earlier diagnosis and ambulatory treatment. Many studies have indicated that patients are treated badly or carelessly when they present at health facilities, and that the necessary drugs or attention may be missing. There is also little emphasis on the possible unpleasantness experienced in taking anti-tuberculosis drugs. In an otherwise good social behavioural account of patient adherence, Sumartojo (1993) mentions the fact that patients may experience unpleasant side effects from taking anti-tuberculosis drugs, but never returns to this point. Frantz Medard, who headed the Harlem Hospital DOT programme from 1992, and himself suffered a year of undiagnosed illness and then 27 months of multidrug therapy, talked of the painfulness of amikacin injections (Garrett, 1994, p. 527). Patients in India mentioned a variety of symptoms after taking drugs (Narayan, 1998).

Patients may complain with reason about the failure of health services to deliver good-quality care, and health workers are often blamed for unprofessional attitudes to work and to patients. Status and gender differentials may exacerbate what are already unequal power relations — especially when the majority of patients are among the poorest members of communities. Focusing on the weaknesses of health workers, however, detracts attention from structural factors which leave them on relatively low wages, with poor levels of support and supervision, irregular drug supplies, feelings of isolation and limited opportunities for continuing education and career enhancement. Health workers are also at risk from developing tuberculosis from their contact with patients (Colditz et al., 1996) and may have difficulties in relating to patients with what is perceived to be, and is experienced as, a stigmatising disease.

Stigma affects behaviour in both seeking health care and adhering to treatment. Bryder (1996), for example, notes that even when notification of the disease became compulsory in England and Wales in the first decades of this century, many tuberculosis sufferers were reluctant to come forward because insurance would be lost if insurance companies knew the patients had consumption. In her study of rural India, Narayan (1998) quotes a mother saying she would not tell the multipurpose health worker, who had responsibility for tuberculosis in her village, that her daughter had tuberculosis because it would lessen her chances of marriage. Another study in Bombay suggested that married women were also discriminated against once it was known they had tuberculosis — being sent back to their parental home, for instance (Nair *et al.*, 1997). Even being declared 'cured' does not remove stigma — patients with leprosy who were successfully treated nevertheless continued to feel stigmatised (Justice, personal communication). Although many famous people are known to have had tuberculosis, from statesman President Nelson Mandela to film actress Vivien Leigh, there are few cases where such people have taken public stances (as have some public figures with AIDS) to mobilise support for overcoming some of the stigmatising effects of being diagnosed to have tuberculosis.

Policy Processes

Identification and design of technically-feasible and cost-effective policies to combat infectious diseases is only one part of a complex policy cycle. Implementing those policies, even when they are relatively uncontroversial, may be constrained by a host of factors, which may or may not be taken into consideration by policymakers. With diseases such as tuberculosis, which are relatively difficult to diagnose and treat, the gap between policy intention and implementation may be great. There may also be considerable debate about the best strategy to implement the policy. For example, a major source of tension in international health aid since the second world war has been between two strategies: one which emphasises *the development of health infrastructures* (as in the primary health care approach described above), and the other which promotes *selective, vertical programmes* to solve health problems. At the international level, the interests promoting the latter approach have always been stronger than those supporting the development of health systems, although not everyone perceives them to be mutually exclusive. Which approach is followed is influenced by political factors such as authority: of those who can enjoin others to provide funds for specific programmes, and whose status is such that promotion of a particular approach will be accepted. It is notable that the major achievements in eradicating smallpox, increasing the coverage of childhood immunisation, controlling river blindness, potentially eradicating polio, and possibly measles after that, have all needed concerted support from well-established, high-status, international organisations (and particular individuals within them) as well as national governments.

It is not surprising that international support has been for selective, vertical programmes based on clear technical approaches. For both organisations and individuals within them there is probably greater satisfaction in pursuing a single goal which may be achievable within the life career of a professional and which can be easily quantified, than helping to build a system which may take a much longer time, and is dependent on many different inputs. This is particularly true when programmes are supported by foreign technical co-operations. It is also easier to capture the imagination of other international participants, sponsors and domestic constituencies to particular issues or diseases than to generalised infrastructure building. Finally, it is much easier to monitor and control resources to such programmes, thus providing the justification for undertaking them in the first place.

Even in the industrialised countries, some have observed that it was, among other factors, the withdrawal of earmarked, or targeted, funds for tuberculosis that led to the re-emergence of the disease (Hopewell, 1994). In most of Europe and the USA, tuberculosis control was organised as a vertical programme within the public health services, and it was only when anti-tuberculosis drugs became widely available, and ambulatory care sanctioned, that tuberculosis became integrated into other health services.

As tuberculosis began to be treated at home, and patient numbers decreased, so public health professionals diverted their attentions to other public health problems and funds for tuberculosis declined. In 1968 New York City spent US$40 million annually to maintain 100 designated tuberculosis beds; by 1978 this had been decreased by up to US$17 million, and the beds had disappeared (Farmer, 1997). Reichman argues that block grants to the states for general public health services, which replaced targeted funding for tuberculosis control, further undermined tuberculosis work in the 1970s. Although he concedes this was not the only factor that led to the "start of a vicious tuberculosis resurgence", he nevertheless sees the recrudescence as "a direct result of the national switch from targeted categorical grants to block grants for tuberculosis control a decade earlier" (Reichman, 1996, p. 176). A block grant is, claims Reichman "extremely desirable to governors, mayors, and health commissioners ... because it gives them access to a spending bonanza of unrestricted federal funds".

While somewhat overstated, block grants do allow public health specialists (who usually advise governors, mayors and other local policymakers) to decide their own priorities according to local needs. Given the widespread post-1950s belief in the public health community that tuberculosis was a disease of the past, it is not surprising that funds went to other public health problem areas.

It is, however, interesting that in the UK the increase in tuberculosis rates was much slower (5% between 1987–1991) compared to the USA which was 20% (between 1985–1992). This may have been due to the UK's national health service, which offered an accessible, universal service, free at point-of-contact, to all its citizens, in sharp contrast to the USA's health policies which excluded some 40 million people. If so, this would support those who believe that building a health service infrastructure is an important part of controlling infectious diseases. However, both having, and then allocating, *sufficient* resources to developing health services is essential. India's national tuberculosis programme launched in 1962 was always conceived as part of the public health services from national to district level, but it was underfunded and had to compete with a strong private sector. Furthermore, building up health infrastructures is perceived to be a national responsibility, and there is, understandably, much less interest on the part of international organisations to devote the sort of long-term, intensive technical assistance and funds that are required for the improvement of such systems.

One of the arguments against vertically-managed and resourced programmes is that they divert resources and attention from integrated services. Narayan (1998) identifies one of the many factors that explain the gap between policy development and implementation of the national tuberculosis programme in India as being the huge resources which were made available by international organisations and the Government of India for the vertically-managed family planning programme of the 1960s and 1970s. Losing physical, economic and human resources to other programmes is well recognised. Millard (quoted in Gounder, 1998) described what happened in a South African context:

> 'During the polio campaign, nurses and transport were withdrawn from the TB services with no warning. It was only for a short time, we were told, and of course a few days without drugs will do no harm, but it is precisely this attitude that is so damaging to the TB programme. The message is clear to patients, supervisors and nursing staff — TB is not important ...'

It is certainly true that, as the number of cases of tuberculosis declined in the industrialised world, specific funding for tuberculosis was diverted or decreased. This diminution was accompanied by a loss of specialist interest in the disease. Many attest to the loss of experienced and committed tuberculosis specialists from the 1960s onwards (Reichman, 1996, Farmer, 1997, Garrett, 1994), not only in the industrialised world where tuberculosis, it seemed, was disappearing, but also in low-income countries, such as India, where it still took its toll. Banerji (1993) notes the downward spiral in output and influence of the 'politically mandated' National Tuberculosis Institute in Bangalore, where international experts such as Halfdan Mahler (before he became Director-General of the WHO) had worked closely with Indian colleagues on research which resulted in the design for a socially-acceptable, integrated National Tuberculosis Control Programme. Narayan (1998) observes that, in the 1980s, tuberculosis specialists in public health were replaced at the district level with public health officers who had much wider responsibilities. Many regional offices of the WHO abolished the post of tuberculosis officer over the same period. By the early 1990s, as resources for tuberculosis began to rise, reports were made of improving tuberculosis surveillance and cure rates as new posts were made and, once more, health workers were appointed specifically to work on tuberculosis (Harries *et al.*, 1996).

Policy Outcome

Although the WHO's declaration of tuberculosis as 'a global emergency' in 1993 was welcomed by many, the Organization struggled to take a leadership role in tuberculosis. Boseley (1998) quotes Grange as saying:

> '*I think the WHO have had a very difficult time ... they have established policies but they just haven't had the global support for TB. I feel the WHO is being asked to do something without the money.... It is the world governments that have to vote the money to the WHO and with the notable exception of the UK, the money has not been forthcoming.*'

The WHO's lack of ability to mobilise sufficient external extra resources may have been influenced by many different factors: the effort and funds the donor community has committed to polio eradication, for example. But there has also been some concern expressed over the rigid design of the WHO's chosen strategy to address the emergency — using Directly Observed Therapy Short Course (DOTS) on a grand scale — and some reservations about the high-profile, public relations approach to advocating its strategy. Glossy publications were seen by many as being a waste of resources.

Many studies of relatively small populations have shown that supervision of medication, whether directly observed by health workers or others, such as family members, can achieve high levels of cure rates. Such programmes tended to be on a relatively small scale and adopted to local community needs, and none has been based on a randomised controlled trial (Volmink and Garner, 1997). While few doubt the effectiveness of supervised treatment, doubts have been expressed about the feasibility of programmes based on large-scale direct observation by health workers. Current enthusiasm for DOTS (which does depend on health worker supervision of medication) stemmed from the positive results attained in the highly-specialised situation and population of New York City and some have questioned the relevance of transferring the New York strategy to cover very large populations such as in India or China. The World Bank has, however, made loans available to national programmes which have adopted the DOTS strategy, and in the 1990s both China and India introduced DOTS programmes. The first reports from China suggest that high cure rates are possible, although with relatively high financial incentives for health workers concerned (Huus, 1993), which may not be affordable or sustainable in all situations. The programme has nevertheless been hailed as a model for programmes elsewhere (China Tuberculosis Control Collaboration, 1996).

In India, where such incentives were not an integral part of the Revised National Strategy on tuberculosis, initial negotiations between the World Bank and the government over terms and conditions were both protracted and perceived as being highly political (Narayan, 1998). For example, many policymakers resented what they saw as foreign interference in national health policy; they perceived consultants to be arrogant and unappreciative of long Indian experience with the disease, and were concerned about the opportunities DOTS gave for corruption. The discussions in India have reflected familiar dilemmas: firstly, the built-in tensions between the needs of externally-funded programmes for targets, short-term goals and rapid results, and the needs of domestic programmes for long-term capacity building, performance enhancement and development, and secondly, the tendency to focus on 'cases' controlled, in order to stem the spread of infection, rather than on patients and their families, whose needs are not always recognised.

Balancing external and domestic demands

In the first case, concerns have been raised about 'bad public policy', which in its haste to implement strategies such as DOTS, reflects some of the worst aspects of vertical programme implementation: an orientation towards rigidity, rapidity, results, and an over-ambitious commitment to eliminating or eradicating the disease. As one of the major infectious diseases which has dominated public health for centuries, tuberculosis cannot be equated with other diseases such as smallpox or polio, where eradication is mooted. Even the elimination of leprosy, caused by the related pathogen *Mycobacterium leprae*, which has been described as 'a real possibility' (Noordeen, 1995, p. 6) is being disputed as research suggests that the number of new cases of leprosy have not diminished even in those areas where the numbers of patients cured has increased dramatically. Understanding the disease is essential to the design of policy and, in the case of both smallpox and polio, much was understood about the disease. Also, the technologies available for treatment were relatively simple, although the strategies for delivering treatment were in sharp contrast. The smallpox campaign was a military-style, vertically-organised, well-funded and orchestrated mass vaccination programme, which was attained at considerable financial cost, commitment and leadership, but was also characterised, at least in its final stages in South Asia, by intimidation and coercion (Greenough, 1995).

It has been suggested that polio eradication was also forced on some countries which did not see it as a primary priority, but was less vertically organised. In the Americas, where it was initiated, it was conceived of as a targeted programme *within* existing primary health services. Ciro de Quadros of the Pan American Health Organisation (PAHO), who spearheaded polio eradication, has been quoted as saying:

> *'In the Americas, when we started polio eradication, we intentionally reinforced one, the immunisation program in general, and two, the health infrastructure, particularly in relation to surveillance, program planning and program management'.* (Gounder, 1998)

How true this experience is for other parts of the world is unclear, and it still raises questions of sustainability since huge financial resources have been raised for polio eradication, and a large number of actors, including Rotary International from the private sector, have been mobilised to participate in its implementation both locally as well as globally.

As argued earlier, vertical programmes are attractive to the international community for many reasons, and if they are promoting eradication or elimination of a disease they have an even greater cachet. Whether they are the *best* public health policies remains hotly debated (Taylor *et al.*, 1997; Cutts and Steinglass, 1998; Gounder, 1998). While some argue that tuberculosis could be eliminated — Enarson (1995, p. 809), for example, has suggested that "the elimination of tuberculosis from human society is theoretically possible" — it is unlikely that this view is widespread. Nevertheless, the demands of donors providing resources for programmes in low-income countries for rapid (and successful) results to satisfy their domestic constituencies cannot be underestimated. This may lead to programme designs which do not allow sufficient flexibility to take account of local conditions and culture (rigidity); which do not allow time for mobilising communities and health workers (rapidity); and which are so focused on reaching targets that falsification occurs and findings are undermined (results). The importance of building understanding and goodwill among health workers and communities is paramount to good implementation practice. Incentives for sustaining diagnosis and control will not have a sustained impact if they are merely financial, although they may help in the short term. Nichter (1995) has highlighted the differences between a dependent community, on whom health solutions are imposed, and a mobilised community, whose members perceive the need and thus *demand* resolution of health problems.

The other criticism of DOTS is that it focuses on cases and on controlling the spread of disease, rather than on concern for individual patients. Critics of large national DOTS programmes have pointed to the lack of attention given to patients' costs — in terms of travel time, unpleasantness of treatment (by health workers, but also from having to take 12 pills daily for two months, and the side effects of the drugs) — and having to live with the daily acknowledgement of stigma. Porter and Ogden (1997, p. 124) question some of the ethics of public health where civil liberties may be undermined by drawing on research in India:

> "Is the autonomy of the average Indian TB patient being respected when he/she is expected to travel long distances, expose himself to public scrutiny, and deplete his small resource base simply to comply to DOTS?"

Some also perceive the policy to treat only sputum-positive patients as unethical and unfair, and a clear indication that the public health concern is with the goal of controlling the spread of disease, rather than seeing patients as sick individuals, whether sputum-negative or positive.

Conclusion

By describing the context, actors and processes that have influenced tuberculosis policy, it is apparent how important political factors have been in the identification and recognition of the problem, and in the development of policies to deal with it. Without recognition by policymakers, issues do not make it to the policy agenda, described by Kingdon (1984, p. 3) as

> "the list of subjects or problems to which government officials and people outside government closely associated with those officials, are paying some serious attention at any given time".

From the late 1950s it is fair to say that tuberculosis disappeared from the policy agenda in industrialised countries, and was relegated to a relatively insignificant position in most developing countries a decade later, even where prevalence was still high. A political explanation for the low attention given to it by government officials in those countries would obviously be unique to each country: but a number of generalised factors would have influenced the way tuberculosis policy was perceived. One clearly was the dominance of western medical perceptions mediated through epistemic communities, which set standards, priorities and interest areas through training, and scientific dissemination. In the 1950s and 1960s, even though many developing countries had established independent nation status, they were still highly influenced by colonial ties through professional education and administration. New political elites were sometimes insulated from the poor in their own countries, and had to cope with the competing calls for attention from aid agencies with different, and changing, agendas.

The reappearance of tuberculosis on the policy agenda of industrialised nations in the 1990s was clearly due to serious concern about its re-emergence, multidrug resistance and spread within and between countries. USAID described its rationale for increasing resources to fight infectious diseases as one of 'self-defence' (Brown, 1997). It was key figures in the epistemic community who alerted the international community, through aggregating and disseminating information on the rising incidence of tuberculosis, but it was largely self-interest that led to increased levels of attention and funds. Farmer (1996, p. 267) quotes from the US Institute of Medicines report on emerging infections:

> *'Diseases that appear not to threaten the United States*
> *directly rarely elicit the political support necessary to*
> *maintain control efforts'.*

What was true for the USA was also true for European and other nations. The role of the World Bank in drawing attention to tuberculosis and, through its authority, encouraging others to do the same, was also important.

Each of the four dimensions of politics mentioned at the beginning of this chapter recurs as a thread interwoven throughout the policy analysis. The *role of power and authority* recurs at all levels of the story, with policy elites playing both positive and negative roles. The epistemic community, or the network of scientists and practitioners, was dominated by those from industrialised countries, whose complacency about the disease from the late 1950s was based on the biomedical model which placed drugs at the centre of the solution. It was, however, this same epistemic community (although different individuals) which put tuberculosis back on the policy agenda at the end of the 1980s, and who argued hard for increase in attention and funding for the disease. Among this network are the giants of international public health, who have played a crucial role in regenerating interest in this 'vicious', 'daunting' and 'fastidious' pathogen. Their primary motivation is not self-interest or fear, but humanitarian and ethical concern. Enarson (1995, p. 810), for example, has said:

> *"We know that if we put our minds to it, we can control*
> *tuberculosis even in the midst of poverty, war and HIV.*
> *This engagement is to the mutual benefit of all partners.*
> *It only remains to put this knowledge into practice by*
> *global solidarity and a charitable spirit".*

In developing countries, where tuberculosis never declined to the same extent as in industrialised countries, and where the disease is overwhelmingly (but not only) a disease of the poor, policy elites have, on the whole, been preoccupied with other issues within the health sector (depending on what period is being studied, and the ideology of the government of the time). Members of the epistemic community, the often highly committed tuberculosis specialists and public health physicians, have retired and, in many countries, tuberculosis has returned to the policy agenda only because policy elites have been persuaded by the 'global emergency' advocacy from the WHO and loans from the World Bank.

Understanding politics as the *public allocation of goods* that are valued, is clearly also reflected in the tuberculosis story: industrialised world concern about multidrug resistance and the contagiousness of tuberculosis has mobilised more, if not sufficient, resources for tuberculosis programmes. Newspaper headlines such as 'TB on the Rampage Again' (Boseley, 1998) try to build public support for re-allocating or expanding resources, but there are always competing demands and alternative priorities, as has been clearly observed with, for example, the polio eradication campaign (Gounder, 1998). Since tuberculosis affects the poorest groups, who are the least powerful, they often depend on others who are more influential to represent their interests or demands. And where low-income countries depend on foreign funds to help support tuberculosis control programmes, there may be a conflict between domestic priorities to build up and sustain health infrastructures and external demands for vertically-organised programmes.

Clearly *negotiations between different interests* are mediated at all levels — from international to local. One of the features of international health in the 1990s is that there are far more actors than there were in the days of, say, smallpox eradication. The potential for alliances and partnerships between the private sector, non-governmental organisations, international organisations and governments is much greater than it used to be, but will be fraught with political consequences flowing from the different cultures, agendas and ways of working of the various interests. At the local level, health managers, health workers and patients also reflect different attitudes, expectations and concerns, which influence behaviour and outcomes. The idea of negotiating agreement over behaviour between these groups is relatively rare, especially in formalised programmes which follow standardised norms and procedures, and among health professionals who use hierarchy and position to impose their will on patients.

Finally, the *resolution of conflict* over policy, rather than between political or economic factions, is a recurring theme in public health. In tuberculosis control this plays itself out in two debates: one is about the tension between integrating, but not marginalising, tuberculosis control within basic health services (which in many countries are in desperate need of improvement), and running the risk of creating a vertical programme which focuses on tuberculosis, but weakens existing health services, and may not be sustainable in the longer run. The other debate centres around conflicting notions that decide on the design of programmes: one informed by biomedical values and the other by socio-political values. The former tends to reflect programmes in terms of outcomes, number of cases treated and cured, following standardised procedures and assuming transportability between countries. The latter tends to see tuberculosis as a disease of poverty, but which cannot wait for economic development to change that situation. Hence, it reflects programmes which take account of patients' living and working conditions, which are flexible, accessible and try to deal with both treatment regimes as well as the stigmatising effects of the disease. Resolving this conflict of values is extremely difficult, because there are positive and negative consequences of both, and there is probably no existing model that satisfies the conditions of either, and attains *and* sustains high success rates.

It is difficult to escape the conclusion that the close link between poverty and tuberculosis has been a major political factor in the way policymakers have responded to the disease, from the recognition of the problem, its serious consideration on the policy agenda, to the implementation of programmes. When the disease has been a threat to social groups other than the disempowered (the poor, drug addicts, or the homeless) such as health professionals, travellers or middle-class AIDS sufferers, policymakers have felt inclined to consider new options for its treatment in order to protect non-poor communities. The unintended consequences of the forces of globalisation — from travel to unregulated and indiscriminate drug prescription — may thus have some gains for the poor, in renewed interest in tuberculosis services. Making those services successful and sustainable as they will need to be over many years, however, will depend on focusing more on patients' needs than on counting cases cured. There are encouraging signs that such thinking is beginning. In a 1997 editorial about tuberculosis control, the authors ask the question, "did the programme fail, or did we fail the programme?" (Dujardin *et al.*, 1997). They conclude that, while there are no miracle solutions, current approaches and research priorities need to focus less on technical aspects and more on comprehensive health services, including the perceptions of health personnel and patients.

References

Banerji, D. (1993) A social science approach to strengthening India's national tuberculosis programme. *Ind. J. Tuberc.* **40**, 61–82.

Bloom, B. and Murray, C. (1992) Tuberculosis: Commentary on a reemergent killer. *Science* **257**, 1055–1064.

Boseley, S. (1998) TB on the rampage again. *The Guardian*, 19 March, p. 2.

Brown, D. (1997) US agency devotes $50M more to fight infectious disease overseas. *Washington Post*. December 18th. p. A15.

Bryder, L. (1996) 'Not always one and the same thing': The registration of tuberculosis deaths in Britain, 1900–1950. *Soc. Hist. Med.* **9**, 253–265.

China Tuberculosis Control Collaboration. (1996) Results of directly observed short-course chemotherapy in 112,842 Chinese patients with smear-positive tuberculosis. *Lancet* **347**, 358–362.

Colditz, G., Brewer, T., Berkey, C., Wilson, M., Burdick, E., Fineberg, H. and Mosterller, F. (1996) Efficacy of BCG vaccine in the prevention of tuberculosis. *J. Am. Med. Assoc.* **271**, 698–702.

Commission on Health Research for Development. (1990) *Health Research: Essential Link to Equity in Development.* Oxford: Oxford University Press.

Cutts, F. and Steinglass, R. (1998) Should measles be eradicated? *Br. Med. J.* **316**, 765–767.

Driver, C., Valway, S., Meade Morgan, W., Onorato, I. and Castro, K. (1994) Transmission of *Mycobacterium tuberculosis* associated with air travel. *J. Am. Med. Assoc.* **272**, 1031–1035.

Dujardin, B., Kegels, G., Buve, A. and Mercenier, P. (1997) Tuberculosis control: Did the programme fail or did we fail the programme. *Trop. Med. Int. Hlth.* **2**, 715–718.

Enarson, D. A., *et al.* (1995) The challenge of tuberculosis: Statements on global control and prevention. *Lancet* **346**, 809–819.

Farmer, P. (1996) Social inequalities and emerging infectious diseases. *Emerg. Infect. Dis.* **2**, 259–269.

Farmer, P. (1997) Social Scientists and the new tuberculosis. *Soc. Sci. Med.* **44**, 347–358.

Fryatt, B. (1995) Editorial: Foreign aid and TB control policy in Nepal. *Lancet* **346**, 328.

Garrett, L. (1994) *The Coming Plague.* New York: Penguin Books.

Gounder, C. (1998) The progress of the polio eradication initiative and prospects for eradicating measles. *Hlth. Pol. Plann.* **13**, 212–233.

Grange, J. (1997) DOTS and beyond: Towards a holistic approach to the conquest of tuberculosis. *Int. J. Tuberc. Lung Dis.* **1**, 293–296.

Greenough, P. (1995) Intimidation, coercion and resistance in the final stages of the South Asian smallpox eradication campaign. *Soc. Sci. Med.* **41**, 633–645.

Haas, P. M. (1992) Introduction: Epistemic communities and international policy coordination. *Int. Org.* **46**, 1–35.

Harries, A. D., Nyong'Onya Mbewe, L., Salaniponi, F., Nyangulu, D., Veen, J., Ringdal, T. and Nunn, P. (1996) Tuberculosis programme changes and treatment outcomes in patients with smear-positive pulmonary tuberculosis in Blantyre, Malawi. *Lancet* **347**, 807–809.

Hopewell, P. (1994) The baby and the bath water. *Am. J. Resp. Crit. Care. Med.* **150**, 895.

Horton, R. (1995) Editorial: Towards the elimination of tuberculosis. *Lancet* **346**, 790.

Huus, K. (1993) 'Ten Get it, Nine Die.' *Newsweek*, May 17, p. 29.

Jamison, D. and Mosley, H. eds. (1992) *Disease Control Priorities in Developing Countries*. Oxford: Oxford University Press for the World Bank.

Justice, J. Personal communication.

Kingdon, J. (1984) *Agendas, Alternatives and Public Policies*. Boston: Little Brown and Co.

Lucas, A. (1998) Personal communication

Lurie, P., Hintzen, P. and Lowe, R. (1995) Socioeconomic obstacles to HIV prevention and treatment in developing countries: The roles of the International Monetary Fund and the World Bank. *AIDS* **9**, 539–546.

Mills, A. and Zwi, A. (1995) Health policy in less developed countries: Past trends and future directions. *J. Int. Dev.* **7**, 299–328.

Morse, S. (1995) Factors in the emergence of infectious diseases. *Emerg. Infect. Dis.* **1**, 7–15.

Mudur, G. (1998) Flawed immunisation policies in India led to polio paralysis. *Br. Med. J.* **316**, 1264.

Nair, D., George, A. and Chacko, K. T. (1997) Tuberculosis in Bombay: New insights from poor urban patients. *Hlth. Pol. Plann.* **1**, 77–85.

Narayan, T. (1998) *A Study of Policy Process and Implementation of the National Tuberculosis Control Programme in India*. Doctoral Thesis, London School of Hygiene and Tropical Medicine.

Nichter, M. (1995) Vaccinations in the third world: A consideration of community demand. *Soc. Sci. Med.* **41**, 617–632.

Noordeen, S. K. (1995) Elimination of leprosy as a public health problem: Progress and prospects. *Bull. Wld. Hlth. Org.* **73**, 1–6.

Packard, R. (1989) *White Plague, Black Labour*. London: James Currey.

Porter, J. and Ogden, J. (1997) Ethics of directly observed therapy for the control of infectious diseases. *Bull. Inst. Pasteur.* **95**, 117–127.

Porter, R. (1997) *The Greatest Benefit to Mankind*. London: Harper Collins.

Reich, M. and Govindaraj, R. (1998) Dilemmas in drug development for tropical diseases: Experiences with praziquantal. *Hlth. Pol.* **44**, 1–18.

Reichman, L. (1996) How to ensure the continued resurgence of tuberculosis. *Lancet* **347**, 175–177.

Ryan, F. (1992) *Tuberculosis: The Greatest Story Never Told*. Bromsgrove, England: Swift Publishers.

Saunderson, P. (1995) An economic evaluation of alternative programme designs for tuberculosis control in rural Uganda. *Soc. Sci. Med.* **40**, 1203–1212.

Sumartojo, E. (1993) When tuberculosis treatment fails. A social behavioural account of patient adherence. *Am. Rev. Res. Dis.* **147**, 1311–1320.

Taylor, C., Cutts, F. and Taylor, M. (1997) Ethical dilemmas in current planning for polio eradication. *Am. J Publ. Hlth.* **87**, 922–915.

Vaughan, J. P., *et al.* (1996) Financing the World Health Organization: Global importance of extrabudgetary funds. *Hlth. Pol.* **35**, 229–245.

Volmink, J. and Garner, P. (1997) Systematic review of randomised controlled trials of strategies to promote adherence to tuberculosis treatment. *Br. Med. J.* **315**, 1403–1406.

Walsh, J. and Warren, K. (1979) Selective primary health care. *N. Engl. J. Med.* **301**, 967–974.

Walt, G. (1993) WHO under stress: Implications for health policy. *Hlth. Pol.* **24**, 125–144.

World Bank. (1993) *World Development Report: Investing in Health.* Oxford University Press: Oxford.

World Health Organization. (1994) *TB: A Global Emergency.* Geneva: World Health Organization. (WHO/TB/94.177)

World Health Organization. (1996) (August) *Consultative Document: Renewal of Health-for-All.* Geneva: World Health Organization. Unpublished document, pp. 26–30.

CHAPTER 5

PUBLIC HEALTH AND HUMAN RIGHTS: THE ETHICS OF INTERNATIONAL PUBLIC HEALTH INTERVENTIONS FOR TUBERCULOSIS

Paul Pronyk and John Porter

> *"Neither science nor activism can be conceived outside or apart from a broader ethical framework, rooted in moral philosophy, capable of giving meaning to our work, of respecting while at the same time moving beyond the particularities and differences that define us".* (Parker 1996)

The scene is a small African country with a population of five million people. Sixty per cent of individuals reside in the rural areas. The life expectancy is 60 years, and the infant mortality rate is five times that of industrialised nations. The literacy rate is 60% and 10% of children under five are chronically malnourished. Access to health care is available to those who can afford it in the urban areas. In rural areas, there are poorly-developed medical and public health infrastructures which, when fully operational, serve half of those residing there.

The country has recently undergone a period of economic readjustment which has resulted in increasing poverty and a widening of the gap between rich and poor. Basic health services in the rural areas have had to face the introduction of cost-recovery user-fees. As a consequence of increasing foreign investment and an emerging cash-economy, many more have entered the work force. Most men in the rural areas now migrate to the cities for seasonal work.

Tuberculosis is endemic. Most of the population has been exposed to *Mycobacterium tuberculosis* based on skin test surveys. In addition, there have been reports of a recent increase in active cases, both in the urban and rural areas. There has been a concurrent rise in the prevalence of HIV based on a limited screening programme.

As a member of the National Tuberculosis Control Programme, you are involved in the development and implementation of a public health strategy to contain the spread of tuberculosis? What are the ethical dimensions of such a challenge?

Introduction

Any attempt to articulate and address the forces mitigating the health of populations is necessarily framed in ethical perspectives. The interactions between exposure and vulnerability, often the direct consequence of specific social, structural and environmental conditions, are enmeshed in human judgements and decisions of value. Tuberculosis, both as a historical scourge and a re-emerging disease, has its roots in the interactions of such proximate social dynamics. Disease control programmes, therefore, need to reflect not only a scientific understanding of the generation and transmission of an infectious pathogen, but also, in the broadest sense, a sensitivity to existing structural relationships and social dynamics, particularly among those most marginalised groups in a population.

As the year 2000 approaches, 50 years after the UN Declaration of Human Rights and 20 years after the Declaration of Alma-Ata (see below), a rediscovery of the significance and strength of these 'ethics' documents is warranted. Both documents provide a focus for public health and for the control of infectious diseases such as tuberculosis.

Ethics

In practice, ethics denotes several mutually interconnected perspectives; namely, the study of ethics, the adherence to ethical guidelines laid down by governments and professional bodies, and the application of ethical principles in daily life. In the study of ethics, philosophers develop theories about the interaction between moral values and the ways in which societies operate. Morals — the values and norms that frame societies' ideas about 'right' and 'wrong' — are inherently cultural constructions. All cultures and societies have moral codes, but because these are culturally and historically contingent, they shift and change over time (Porter and Ogden, 1997).

Beaufort and Dupuis (1988) have suggested that the ethical process might be used to clarify concepts, analyse and structure arguments, weigh alternatives and provide advice on an 'appropriate' course of action. Another way of looking at an ethical argument is that it can assist us in identifying the obstacles that prevent us from acting 'morally'. Once these obstacles have been identified, it is easier to find ways of overcoming them.

The four principles which currently dominate ethical debates are: respect for autonomy, beneficence, non-maleficence and justice (Beauchamp and Childress, 1983). These principles — plus attention to their scope (i.e. how and to whom they apply) — provide the basis for a rigorous consideration and resolution of ethical dilemmas. Although they do not provide 'rules', these principles can help public health workers to make decisions when moral issues arise. In effect they attempt to make a common set of moral commitments more visible and more accessible (Gillon, 1994). These principles are considered to be *prima facie*: they are binding unless they conflict with other moral principles.

Though generally accepted as useful guidelines when facing ethical questions among individuals (between a patient and provider, or between an individual and a government structure), the application of these principles to larger questions of research or policy may be less clear cut. For example, recent controversies regarding the testing of new drugs or vaccines in poor communities of underdeveloped countries, where minimum standards of care are often unmet, raises questions that are more murky (Halsey *et al.*, 1997). Whose interests are being served through the research? Will the product being developed be realistically affordable and accessible to these communities once the study is over? How does the research address the fundamental needs and health priorities of a community?

When framing the ethical dimensions of the public health process more generally, issues and interests operating on many levels necessarily intermingle — from local, national and international, to the personal, professional and legal. Nothing is primarily black or white. Ethical questions that arise around the case of tuberculosis control are inextricably related to an emerging discourse on the nature and scope of public health paradigms.

What is Public Health?

Public health is "fulfilling societies' interest in assuring the conditions in which people can be healthy" (Institute of Medicine, 1988). There is growing appreciation that the mechanisms underlying disease transmission require wider analysis than that encompassed by prevailing approaches to the control and elimination of infectious disease (Krieger and Zierler, 1996; Shy, 1997; Wing, 1994; Susser and Susser, 1996). New perspectives in public health attempt to shift the debate from the assumption that health happens by eliminating diseases like tuberculosis, to a public health paradigm founded on the *creation* or production of health (Kickbusch, 1997). This is more than a semantic distinction if public health is to be understood as a broadly-organised social response to both the production of health and the consumption of health services. Operating both in the mainstream and perhaps more notably at societies' fringes (i.e. with society's most vulnerable groups), it is ultimately a product of how we have come to understand ourselves — integrating perspectives on class, culture, science and politics.

In this context, ethics are inescapable. Implicit is the need to incorporate a diversity of interests, and to effect collaborative efforts with those outside the traditional health sector. Such constructs acknowledge that health and disease are often the endpoints of complex social and environmental interactions, rarely respecting disciplinary boundaries.

We are presently immersed in an era of profound historical transition, the impact of which on human health and well-being is the subject of substantial research and speculation. The US Institute of Medicine has put forward six factors that are predicted to have the most influence on health over the next 20 years: human demographics and behaviour; technology and industry; economic development and land use; international travel and commerce; microbiological adaptation and change, and the breakdown of public health measures (Institute of Medicine, 1988). All six factors are clearly related to the control of tuberculosis. There is, for example, already evidence of rapid microbiological adaptation in *M. tuberculosis* with the development of drug resistance (Porter and Ogden, 1997), high case prevalence among economically-disadvantaged populations and immigrants (Bayer and Dupuis, 1995) and evidence of poorly-funded public health infrastructures leading to low cure rates and the emergence of drug resistance (Gittler, 1994).

It is clear that a coherent public health approach to tuberculosis control must be concerned with an understanding of the variety of forces mitigating the burden of this disease in a population. Through this focus and concentration, it then becomes possible to explore those factors necessary to provide the conditions in which people do not acquire tuberculosis.

The Public Health Declarations: Human Rights, and Alma-Ata

Human rights

The first legal texts concerning the right to health did not emerge until the 20th century (Susser, 1993). The preamble of the World Health

Organization's (WHO) Constitution of July 22, 1946, states that, "the enjoyment of the highest attainable standards of health is one of the fundamental rights of every human being without distinction of race, religion, political belief, economic or social condition". Similarly, Article 25 of the Universal Declaration of Human Rights of December 14, 1948, begins with the assertion that, "everyone has the right to a standard of living adequate for the health and well-being of himself and of his family, including food, clothing, housing and medical care and necessary social services...". In essence, the Declaration advocates equal access to those factors well recognised as basic prerequisites for health.

The document emerged in the aftermath of World War II, as a testimony and multi-nation recognition of the inherent dignity and inalienable rights of all, which are considered to be the foundation for freedom, justice and peace. It is an attempt to find a "common ground," and to assist countries in working together to address common rights and duties. Rights rest on certain assumptions: on the dignity, worth, value and respect of a human being; on the importance of communities, social networks, and governnments; and on accountability within these structures. As such, the right to health cannot feasibly entail a set of individual contracts to ensure a healthy state for each person (Susser, 1993). It is more of a societal commitment that necessarily entails equity between groups as a fundamental principle.

The Alma-Ata Declaration

At the International Conference on Primary Health Care held at Alma-Ata in 1978, a declaration that radically challenged prevailing thinking on the interaction of health and disease was produced (World Health Organization, 1978). Known subsequently as the Alma-Ata Declaration, it was, in essence, an affirmation of the fundamental relationship between equity, justice and health, in an increasingly interdependent world (Pronyk, 1997). It explicitly recognised the links between health care and sustainable economic and social development in the 'spirit of self-reliance and self-determination'. As such, it aspires to address the root causes of disease and those preconditions necessary for the well-being of populations. In this respect, Alma-Ata articulates the broad concept of public health described earlier.

The first article of the Alma-Ata declaration reaffirms that health, as 'a state of complete physical, mental and social well-being, and not merely an absence of disease or infirmity', is a fundamental right and that the attainment of the highest possible level of health is an imperative whose realisation requires the action of many other social and economic sectors in addition to the health sector. Articles six to eight state the unacceptability of existing gross inequalities in health status, as well as in economic and social development, and emphasise the right and duty for people to participate both individually and collectively in the planning and implementation of their health care. The articles then affirm the responsibility of governments in providing adequate health and social measures, and finally point to primary health care as an essential component. The declaration, however, recognises that primary health care alone, without corresponding economic and social advances, is a hollow aspiration.

Ethics Unites all the Declarations and is at the Core of Public Health

Common themes recur throughout these important 'historical' documents: equity, the need for collaborative and multi-disciplinary approaches, self-reliance and self-determination. The strength of these imperatives has re-emerged in the context of other international discourse. Current perspectives on biodiversity and ecosystem health underscore the importance of equity and sustainability in priority-setting (McMichael, 1996). Their relevance to health and human development pervades international declarations and UN documents (World Health Organization, 1996; United Nations Development Programme, 1994; 1996). The recent Habitat II conference, for example, placed equity, sustainability and civic engagement as the foremost preconditions to health in human settlements (Korten, 1996). As such, they form broadly agreed upon parameters with which to frame, address and evaluate much of the public health process. In a sense, they serve as quasi-legal and moral prerogatives that might assist in applying ethical structure to questions of research, programme development, or policy formulation.

Though many acknowledge that these documents are reflective of international consensus, and that their bearing on the health of populations is profoundly important, how might they assist in making 'real world' decisions? How are we able to put these themes into practice? It is evident from these declarations that we know what we want, but we do not know how to get there. There exists a profound need to diminish abstraction in the interests of moving forward.

Ethics and the Control of Tuberculosis

Tuberculosis control — An overview

Current tuberculosis control strategies concentrate on reducing the transmission of pulmonary tuberculosis through infected sputum (sputum-positive cases) by finding cases of sputum-positive tuberculosis and treating them until they become sputum negative and are eventually cured. The regimen of short course anti-tuberculosis lasts for six months, with four drugs (rifampicin, isoniazid, pyrazinamide and ethambutol) being taken for the first two months and two drugs (rifampicin and isoniazid) for the subsequent four months. If the patient does not take the full course of medication correctly, there is the danger that drug resistance will develop. In response to low cure rates and the threat of increasing drug resistance, directly observed therapy, short course (DOTS) has become the cornerstone of the World Health Organization Global Tuberculosis Programme (Harries and Maher, 1996). The components of this programme are listed in Table 1.

The World Health Organization DOTS strategy has achieved excellent results in New York and other parts of the USA (Frieden, 1995; Morse, 1996) and in China (Zhao Feng-Zeng *et al.*, 1996). In other

Table 1.   The components of the WHO Global Tuberculosis Control Programme.*

1   Government commitment to a national tuberculosis programme.
2   Case detection through 'passive' case finding (sputum smear microscopy for pulmonary tuberculosis suspects presenting at a health care facility).
3   Short course chemotherapy for all smear positive pulmonary tuberculosis cases, under direct observation for at least the initial phase of treatment (DOT).
4   Regular, uninterrupted supply of all essential anti-tuberculosis drugs; and a monitoring system for programme supervision and evaluation.

*Source: WHO, 1994; WHO, 1995; Harries and Maher, 1996.

parts of the world, however, questions have been raised as to whether DOTS is the most effective way to control tuberculosis (Juvekar *et al.*, 1995; Gangadharam, 1994), whether it can and should be perceived as a panacea (Makubalo, 1996) and even whether it is ethical (Bayer and Dupuis, 1995; Porter and Ogden, 1997).

Defining the issues — Ethics

Programmes and policies aimed at the control of tuberculosis bring multiple ethical perspectives to light. One cannot thoughtfully examine such issues without regard to the broader framework which informs public health and infectious disease control more generally.

Framing the picture

The theoretical basis for the World Health Organization Global Tuberculosis Programme, and for much of public health, derives from particular historical and scientific foundations. The process of clinical and basic science and the tools of epidemiological research have combined to help us understand the world around us. These dynamics interact with an array of competing interests and social forces in the formulation and orchestration of public health policy. The framework in which empirical evidence is gathered then ultimately defines the limitations of its ability to influence larger social and political decisions (Wing, 1994; Krieger, 1994; Rothman and Poole, 1985).

Prevailing biomedical approaches attempt to understand and isolate micro-level interactions, and emphasise individualistic conceptions of causation and cure (Fee and Krieger, 1993). By contrast, modern epidemiology attempts to define and model patterns of risk based on empirically-derived data (Wing, 1994). In the case of tuberculosis, population-level risk is generally defined by the proportion of susceptible individuals who come into contact with active cases. As such, public health programmes generally emphasise the identification and treatment of individuals with active disease, the prevention of latent disease from becoming active, and, to a lesser extent, the prevention of initial infection (Bayer and Dupuis, 1995). The empirical methods which form the basis of control efforts are attractive to policy makers as they are scientifically generated, concrete and open to evaluation by measures such as the amount of drugs or vaccines dispensed, the number of patients screened, or the proportion of cases cured.

Much of the ethical discourse surrounding the control of tuberculosis juxtaposes the rights of the individual and that of the community at large (Bayer and Dupuis, 1995). It acknowledges the autonomy and self-determination of the individual, but places limits on this freedom when there exists the potential for harm to others — as an individual with active tuberculosis might infect others in the community. It is in this situation that 'the state' or institutions of public health may intervene. Questions arise such as how an individual might maintain his or her dignity and worth, while at the same time protect the community of which that person is a part. Issues of involuntary quarantine and the requirement of patients with active disease to take their pills in the presence of an observer (directly observed therapy) serve to test the moral and legal application of public health principles (Annas, 1993).

Despite its claims of scientific objectivity and impartiality, the ethical dimensions of the present public health and policy discourse are often revealed through the weight of those questions that it is unable to address. For example, is curing tuberculosis in individuals sufficient as a strategy for the overall control of tuberculosis in a population? What are the relationships that exist between risk factors that serve to increase the chance of developing tuberculosis? How do particular social and historical relationships serve to generate unhealthy exposures? Does the scientific and public health process itself contribute to inequity and, if so, how might these imbalances be reinforced by disease control measures? Are there alternative ways of approaching public health interventions that would redress, rather than reinforce, these kinds of imbalances and inequalities? (Bayer *et al.*, 1993; Bayer and Dupuis, 1995; Porter and Ogden, 1997).

An inability to address such issues, which are fundamental to understanding population risk and vulnerability, results in inadequate research questions, insufficient programmatic responses and stunted policy formulation. It is in this shortcoming in the scope of the public health agenda, to which the current priority-setting process may be ethically and morally complicit. In effect, the deficiency of an adequate and informed ethical process may result in bad public health.

The 'Right to Health'?

In examining the burden of tuberculosis in populations, the work of McKeown and colleagues based on data from the past two centuries highlights the importance of social and economic improvement alone in reducing rates of disease. It was shown that improvements in living standards were in themselves responsible for much of the historical decline in rates of tuberculosis (McKeown and Record, 1962; McKeown *et al.*, 1975). More recent data similarly confirm that tuberculosis rates are generally highest among the poor and marginalised. Such groups face a higher burden of disease in relation to conditions of homelessness, substance abuse, psychological stress, poor nutritional status, and congregate residence in shelters or incarceration facilities (Bayer and Dupuis, 1995; Gittler, 1994). Such conditions also intensify the vulnerability to HIV infection, which substantially amplifies the risk for active tuberculosis among groups with previously latent infection. Access to health services is also often limited for such groups. An epidemiology founded on the identification of risk factors for tuberculosis in individuals and biomedical approaches to treating active cases and their contacts do little to address the fundamental importance of such issues. Furthermore, is a public health agenda founded on predominantly such principles ethical?

Such issues are certainly complex. Rose argues that an overemphasis on individuals deemed to be 'high risk', as defined by independent variables such as economic status, place of residence (common lodging house or prison), or a personal history of drug use, may be short-sighted. He postulates that disease in populations is more a reflection of the mean-level of risk in that society, rather than simply a product of cumulative, individual choices (Rose, 1985). Those with active tuberculosis are a reflection of that proportion of individuals on the 'high end' of the normative distribution. Some populations are clearly at higher risk of tuberculosis than others. Is this a product simply of cumulative individual choices, or are there larger social and structural issues that, once articulated, might be more effectively addressed? Rose argues that without a concerted effort to reduce the mean population risk (shift the curve to the left), the best a programme may hope to achieve is a temporising effect. For example, case studies in South Africa detailing the relationship between tuberculosis, poverty, and the migration of labour to work in the mines — where overcrowding, poor ventilation and an absence of UV light create an optimum environment for tuberculosis dissemination — highlight the complexity of such issues (Packard, 1989). A control programme targeting only those with active disease, without taking steps towards reducing the 'mean risk' for all workers — through measures such as legislation, education, work-place safety — is clearly insufficient. Such environments are simply microcosms which well illustrate similar structural forces influencing the wider burden of tuberculosis in populations.

In 1993, the WHO declared tuberculosis a 'global health emergency' based on new evidence that this disease is responsible for more annual deaths worldwide than any other infectious disease (Kaye and Frieden, 1996). Great strides in improving those structural conditions that engender health will certainly not evolve overnight, and many feel that responsibility for them lies outside the direct purview of health sector interventions. In addition, there is a profound human need to feel as if we are doing something for patients and communities. Though the strengths of biomedical approaches are well substantiated, are they alone sufficient to control tuberculosis? Shifting the emphasis to the structures and processes that engender health may require new tools and perspectives. Ethics necessarily intermingles with all elements of the priority-setting process — on personal, professional, and organisational dynamics. As such, it has the potential to prompt a re-examination of the way science interacts with society in the development of more effective and ethical public health. The tenets of the Human Rights Declaration and Alma-Ata have the potential to serve as useful tools to guide this process.

Equity

Equity entails treating no portion of the population in a disproportionate manner. Inequity, then, is a descriptive term used to denote existing differences between groups or individuals in the distribution of or access to resources. Inequity, however, denotes the reasons behind and responsibilities for underlying conditions of inequality. As such, it is inherently a statement of justice (Stephens, 1997).

The United Nations Development Programme (UNDP) describes equity in terms of the opportunities that allow individuals "to enlarge their human capabilities to the full and put those capabilities to their best use in all fields — economic, social, cultural, and political" (United Nations Development Programme, 1994). As such, it is the availability and universal access to adequate health and social measures which form the preconditions for leading "socially and economically-productive lives" (World Health Organization, 1978). Susser (1993) suggests that there are at least four constituents of an equitably distributed health right: equal access to appropriate services, equity in health states, evaluative mechanisms, and equitable socio-political arrangements that give a voice to all groups in sustaining equity in health.

That social equity is an essential component to the health and well-being of populations is unquestionable (Kawachi and Kennedy, 1997). There is a growing body of literature confirming the relationship between inequality, disease rates and a host of other detrimental social parameters (Davey-Smith, 1996; Rodgers, 1979; Waldman, 1992; Wilkinson, 1994; Kaplan *et al.*, 1996). In addition to the importance of equity in the context of access to basic needs, it serves as a proxy for far more complex human relationships. Such conditions of equity form the basis of health both within nations and between them (Wilkinson, 1996). Susser (1993) concludes his article on 'Health as a Human Right' by stating "Equity will elude any society that does not weigh the questions before it in terms of their higher professional values — that is, the right to health of the people at large".

Inequity within societies determines, to a great extent, those populations vulnerable to tuberculosis. It colours the relationships between patient and provider and between the public health system and communities more generally. Individual interactions so often singularly encapsulate many dimensions of existing inequities — for example, between a poor illiterate woman and her child with tuberculosis and a male physician from the dominant social, economic and linguistic class. Similar relationships are also reflected on the level of interactions between institutions and high-risk communities. Any ethical position justifying potentially coercive disease control measures must be sensitive to this reality. It underscores the importance of addressing root causes in addition to the immediate symptoms of tuberculosis.

Dominant paradigms of disease causality in individuals with definable risks tend to obscure the relationship between equity and health (Farmer, 1997, Wilkinson, 1996). Poor housing, illiteracy, or income level may each be noted and controlled for as 'independent variables'. It is, however, the complex interaction between variables and how they are perceived within a particular social and cultural framework that impart significance. By implication, then, there are certain properties of society as a whole that critically influence the health of that society.

One might argue that DOTS is a reaction to the failure to address the wider issues of poverty and social inequality by the international community (Annas, 1993). The cruel irony is that failures of this kind can lead to increased social control and coercion. Rather than confronting squarely their responsibility to recast their approaches to treatment, tuberculosis control programmes place the onus on patients to comply with increasingly rigid regimens. Clearly, the threat of increasing drug resistance and the potential lack of new drugs for treating tuberculosis is a frightening prospect. Yet programmers and policy makers have a choice in how to respond: they can close ranks and force people to comply with a programme they deem appropriate, or they can engage with a process by which communities are enabled to identify tuberculosis control measures that are appropriate to them. In situations where access to the most basic material and social resources are seriously constrained, the ethics of DOTS is no less contentious (Porter and Ogden, 1997).

Finally, equity as a matter of personal ethics or professional norms, demands more than simply access to health and other services among socially marginalised groups. It entails a critical self-awareness of the social and historical context of one's own work and perspective. Implicit is an open-minded willingness to be educated by and socialised to the complex dimensions of life in those communities where tuberculosis is endemic.

Civic engagement

Alma-Ata's call to civic engagement and popular participation has been a largely neglected facet of tuberculosis control. This pertains to all aspects of the priority-setting process — from the formulation of research imperatives, to the interpretation and presentation of results, to the orchestration of public health policy. In HIV/AIDS, the presence of an active civic movement leaves an "indelible stamp on what takes place ... and serves as a constant reminder of how the research/policy affects the lives of individuals" (Heymann, 1995). In addition, such participation may foster a better understanding of, and adherence to, treatment protocols by patients, and may assist in obtaining good results under many different circumstances.

At present, communities are often left to manage or implement the policy decisions that others have determined to be best for them (Loewenson, 1993). Issues pertaining to the cultural and historical relevance of interventions are muted in the face of standardised approaches to disease control (Porter and Ogden, 1997). This is in spite of the fact that active community participation often leads to creative, innovative and more 'common sense' solutions, with equity and common values high on the agenda (Stephens, 1997; Gaye and Diallo, 1997). Public health approaches that support "collective empowerment and community mobilisation" provide the structural foundation for the success of such efforts (Parker, 1996).

Intersectoral collaboration

As tuberculosis has its roots in complex social, economic and political realities, efforts to work between disciplines and sectors is essential. It is well recognised that no single approach or single discipline has the capacity to meet adequately the challenges of re-emerging infectious diseases such as tuberculosis (Morse and Hughes, 1996). In addition, the same factors that place communities at risk for tuberculosis also amplify the risk of HIV, diarrhoeal disease, and malaria, to name a few (Pronyk, 1997; Environmental Health Project, 1996).

Strict disciplinary structures can be witnessed in all aspects of the priority-setting process — from attendance at meetings and conferences, to the organisation of universities, governments and international bodies — each with its own distinct budget allocation and research methods. Such structures place constraints around everything from the attendance at conferences and meetings, to budget allocation, to the choice of research methods — which are often neither understood nor respected by those outside the field.

Bridging the rigid academic and institutional disease-oriented focus and moving towards integrated and collective disease-control models has the potential to address those common conditions underlying ill-health (Stephens, 1997; United Nations Development Programme, 1994; see also Chapter 20). Efforts to work between disciplines bring multiple academic, social and historical perspectives to bear on an issue and assist in providing alternative approaches that address the root-causes rather than the symptoms of ill-health. Rather than reducing a problem down to its smallest elements to be analysed individually, new approaches look for broader dimensions common to many issues. Programmes founded on such premises may support the long-term needs of communities and have diffuse impact on many fronts. As such, they have the potential to underscore and impact upon those large-scale social forces which influence unequally-positioned individuals and groups in increasingly interconnected populations. Through a diversity of perspectives and expertise, such collaborative effort serves to expand the scope of what is possible.

Conclusions

The 'ethics' documents of the Universal Declaration of Human Rights and the Alma-Ata Declaration demonstrate that the human family knows what it wants, but does not know how to achieve what it wants. Currently, in public health, we seem to be unable to find an appropriate way forward. This is well demonstrated in this chapter which has produced more questions than it has answered. Could, for example, ethical considerations help to address the issues of tuberculosis faced by the small African country mentioned at the beginning of this chapter? What is this 'process' that we are looking for and how are we going to develop it? In public health terms we are looking for ways to 'create health', to create 'healthy communities' and by doing so, more appropriate ways of controlling tuberculosis.

The content of this chapter suggests that the core discipline needed to help us find this 'way forward', this 'process', is ethics. In reading policy and strategy documents on tuberculosis control (e.g. World Health Organization, 1974; 1982; 1988) certain words appear consistently: integration, commitment, collaboration, communication, consideration, involvement, community, value, participation, relationship... All these words relate to how we interact as human beings and how we relate to each other. This issue of relatedness is what ethics is about. Ethics is "learning to live together" (Bonhoeffer, 1971, p. 237) and we need to see health as being inseparable from the local moral order of our everyday worlds (Kleinman and Kleinman, 1997, p. 115).

We are proposing that a first stage in the development of our process is to use the concepts of equity, civic engagement and inter-sectoral collaboration contained within the Declaration of Human Rights and the Alma-Ata Declaration, to address the current perspective of tuberculosis control in order to re-frame the picture and to expand the current biomedical perspective. In re-framing the picture, we will find different and more creative approaches to our current 'old' methods of disease control (See Chapter 19).

But equity, civic engagement and inter-sectoral collaboration are in themselves difficult concepts to understand and act on. A concept of 'civic engagement', for example, can only be achieved if each of us is willing to engage in a communal act of inter-relating with other people and being willing to witness and accept other people's perspectives. The concept of 'community', inter-personal relatedness, and the social origins of disease are largely left out of the biomedical discourse and, consequently, are less of a way of life in western industrialised countries compared to countries in Asia (Kleinman and Kleinman, 1997, p. 101). The Eastern philosophies and ways of life have much to teach the West about autonomy, community and divinity (Shwedar *et al.*, 1997). This communal inter-relating needs to occur not only in communities affected by tuberculosis, but also among the groups relating to these communities, and among the organisations that employ health care workers and researchers to work with these communities.

In using these ethical concepts of equity, civic engagement and inter-sectoral collaboration to guide our way forward, we will inevitably produce conflict and problems. These problems need to be seen as positive and must be dealt with positively. This is the art of making difficult problems soluble, a process which Medawar (1984) called the 'art of the soluble'. After all, it is through tackling problems that we find a process of engagement and integration between people with tuberculosis, their communities, districts, states, governments and the international community.

References

Annas, G. J. (1993) Control of tuberculosis — The law and the public's health. *N. Engl. J. Med.* **328**, 585–588.

Bayer, R. and Dupuis, L. (1995) Tuberculosis, public health and civil liberties. *Annu. Rev. Publ. Hlth.* **16**, 307–326.

Beauchamp, T. L. and Childress, J. F. (1983) *Principles of Biomedical Ethics*, 2nd edn. Oxford: Oxford University Press.

Beaufort, I. D. and Dupuis, H. M. (1988) *Handbock Gezondheidsethick.* Assen/Maastricht: Van Goreurn.

Bonhoeffer, D. (1971) *Ethics.* London and New York: McMillan.

Davey-Smith, G. (1996) Editorial: Income inequality and mortality: Why are they related? *Br. Med. J.* **312**, 987–988.

Environmental Health Project. (1996) *Prevention: Environmental Health Interventions to Sustain Child Survival.* Applied Study No. 3. Washington DC: USAID.

Farmer, P. (1997) Social inequalities and emerging infectious disease. *Emerg. Infect. Dis.* **2**, 259–269.

Fee, E. and Krieger, N. (1993) Understanding AIDS: Historical interpretation and the limits of biomedical individualism. *Am. J. Publ. Hlth.* **83**, 1477–1486.

Frieden, T. R., Fujiwara, P. I., Washko, R. M. and Hamburg, M. A. (1995) Tuberculosis in New York City — Turning the tide. *N. Eng. J. Med.* **333**, 229–233.

Gangadharam, P. R. J. (1994) Editorial: Chemotherapy of tuberculosis under program conditions. *Tubercle. Lung. Dis.* **75**, 241–244.

Gaye, M. and Diallo, F. (1997) Community participation in the management of the urban environment in Rufisque (Senegal). *Environment and Urbanization* **9**, 9–29.

Gillon, R. (1994) Medical ethics: Four principles plus attention to scope. *Br. Med. J.* **309**, 184–188.

Gittler, J. (1994) Controlling resurgent tuberculosis: Public health agencies, public policy and law. *J. Hlth. Politics Policy Law* **19**, 107–143.

Halsey, N. A., Sommer, A., Henderson, D. A. and Black, R. E. (1997) Ethics and international research. *Br. Med. J.* **315**, 965.

Harries, A. D. and Maher, D. (1996) *Tuberculosis/HIV: A Clinical Manual.* Geneva: World Health Organization (TB/96.200).

Heymann, S. J. (1995) Patients in research: Not just subjects but partners. *Science* **269**, 797–798.

Institute of Medicine. (1988) *The Future of Public Health.* Washington, DC: National Academy Press.

Juvekar, S. K., *et al.* (1995) Social and operational determinants of patient behaviour in lung tuberculosis. *Ind. J. Tuberc.* **42**, 87–94.

Kaplan, G. A., Pamuk, E. R., Lynch, J. W., Cohen, R. D. and Balfour, J. L. (1996) Inequality in income and mortality in the United States: Analysis of mortality and potential pathways. *Br. Med. J.* **312**, 999–1003.

Kawachi, I. and Kennedy, B. (1997) Health and social cohesion: Why care about income inequality? *Br. Med. J.* **314**, 1037–1040.

Kaye, K. and Frieden, T. K. (1996) Tuberculosis control: The relevance of classic principles in an era of acquired immuno deficiency syndrome and multidrug resistance. *Epidemiol. Rev.* **18**, 52–63.

Kickbusch, I. (1997) New Players for a new era: Responding to the global public health challenges. *J. Publ. Hlth. Med.* **19**, 171–178.

Kleinman, A. and Kleinman, J. (1997) Moral transformations of health and suffering in Chinese society. In: Brandt, A. M., Rozin, P., eds. *Morality and Health.* New York and London: Routledge. pp. 101–118.

Korten, D. (1996) Civic engagement in creating future cities. *Environment and Urbanization* **8**, 35–49.

Krieger, N. (1994) Epidemiology and the web of causation: Has anyone seen the spider? *Soc. Sci. Med.* **39**, 887–903.

Krieger, N. and Zierler, S. (1996) What explains the public's health — A call for epidemiologic theory. *Epidemiology* **7**, 107–109.

Loewenson, R. (1993) Structural adjustment and health policy in Africa. *Int. J. Hlth. Serv.* **23**, 717–730.

Makubalo, L. E. (1996) Editorial. *Epidemiological Comments* **23**, 1.

Medawar, P. (1984) *Pluto's Republic* (incorporating the 'Art of the Soluble'). Oxford: Oxford University Press.

McKeown, T. and Record, R. G. (1962) Reasons for the decline of mortality in England and Wales during the nineteenth century. *Population Studies* **16**, 94–122.

Public Health and Human Rights 119

McKeown, T., Record, R. G. and Turner, R. D. (1975) An interpretation of the decline of mortality in England and Wales during the twentieth century. *Population Studies* **29**, 391–422.

McMichael, A. J. (1996) *Global Environmental Change and Human Health: Scales of Impact; Population Vulnerability; and Research Priorities.* Beijer Discussion Paper Series 84.

Morse, D. I. (1996) Directly-observed therapy for tuberculosis: Spend now or pay later. *Br. Med. J.* **312**, 719–720.

Morse, S. and Hughes, J. M. (1996) Developing and integrated approach to emerging infectious diseases. *Epidemiol Rev.* 18, 1–3.

Packard, R. (1989) *White Plague, Black Labour: Tuberculosis and the Political Economy of Health and Disease in South Africa.* Pietermaritzburg: University of Natal Press.

Parker, R. G. (1996) Empowerment, community mobilization and social change in the face of HIV/AIDS. *AIDS* **10** (suppl III), s27–s31.

Porter, J. D. H. and Ogden, J. A. (1997) Ethics of directly observed therapy for the control of infectious diseases. *Bull. Inst. Pasteur* **95**, 117–127.

Pronyk, P. M. (1997) *The Control of Infectious Diseases: Re-examining Alma-Ata.* MSc thesis, London School of Hygiene and Tropical Medicine.

Rodgers, G. B. (1979) Income and inequality as determinants of mortality: An international cross-sectional analysis. *Population Studies* **33**, 343–351.

Rose, G. (1985) Sick individuals and sick populations. *Int. J. Epidemiol.* **14**, 32–38.

Rothman, K. J. and Poole, C. (1985) Science and policy making (editorial). *Am. J. Publ. Hlth.* **75**, 340–341.

Shwedar, R. A., Much, N. C., Mahapatra, M. and Park, L. (1997) The big three of morality (autonomy, community, divinity) and the big three explanations of suffering. In: Brandt, A. M., Rozin, P., eds. *Morality and Health.* New York and London: Routledge.

Shy, C. M. (1997) The failure of academic epidemiology: Witness for the prosecution. *Am. J. Epidemiol.* **145**, 479–484.

Stephens, C. (1997) *Environment, Health and Development: Addressing Complexity in The Priority Setting Process.* Geneva: World Health Organization Office of Global and Integrated Environmental Health.

Susser, M. (1993) Health as a human right: An epidemiologist's perspective on the public health. *Am. J. Publ. Hlth.* **83**, 418–426.

Susser, M. and Susser, E. (1996) Choosing a future for epidemiology I: Eras and paradigms. *Am. J. Publ. Hlth.* **86**, 668–673.

United Nations Development Programme. (1994) *Human Development Report.* Geneva: United Nations Development Programme, p. 4.

United Nations Development Programme. (1996) *Human Development Report.* Geneva: United Nations Development Programme.

Waldman, R. J. (1992) Income distribution and infant mortality. *Quart. J. Econ.* **107**, 1283–1302.

Wilkinson, R. G. (1994) *Unfair Shares*. Ilford: Barnardo's.
Wilkinson, R. G. (1996) *Unhealthy Societies: The Afflictions of Inequality*. New York and London: Routledge.
Wing, S. (1994) Limits of epidemiology. *Medicine and Global Survival* 1, 74–86.
World Health Organization. (1974) *Tuberculosis: Ninth Report of the WHO Expert Committee* (Technical Report No. 552). Geneva: World Health Organization.
World Health Organization. (1978) *Declaration of Alma-Ata. International Conference on Primary Health Care*, Alma-Ata, USSR, 6–12 September 1978. Geneva: World Health Organization.
World Health Organization. (1982) *Tuberculosis Control. Report of a Joint IUAT/ WHO Study Group* (Technical Report No. 571). Geneva: World Health Organization.
World Health Organization. (1988) *Tuberculosis Control as an Integral Part of Primary Health Care*. Geneva: World Health Organization (Publication No. 88/7778).
World Health Organization. (1996) *World Health Report*. Geneva: World Health Organization.
Zhao, F.-Z., *et al.* (1997) Results of directly-observed short course chemotherapy in 112, 842 Chinese patients with smear positive tuberculosis. *Lancet* **347**, 358–362.

PART II

THE CURRENT INTERNATIONAL STRUCTURE

CHAPTER 6

TUBERCULOSIS IN HIGH-PREVALENCE COUNTRIES: CURRENT CONTROL STRATEGIES AND THEIR TECHNICAL AND OPERATIONAL LIMITATIONS

Klaus Jochem and John Walley

Introduction

The current international approach to tuberculosis control follows the paradigm of a disease control programme managed by public health services. This chapter focuses on the principal medical interventions for the control of tuberculosis, summarised in Fig. 1, and some of the technical and operational issues of service delivery in developing countries. The implication is that broader social and policy issues need to be addressed if effective care for tuberculosis patients is to be part of a general commitment to improved health, and not a sometime achievement of a disease control programme hostage to donor funding and susceptible to the vagaries of priority setting in the health sector — arguments taken up explicitly in other chapters.

Control Strategies Involving Medical Interventions

BCG vaccination

Since its introduction in 1921, bacille Calmette–Guérin (BCG) has been the most widely used of all vaccines. Its efficacy has been a subject of

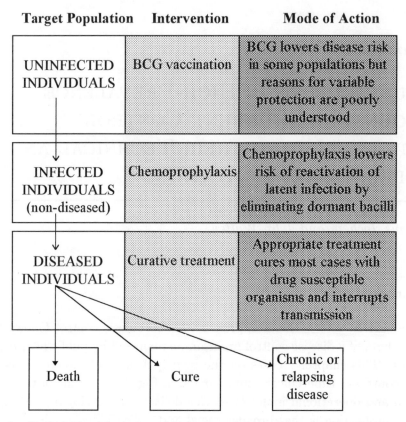

Fig. 1. Basic epidemiological model of tuberculosis showing target populations and mode of action of medical interventions.

controversy since the late 1950s when large discordances were observed in major trials, ranging from a negative efficacy in the large Chingleput trial in South India to a maximum efficacy of 80% in clinical trials in the UK and the USA (Bloom and Fine, 1994). Though nutritional status can affect immune responses (Adeiga et al., 1994), the most plausible interpretation of variable protection has been differential exposure to environmental mycobacteria, or heterologous immunity involving common mycobacterial antigens, the higher exposure in tropical zones masking the protective benefit of BCG vaccine (Fine, 1995).

Another problem in the interpretation of vaccine efficacy has been the changes in BCG strains over time. The sub-culturing of BCG for its maintenance and a bias for selecting daughter strains with low incidences of side effects, but still able to stimulate tuberculin reactivity (falsely considered a proxy for protection), may have resulted in a progressive loss of those antigens important for protective immunity against tuberculosis. There is, for example, some evidence that daughter strains used in later BCG trials were of lower efficacy than those used earlier (Behr and Small, 1997).

It is thought that the protective effect of BCG vaccination, where observed, is due to a decreased risk of primary complex formation and haematogenous spread following a first infection, but that once there has been exposure to *M. tuberculosis* (or to environmental mycobacteria stimulating heterologous immunity) then the immune environment within the host changes and subsequent vaccination provides no additional protection against the risk of disease from re-infection (Ten Dam and Pio, 1982). This explanation is based on the evidence of a protective benefit against the serious forms of childhood tuberculosis in developing countries (Colditz *et al.*, 1995) and the benefit demonstrated in child contacts of infectious cases in the UK (Vynnycky and Fine, 1997) alongside the epidemiological evidence that BCG appears to have no impact on the annual risk of infection or the incidence of infectious pulmonary tuberculosis, which is almost exclusively a disease of adults (Styblo and Meijer, 1976). A review of BCG trials to evaluate the duration of protection found no evidence for protection after ten years (Sterne *et al.*, 1998). On the assumption that BCG has a 40–70% effectiveness in preventing tuberculosis mortality in children under the age of 15, then its potential impact on reducing tuberculosis deaths could be about 4-7% (Murray *et al.*, 1990).

In Malawi, a second dose of BCG showed no benefit in preventing tuberculosis (Karonga Prevention Trial Group, 1996) but no protective effect was demonstrated for a first dose either, though BCG did confer protection against leprosy. There is an ongoing study in Brazil to test the benefit of second dose in school-aged children (Sterne *et al.*, 1998). If a second dose of BCG has potential benefit only in those not exposed to M. *tuberculosis* (or to environmental mycobacteria conferring heterologous immunity) following their initial dose, then the potential benefit of re-vaccination will depend on the cumulative incidence of mycobacterial exposure at the age chosen for re-vaccination.

In view of the variability of the efficacy of BCG, there is a general consensus that current vaccine strategies have a very limited impact on the world-wide tuberculosis burden (Fine, 1995). New vaccine approaches using plasmid DNA vector technologies, recombinant or mutant BCG and specific mycobacterial sub-units are being developed in the hope that higher levels of protection can be induced (reviewed by Orme (1997) and Grange (1997)).

Chemoprophylaxis

The effectiveness of preventive therapy with isoniazid in reducing the risk of active tuberculosis in infected individuals has been demonstrated in numerous controlled trials. Early trials showed a wide range of protection from a 12-month regimen of isoniazid (25–92%) with most of the differences in effectiveness attributable to differences in adherence (Ferebee, 1969). A placebo-controlled study involving almost 28,000 subjects with positive tuberculin reactions and fibrotic lesions on chest radiography recruited from dispensaries in seven European countries showed 31, 69 and 93% reductions in culture positive tuberculosis after five years of follow up among persons who completed, respectively, three, six and 12 months of therapy, though the additional benefit of a 12-month over a six-month course was demonstrated only in those with fibrotic lesions greater than 2 cm^2 (International Union Against Tuberculosis Committee on Prophylaxis, 1982). A study among the Inuit in Alaska indicated that the duration of protection conferred by preventive therapy taken for 12 months is at least 19 years and can be presumed to be lifelong in the absence of re-infection (Comstock *et al.*, 1979). In addition to tuberculin reactors with fibrotic lesions on chest radiography and HIV-infected persons, discussed below, recent skin-test converters among contacts of active cases, tuberculin-positive patients with silicosis and tuberculin-positive children and adolescents are also at increased risk for active tuberculosis and are, therefore, preferential candidates for preventive therapy (Hong Kong Chest Service/British Medical Research Council, 1992; American Thoracic Society/Medical Section of the American Lung Association, 1994).

Since only a small proportion of infected persons will develop active tuberculosis in the absence of other risk factors, recommendations for chemoprophylaxis in low-income countries in the pre-HIV era have been limited to household contacts of smear-positive cases under the age of five, a group easy to identify and at highest risk for serious disease. This restrictive policy has been questioned because of the negligible impact it has on the population incidence of tuberculosis. While household contacts may be at highest risk of infection from a particular case of smear-positive tuberculosis, most children in developing counties acquire their infection outside the home. In a study conducted in a shanty town in Lima, Peru, where 34% of children between the ages of six months and 14 years were tuberculin positive, the proportion of infected children that would be detected by a strategy of household contact tracing was estimated at less than 1% (Madico *et al.*, 1995). As expected, the relative importance of community-acquired infection versus within-household infection increased with age. On the basis that between five and 15 children would need to receive prophylaxis to prevent one case of active tuberculosis, the authors propose that a school-based programme of tuberculin screening and prophylaxis for tuberculin-positive children could still be a cost-effective strategy to reduce tuberculosis incidence in urban areas where community transmission rates are high and wide programme coverage is feasible. Community-wide preventive therapy was used among Inuits in Alaska in the 1960s and there was a four-fold decrease in incident cases during six years of follow up among those given preventive therapy (Comstock *et al.*, 1967).

Since 1986, American public health guidelines have recommended a 12-month regimen of isoniazid prophylaxis for HIV-positive persons with a tuberculin reaction greater than 5 mm (Centers for Disease

Control, 1986). In 1991, these recommendations were extended to include those with skin test anergy but with risk factors for tuberculosis (Centers for Disease Control, 1991). In 1993, the World Health Organization (WHO) and the International Union Against Tuberculosis and Lung Disease (IUATLD) issued a joint statement recommending preventive therapy for HIV-infected persons with positive tuberculin reactions where evaluation for active tuberculosis and monthly follow up for adverse treatment effects was feasible (World Health Organization/IUATLD, 1993). The effectiveness of self-administered preventive therapy in HIV-infected adults was tested in a randomised placebo-controlled clinical trial in patients enrolled at medical clinics and counselling centres for persons with HIV type-1 infection in Kampala, Uganda (Whalen et al., 1997). The adjusted relative risks of tuberculosis among tuberculin-positive subjects when compared to placebo on an intention-to-treat analysis after a mean follow up of 15 months are shown in Table 1. A small benefit of preventive therapy with isoniazid was demonstrated in subjects with anergy to both tuberculin and Candida after a mean of 12 months of observation but this was not statistically significant. The incidence and grade of adverse events, as well as the proportion discontinuing therapy increased with the number of drugs in the preventive regimen. Short-term survival did not differ significantly between the placebo and treatment groups. However, because the all-cause mortality rate in the placebo group was almost three times higher than the tuberculosis incidence rate in this population, larger trials would be needed to demonstrate a survival benefit if this benefit is conferred through a reduction in tuberculosis-attributable case fatality.

Intermittent regimens or short course regimens for dually infected subjects have been evaluated in other settings. A six-month biweekly regimen of isoniazid and a two-month biweekly combination of rifampicin and pyrazinamide were compared in a four-year follow up study in Haiti among tuberculin-positive adults (Halsey et al., 1998). The risk of tuberculosis during the first ten months after entry was 3.7% among participants who received rifampicin and pyrazinamide compared

Table 1. Self-administered preventive therapy. The adjusted relative risks of tuberculosis among tuberculin-positive subjects when compared to placebo on an intention-to-treat analysis after a mean follow up of 15 months.

Regimen	Relative risk	95% confidence intervals
Six-month daily isoniazid	0.32	0.14–0.76
Three-month combined formulation of isoniazid and rifampicin	0.41	0.19–0.89
Three-month combined formulation of isoniazid, rifampicin and pyrazinamide	0.43	0.20–0.92

to 1.0% ($p = 0.03$) among participants who received isoniazid, and 5.4% versus 5.1%, respectively ($p = 0.9$), at 36 months after entry. The better protection among recipients of isoniazid during the first ten months was most likely secondary to the longer duration of chemoprophylaxis. There were no significant differences in total mortality. A two-month daily combination of rifampicin and pyrazinamide was compared to a 12-month daily regimen of isoniazid in a four-country randomised trial sponsored by the National Institute of Allergy and Infectious Diseases, the Pan American Health Organization and the US Centers for Disease Control. Preliminary results of the study were presented at the Fifth Conference on Retroviruses and Opportunistic Infections in Chicago in February 1998 and showed that subjects were more likely to complete the shorter regimen, with completion rates of about 80%, compared to less than 50% for patients assigned to the 12-month regimen.

Though not yet evaluated in preventive trials against tuberculosis, rifabutin has been recommended for the prevention of *M. avium* infection in severely immunocompromised HIV-infected patients, and in June 1998 it was granted accelerated approval by the US Federal Drug Agency for use in the treatment of pulmonary tuberculosis. The use of anti-microbial agents with activity against a variety of opportunistic pathogens, or multiple opportunistic pathogen prophylaxis (MOPP), in HIV-infected patients is gaining acceptance because of the potential for better patient compliance, reduced toxicity, fewer drug interactions, and lower cost (Chaisson, 1996). Rifabutin is a potential candidate drug for MOPP as it may be effective for other bacterial infections and toxoplasmosis.

Preventive therapy for tuberculosis in HIV-infected persons was carefully reviewed in 1995 by O'Brien and Perriëns in a paper appropriately subtitled 'the Promise and the Reality'. Though more recent results are available from controlled trials, the operational and cost-effective questions surrounding tuberculosis preventive therapy in HIV-infected persons in developing countries remain unchanged. A study of the feasibility and acceptability of offering preventive chemotherapy from a HIV counselling and testing centre in Kampala identified many factors causing attrition, including limited motivation of counsellors to discuss tuberculosis, insufficient availability of medical screening, physical separation of different services, and frequent tuberculin test negativity (Aisu et al., 1995). Because of the difficulty in diagnosing tuberculosis in patients with advanced HIV infection, there is concern that resistant bacilli will be selected due to the incomplete exclusion of active tuberculosis cases among those offered chemoprophylaxis. Another issue is the appropriate criteria for identifying candidates for preventive therapy in different settings. In Thailand, HIV-positive persons had markedly decreased tuberculin reactivity; skin test reactions to mumps and Candida antigens did not predict tuberculin reactivity and were present in more than half of HIV-positive persons with CD4+ cell counts less than 200 cells per ml, a marker of advanced immunosuppression. In this setting, tuberculin and anergy skin tests have a low predictive value in HIV-infected persons and a limited utility in identifying HIV-positive candidates for tuberculosis preventive therapy (Yanai et al., 1997).

While the cost for a six-month course of isoniazid prophylaxis is much lower than the cost of treating a case of active tuberculosis (see Chapter 10), the costs of broader implementation would be significant. Moreover, the entry point for preventive therapy is HIV voluntary counselling and testing, services which themselves are costly to implement.

Modelling studies suggest that in high HIV prevalence settings, the broad application of preventive therapy to dually infected adults could have a significant impact on reducing tuberculosis incidence (Heymann, 1993). The bitter irony is that the greatest potential impact is in those communities most severely affected by the dual epidemics and, partly as a consequence, least equipped to implement such programmes. Community-based screening for HIV infection within a tuberculosis control programme was evaluated during the preventive therapy trial in Haiti cited above, suggesting that this might be an effective way to target screening for both infections (Desormeaux *et al.*, 1996). Over a two-year period, adults in Cité Soleil were recruited by community health workers at their homes and in clinics for individual, clinic-based counselling and testing for HIV and tuberculosis. All subjects screened for HIV were offered post-test counselling, those with active tuberculosis were treated, and those with dual infection were offered the opportunity to participate in the tuberculosis preventive therapy trial. Among the 10,611 individuals screened for HIV, representing 10% of the adult population in Cité Soleil, 15.4% were HIV infected — a higher prevalence when compared to other groups screened for HIV in the same community, suggesting that those at higher risk for HIV infection selectively sought or accepted tuberculosis clinic screening. Infection by the tubercle bacillus was found in 67.5% of the 7,309 residents who completed tuberculosis screening, 781 (16.3%) of whom were co-infected with HIV. Active tuberculosis was detected in 242 persons (2.3%) who, as a result of the screening programme, were identified earlier in the course of their disease.

Curative treatment

As early as the middle 1950s it was evident that multiple drug therapy could cure most patients infected with drug-susceptible bacilli (Crofton, 1962). Since that time, numerous clinical trials, many carried out under collaborative research arrangements with the British Medical Research Council in East Africa, Hong Kong, Madras and Singapore, have shown that for regimens containing rifampicin, isoniazid and pyrazinamide, the minimum effective duration of treatment for smear-positive patients is six months, and that twice and thrice weekly regimens are as effective as daily regimens (Fox, 1981; Iseman and Sbarbaro, 1987; World Health Organization, 1997b; American Thoracic Society/Medical Section of the American Lung Association, 1994). In patients with susceptible organisms who complete a full course of therapy, five-year relapse rates of less than 5% can be achieved (Hong Kong Chest Service/British Medical Research Council, 1987; Singapore Tuberculosis Service/British Medical Research Council, 1988).

As discussed in Chapter 10, tuberculosis is among the most cost effective of all chronic diseases to treat. While cost effectiveness studies compare cost and outcomes under different regimens or service models, absolute rather than relative cure rates achieved under programme conditions are critically important for the prevention of multidrug resistance. Resistance to known anti-tuberculosis drugs develops spontaneously at defined rates during bacterial replication varying between 10^{-3} and 10^{-10} depending on the drug, but the frequency of resistance among strains of M. tuberculosis not exposed to anti-tuberculosis drugs is negligible because of the preponderance of drug-susceptible bacilli. In the presence of anti-tuberculosis drugs there is a selective pressure for resistant organisms to become predominant and single or multidrug resistance will occur in a patient who is given an inadequate regimen or substandard drugs, or does not take each drug as prescribed. The emergence of drug resistance is the major threat to the effectiveness of treatment programmes world wide and the magnitude of this global problem is reviewed by Cohn et al. (1997) and the World Health Organization (1997c). See also Chapter 1.

Though effective treatment regimens exist today for most tuberculosis patients, and are equally effective in HIV-infected persons with drug-susceptible strains, there is ongoing research to develop new drugs to treat multidrug-resistant tuberculosis and to shorten the duration of treatment, perhaps the single most important treatment-related determinant of adherence (Haynes, 1979). Reducing treatment duration is also a goal of current trials using immunotherapy as an adjunct to chemotherapy. One approach has been to modulate the immune response by concurrent vaccination with mycobacterial antigens along the same principle of using BCG as an immunostimulant in cancer therapy (Grange *et al.*, 1995; Cocito and Maes, 1998). Small pilot studies and anecdotal reports suggest that use of a heat-killed preparation of *M. vaccae* may be of beneficial (Onyebujoh *et al.*, 1995; Corlan *et al.*, 1997a; Corlan *et al.*, 1997b; Skinner *et al.*, 1997), and more extensive studies are ongoing in Zambia and Malawi. The other approach has been to enhance the immune response by the concurrent administration of cytokines important in the cellular immune response to *M. tuberculosis*, including interleukin-2 (Johnson *et al.*, 1995; Johnson *et al.*, 1998) and interleukin-12 (Skinner *et al.*, 1997; Altare *et al.*, 1998).

Service Delivery in High Prevalence Countries

Technical issues in case-finding

In the context of high-prevalence countries, the term *case-finding* refers to the detection of infectious cases of pulmonary tuberculosis who are the reservoir for transmission and who account for most tuberculosis-attributable deaths (Styblo and Salamao, 1993). Numerous studies confirm that the patients most likely to infect others are those excreting a sufficient number of bacilli to be visible on direct microscopic examination of sputum (reviewed by Rouillon *et al.*, 1976).

The international recommendation to make examination of the sputum of chest symptomatics self-presenting to health facilities the principle strategy of tuberculosis case-finding in low-income countries is based on the specificity of microscopic examination for acid-fast bacilli in identifying *M. tuberculosis*, its ability to identify infectious patients, its low cost and good performance under field conditions, and the crucial fact that infectious pulmonary tuberculosis is a symptomatic disease of adults who can be expected to seek relief and can therefore be identified by a symptom screen. In low-prevalence countries, where case notifications are more complete, bacteriologically-confirmed pulmonary disease accounts for less than 15–30% of tuberculosis cases in children under the age of 15, and the majority of such cases are positive by culture only and therefore minimally infectious (Barnett and Styblo, 1977; Styblo, 1991). Data from Norway and the USA concur that less than 10% of all tuberculosis cases under the age of 15 are smear-positive (Galtung Hansen, 1955; Murray et al., 1990). Data from national programmes in Africa and prevalence surveys in India likewise show that smear- and culture-positive pulmonary tuberculosis is uncommon in children (Murray et al., 1993; Chakraborty, 1996).

The majority of patients with infectious pulmonary tuberculosis are thus adults and perhaps 70–90% of these experience symptoms, the most common being chronic cough (Banerji and Andersen, 1963; Toman, 1979). The validity of symptom screening to identify pulmonary tuberculosis was indirectly confirmed in a recent evaluation of initial screening methods for identifying persons for further bacteriological examination in a peri-urban area of Bangalore: the prevalence rates of smear-positive or culture-positive disease were similar whether subjects were selected for bacteriological examination by mass miniature radiography or by symptom screening (Chakraborty et al., 1994). General health workers and qualified sociological investigators were equally successful in identifying symptomatics. In the Khon Kaen province of Thailand, symptom screening detected as many smear-positive cases as a sputum survey of the entire adult population (Elink Schuurman et al., 1996).

The usefulness of cough as a cardinal symptom for screening varies between populations depending on the prevalence of chronic cough and tuberculosis. In the highlands of Papua-New Guinea, to take an extreme example, chronic cough is apparently so prevalent that, if taken alone as the case definition of a tuberculosis suspect, an estimated 1,400 patients would need to be investigated to detect a single case of smear-positive tuberculosis (Pust, 1982). Where tuberculosis patients use general health services, the ratio of suspects to smear-positive cases is closer to ten, a figure recommended by the IUATLD as a guide to estimating supply requirements for smear microscopy services (Rieder and Enarson, 1995).

The specificity of microscopy for acid-fast bacilli in diagnosing tuberculosis is potentially lowered by environmental bacteria in clinical specimens, but this is uncommon, at least in countries with a high tuberculosis prevalence (Aber *et al.*, 1980; Braun *et al.*, 1992). False positives occur either because of contaminated stains or water, poor staining technique, reuse of scratched slides and the inexperience of technicians. Quality control of smear microscopy carried out in Rwanda in 1992–93 showed that rates of false positives were higher in centres where the case load was so low that technicians only rarely saw true positives (Van Deun and Portaels, 1998).

The sensitivity of smear examination, in relation to the 'gold-standard' of culture, a procedure which itself has variable sensitivity depending on the number of specimens examined from the same patient, is of greater concern. In a study of 270 patients with as many as 7–17 cultures carried out in the USA between 1968 and 1973, the first smear and culture only detected 47.4 and 74.1% respectively of those ultimately found positive on culture (Blair *et al.*, 1976). In contrast, in a study in India carried out in the 1950s, 76.7% of patients subsequently culture positive on at least one of four specimens were found to be positive on the first smear (Andrews and Radhadrishna, 1959). The sensitivity of a single smear in relation to one or several cultures is variable depending on the nature of the specimen (the positivity of morning specimens is higher than spot specimens) and the conditions under which the specimen is collected (under programme conditions patients may be examined later in the course of their illness than during a prevalence survey). The sensitivity of smear examination in detecting infectious tuberculosis as opposed to all pulmonary disease can not be directly evaluated, since infectiousness is a continuum. Data from Canada showed, however, that 1,609 of 1,668 (96.5%) infections occurring among 13,472 identified contacts of pulmonary tuberculosis followed exposure to smear-positive cases (Grzybowski *et al.*, 1975), confirming that, in that setting, smear examination identified most cases responsible for transmission among identified contacts.

The sensitivity of smear examinations for identifying all cases of pulmonary disease is lower in tuberculosis patients infected with the human immunodeficiency virus (HIV) in whom smear-positivity is inversely related to the degree of immunosuppression, presumably due a reduction in tissue necrosis and, consequently, in the number of acid-fast bacilli in sputum (Barnes et al., 1991). Where sensitivity has been correlated with the degree of immunosuppression and radiographic findings, the sensitivity of smear examination in less severely immunocompromised adults is similar to that in immunocompetent adults with reactivation tuberculosis (Theuer et al., 1990). In patients with severe immunosuppression and atypical X-ray findings, the sensitivity is lower (Klein et al., 1989). In a study in which two or three sputum specimens were collected from consecutive patients presenting to a district hospital in Haiti and examined by microscopy and culture, the sensitivity of smear examination was 66% (40/61) in HIV-seropositive patients with at least one positive culture for M. tuberculosis on two specimens, versus 79% (155/196) among HIV-seronegative patients. A positive smear predicted M. tuberculosis in 80% of seropositive patients compared to 90% of seronegative patients. A ten-year review of tuberculosis cases presenting to the Queen Elizabeth Central Hospital in Blantyre, Malawi, where HIV seroprevalence among pregnant women presenting to the antenatal clinic had already reached 31.6% in 1993, showed that the proportion of smear positives among adult pulmonary tuberculosis patients declined from 89% in 1986 to 62% in 1995 (Harries et al., 1997a). The proportion of extrapulmonary tuberculosis cases increased from 11% to 33% over the same period, and HIV seroprevalence among tuberculosis patients was in the order of 75% by the end of the study period (Harries et al., 1995). Though the authors suggest that there may have been some overdiagnosis of smear-negative pulmonary and childhood tuberculosis, it is nonetheless clear that where HIV prevalence is high, patients who registered for treatment on the basis of a positive smear form a much smaller proportion of the total caseload than before the HIV epidemic, and that the use of other diagnostic tests has increased. The focus on smear-positive disease as the highest public health priority, while still logical in principle, no longer reflects the actual clinical activities related to tuberculosis case management where HIV is common, even in the poorest countries.

Despite the relatively low technology of smear microscopy as a diagnostic test, it nevertheless requires a significant investment in equipment, supplies, trained personnel and a system of supervision and quality control (Collins *et al.*, 1997). For the period 1988–89, before the WHO declared tuberculosis a global emergency, it was estimated that in developing countries, services for the diagnosis and treatment of tuberculosis covered on average only 46% of the population, ranging from a low of 24% in Africa to 88% in the Western Pacific (Kochi, 1991). In a more recent review of world-wide tuberculosis control activities, case-detection rate estimates were calculated as the ratio of notified cases in 1995 to the expected incidence of smear-positive tuberculosis based on the annual risk of infection method (Styblo, 1985; see Chapter 1) published in the World Bank's 1993 World Development Report (World Bank, 1993) and adjusted for 1995 populations. Data from 180 of 216 countries who responded to the survey gave an aggregate estimate of 35% as the proportion of smear-positive cases notified by public-sector treatment programmes (Raviglione *et al.*, 1997). While, due to under-reporting, this figure almost certainly underestimates the proportion of incident cases actually started on treatment in countries such as India where private services are heavily used (Pathania *et al.*, 1997), a large proportion of tuberculosis cases clearly remain undiagnosed.

The relation between service coverage and case-detection is never straightforward, particularly for a stigmatised disease such as tuberculosis where social barriers to care-seeking and public confidence in the ability and willingness of health service staff to provide compassionate care will determine service usage. Moreover, local perceptions of tuberculosis may not coincide with the vocabulary of health providers, and the effectiveness of symptom questioning in identifying pulmonary tuberculosis suspects early in the course of their disease is compromised if local categories for the signs and symptoms of tuberculosis are not used when questioning patients or attempting to raise community awareness

(Liefooghe *et al.*, 1997; Nichter, 1994). These communication issues are discussed in Chapter 21.

Complex social factors aside, the list of technical and operational limitations of smear microscopy remains long (Chaulet and Zidouni, 1993). The existence of facilities and trained personnel is no guarantee that a strategy of case-detection by symptom screening and smear microscopy is effective in detecting cases early. In Malawi in 1995, an evaluation of the management of patients with cough attending out-patient services suggested that less than 20% of those with chronic cough who should have had their sputum examined were actually tested (Harries *et al.*, 1996). This was in a hospital in which the annual tuberculosis caseload increased from 657 in 1986 to 2,734 in 1995 (Harries *et al.*, 1997a). Studies in Kenya carried out in the 1970s and 1980s showed that, despite repeated visits to health facilities, many suspects were not examined for tuberculosis (Aluoch *et al.*, 1982).

Patients with cough impose a large burden on out-patient and laboratory services. A review of computerised laboratory registers from 42 laboratories in Benin, Malawi, Nicaragua and Senegal showed that the average number of suspect smears to identify one case of smear-positive tuberculosis ranged from an average of 8.0 in Benin to 49.8 in Nicaragua (Rieder *et al.*, 1997). The percentage of cases among suspects varied inversely from 5.2 in Nicaragua to 32.1 in Benin. It should be noted that the figures reported are country averages and that the range among laboratories in a particular country was wider. On a routine basis, a good laboratory technician can be expected to process a maximum of 25 slides a day, though the actual number of slides that can be handled depends on the likelihood of positives among submitted specimens (since negative slides consume more time) and the cut-off for positivity (the scale of the American Thoracic Society, for instance, requires the examination of 300 fields to classify a smear as negative, whereas the IU-ATLD and the WHO scales classify a smear as negative if no bacilli are seen in 100 fields). Whatever the classification system used, time spent on detecting a positive case is high where routine Ziehl–Neelsen staining is used.

The discrepancy between the protocol and reality of case-finding is well demonstrated by a prospective study of case-finding by smear microscopy at the district hospital in Lilongwe, Malawi (B. Squire, personal communication). For six months in 1995, all out-patient tuberculosis suspects submitting a first sputum in the morning clinic were followed to determine whether they submitted further specimens, collected their results and started treatment. Chest radiography was used only for those smear negative on three specimens. Of 499 suspects asked to give a first spot specimen, only 37% submitted three specimens and collected their results. Among all suspects, 69 smear positives were identified, 63 of these on the first smear. Within six months, only 28 had collected their results and were registered for treatment, though four others in the cohort were eventually started on treatment by another route. Of the remaining 37 smear positives (54%), 21 collected a positive result but did not register for treatment, and 16 did not collect their results. There are many possible reasons for drop-outs at each stage, but in this particular setting the case-finding strategy of asking patients to submit repeated sputa and collect the laboratory results is clearly ineffective. A contributing factor was certainly the laboratory delay, a consequence of an average of 50 specimens submitted each day and only one microscopist allocated for two half days per week. This situation is not atypical of district laboratories in countries such as Malawi where, largely due to the HIV epidemic, tuberculosis services are overwhelmed. Along with increased delays in diagnosis, the overburdening of laboratory services results in low staff morale, increases in infection risk and in the likelihood of laboratory error.

Pending a simpler equally-reliable test, smear examination remains the only practical method of bacteriological confirmation in most low income countries. Operational research is now focused on decreasing the burden of smear microscopy without compromising its effectiveness as a case-finding strategy. Several studies have revealed that, while repeated examinations certainly increase the sensitivity of smear microscopy, the increase in yield after the second examination is small (Harries *et al.*, 1996; Ipuge *et al.*, 1996).

The case definition for a tuberculosis suspect can have a significant impact on the number of patients referred for smear examination. The Indian National Tuberculosis Programme has a case definition for a tuberculosis suspect based on chronic cough for three weeks or longer. In Malawi, non response to a course of broad-spectrum antibiotics is included in the case definition of a tuberculosis suspects at most district hospitals and at one large hospital the suspect definition includes weight loss as a third criteria. Each additional criteria, while decreasing the sensitivity of the suspect definition, improves the sensitivity of smear examination by increasing the prior predictive value, thus optimising the use of laboratory facilities. In a comparison of suspect screening strategies at the Queen Elizabeth Hospital, Blantyre, Malawi, 62% of adults referred for smear examination on the basis of a symptom screen did not in fact meet all of the three criteria for a pulmonary suspect, effectively doubling the laboratory workload related to suspect smear examination (Harries *et al.*, 1997b). This study compared the effectiveness of two different screening strategies, as shown in Table 2. The authors point out that with both screening strategies a significant proportion of patients with normal or minimally normally chest X-rays has smear or culture evidence of tuberculosis, observations that have been made in other settings (Greenberg *et al.*, 1994; Simooya *et al.*, 1991). Equally important is the fact that smear examination alone under strategy A identified only 111 (50%) of those with either smear or culture evidence of tuberculosis. Without the availability of radiology for the evaluation of smear-negative suspects, 70 patients (32%) would not have been placed on treatment at this evaluation. Though smear specimens were examined using the Ziehl–Neelsen method used in most peripheral laboratories, the usual method employed in the high-volume setting of the Queen Elizabeth Hospital is fluorescent light microscopy using auramine-phenol staining, a technique which can significantly reduce technician time. Sensitivity can also be improved by concentration methods such as centrifugation or sedimentation (Gebre *et al.*, 1995), but these have field limitations.

Table 2.   Comparison of two screening strategies on 402 enrolled patients.

Strategy	Identified as having pulmonary tuberculosis	Bacteriological evidence of tuberculosis*	Patients that would have been missed*
A. Smear examination of three sputum specimens followed by chest X-ray for patients with negative smears	243	181 (74%)	40 (18%)
B. Screening by chest X-ray followed by smear examination in those with an X-ray compatible with tuberculosis	230	168 (73%)	53 (24%)

*Percentages refer to the proportion of those with smear or culture evidence of tuberculosis.

While operational research has demonstrated that decentralisation of smear microscopy is technically and organisationally feasible, the motivation and performance of laboratory technicians is rarely given the same attention as the clinical care aspects of tuberculosis control (Collins *et al.*, 1997). Where tuberculosis programmes have been integrated into primary health services, the organisation of a smear microscopy network is often left to general laboratory services, and specialised supervisory activities may lapse. Despite a relatively simple technology with a low average cost in high-volume settings, the labour intensive nature of routine smear-microscopy carries significant costs in terms of primary training, supervision and quality control. Surprisingly, there are no field-tested guidelines on the organisation of large-scale quality control systems. Where it exists, quality control often consists of re-examining all positive and a proportion of negative smears, usually 10%, and identifying false negatives and false positives on the basis of the second reader's assessment. Such systems cannot detect missed cases due to poor staining and assume that discrepancies are always the error of the peripheral laboratory; rarely is a distinction made between errors of classification and errors of quantification, or statistical sampling techniques applied in selecting slides for re-testing. Recently, more scientific quality control systems based on lot quality assurance sampling methods and aimed at detecting true misclassification by re-staining the original smear have been developed (Van Deun and Portaels, 1998). The complexity of a valid quality control system for smear microscopy underlines that even this relatively simple test is only as good as its practitioners and the system that supports their work.

Operational problems in service delivery

The tuberculosis control programme model currently promoted by the IUATLD and the WHO for low-income countries was developed in the 1980s by Karel Styblo, initially in Tanzania and later in six other African countries and Nicaragua under the Mutual Assistance Programme of the IUATLD (Enarson, 1991; Kochi, 1991; Styblo and Salomao, 1993). These programmes were initially based on long-course regimens but cure rates were only slightly better than 50% until the introduction of modern short course regimens when cure rates of over 75% were achieved (Enarson, 1991). In addition to a secure supply of drugs, diagnostic materials and a network of quality-assured microscopy centres, a key component of the IUATLD model programmes was the interlinked system of patient cards, treatment registers and reporting forms, designed to facilitate the evaluation of treatment results by quarterly cohorts and now used in IUATLD- and WHO-assisted programmes world wide. Styblo demonstrated that programmes achieving good treatment outcomes could be implemented in low-income settings with sustained technical assistance. The actual model of service delivery developed in Tanzania and other African countries reflected the organisation of curative health services in Africa with a relatively centralised health system focused on the district hospital. Given the general availability of hospital beds before the AIDS epidemic, the use of streptomycin injection in the intensive phase, and the difficulty of organising supplies and supervising programmes at peripheral facilities, it is not surprising that diagnosis and treatment in the IUATLD-supported programmes in Africa was largely based at the district hospital, with the intensive phase of treatment given as in-patient therapy, thereby ensuring daily patient contact without any changes to the normal work routine of the health staff.

A strong management structure for the organisation of tuberculosis services in high-prevalence countries is emphasised by the IUATLD. The provision of diagnostic and treatment services should be based on a 'unit of management' covering a population between 50–150,000, according to the incidence of tuberculosis (Enarson *et al.*, 1996). If microscopy facilities are established for smaller population units, for instance, a low volume of suspect slides and less frequent supervision of laboratories will generally result in a deterioration of quality. Likewise, if the unit of management is too small or too large, the programme becomes either inefficient or unmanageable in respect to the regularity of supplies, defaulter tracing, staff supervision and programme evaluation.

The IUATLD model was evaluated by the Health Sectors Priority Review of the World Bank in 1989 and assessed as one of the most cost-effective health interventions in developing countries and adopted by the WHO as the appropriate model for tuberculosis control in low-income countries (Murray *et al.*, 1990, 1991). In 1991, it was adapted for ambulatory care and piloted in China under WHO auspices and rapidly expanded with World Bank support; by 1994 more than 100,000 new smear positive patients had been enrolled (China Tuberculosis Control Collaboration, 1996). In the face of increasing incidence of tuberculosis secondary to the HIV pandemic and the recognition of this disease as the most important cause of preventable adult morbidity and mortality in developing countries (Murray *et al.*, 1990; World Bank, 1993), a global tuberculosis strategy was endorsed by the 44th World Health Assembly in 1991 and the disease was declared a global emergency by the WHO in 1993. The tuberculosis control policy package endorsed by the WHO follows the IUATLD model in stressing the need for government commitment to the establishment of National Tuberculosis Programmes, the assurance of regular drug supply, case-finding through smear microscopy, health worker supervision, evaluation of treatment outcomes, and supervised treatment at least during the intensive phase (World Health Organization, 1994a). The WHO promotional campaign, in adopting DOTS (directly observed therapy, short course) as the slogan for its revised strategy for tuberculosis control, has, however, focused on treatment supervision (World Health Organization, 1996, 1997a).

Before its world-wide promotion by the WHO, directly observed therapy (DOT), in which a health care provider or another responsible person watches as the patient takes his medications (Etkind, 1993; Centers for Disease Control, 1994), had already been widely used in a variety of settings. In response to the problem of treatment compliance among ambulatory patients in the British Medical Research Council trials in Madras almost 40 years ago, supervised therapy was introduced, first on a daily and then on an intermittent basis (Fox, 1958; Tuberculosis Chemotherapy Centre Madras, 1964). In Hong Kong in the 1960s, large numbers of patients were treated by an ambulatory care programme that evolved to include the direct supervision of oral as well as injectable drugs (Moodie, 1967). In India, it was shown that self-administration was not reliable even when patients kept regular clinic appointments and when efforts were made to involve the family in treatment supervision (Fox, 1961), and in rural Hong Kong there was an 85% treatment completion rate among those on DOT compared to 55% among those on self-administered therapy (Hong Kong Chest Service/British Medical Research Council, 1984). In Cuba, treatment has been administered by DOT since 1970 and is associated with a decline in annual tuberculosis incidence to less than 5 per 100,000 over 20 years (Gonzalez et al., 1994), a low rate for the region. In Beijing, DOT was implemented in 1978 and short course regimens were introduced in 1988. National prevalence surveys carried out in China in 1979 and 1990 showed a decline in smear-positive prevalence from 127 per 100,000 to 16 per 100,000 in Beijing (Zhang and Kan, 1992), but almost no change for the country as a whole, which in 1990 had a smear-positive prevalence of 134 per 100,000 (Ministry of Public Health of the People's Republic of China,

1992). Fully supervised outpatient treatment was also successfully implemented in a large open refugee camp on the Thai-Cambodian border (Miles and Maat, 1984) and under war conditions in Nicaragua (Cruz *et al.*, 1994).

In the USA, the promotion of DOT followed only after public concern about the rising number of cases after 1985, outbreaks in health care facilities, and an increase in drug-resistant disease (Bayer and Wilkinson, 1995), although the use of supervised treatment had been officially recommended for specific patient groups for more than a decade (American Thoracic Society, 1980; McDonald *et al.*, 1982) and advocated as a universal policy by some experts for even longer (Sbarbaro, 1980; Sbarbaro, 1988). In 1993, DOT was recommended as the standard of care for pulmonary tuberculosis by the Advisory Council for the Elimination of Tuberculosis of the Centers for Disease Control (1993) and soon after by the American Thoracic Society/Medical Section of the American Lung Association (1994). The Advisory Council stipulated that DOT should be implemented where treatment completion rates were below 90% and made this the basis of co-operative agreement applications from health departments seeking federal funds for tuberculosis elimination. The implementation of tuberculosis programmes using DOT in the USA has been associated with local decreases in case rates, relapse rates and drug resistance (Weis *et al.*, 1994; Frieden *et al.*, 1995, Chaulk *et al.*, 1995).

Evidence for the importance of close patient supervision during tuberculosis treatment is strong. Whatever the medical condition, regular therapy must compete with other demands on a patient's time, its importance may be poorly communicated by health providers, and regularity may not accord with norms or expectations of the patient's family or social milieu (Haynes, 1979). Despite these general obstacles to successful treatment completion, non adherence has few predictors, whether demographic characteristics, occupation, income or level of education are examined (Haynes *et al.*, 1979). A recent systematic review of randomised controlled trials on interventions to improve adherence to prescribed treatments for a range of conditions (studies evaluating

interventions to improve adherence to tuberculosis treatment did not
meet the selection criteria) showed that effective interventions for long-
term care were complex, including various combinations of more con-
venient care, information, counselling, reminders, self-monitoring, rein-
forcement, family therapy, and other forms of supervision, but that even
the most effective interventions did not lead to substantial improvements
in adherence (Haynes *et al.*, 1996). Notwithstanding the accumulated
experience of successful tuberculosis treatment programmes both in developed and developing countries which favoured the use of DOT as a
component of service delivery, when the WHO launched its aggressive
marketing campaign recommending universal DOT as the central strategy for effective tuberculosis services world wide, there had been no
comprehensive review of the evidence to support this recommendation
(Volmink and Garner, 1997; Chaulk and Kazandjian, 1998).

While there is little disagreement that low rates of treatment completion among diagnosed patients is the most important cause of failure
of tuberculosis treatment programmes in developing countries, there is
considerable debate on the relative importance of provider versus patient
factors contributing to non-adherence (Chaulet, 1987), on the appropriateness of a universal policy of DOT, on the feasibility and acceptability
of DOT in different settings, and on the provider and patient costs of
different DOT options. The promotion of a universal DOTS strategy
implies that adherence sufficient to achieve cure can only be assured by
direct observation, and that patients cannot manage compliance without the supervision of a second party. This view has been challenged
on the basis of experience of treatment programmes that have achieved
good cure rates without DOT, as well as on philosophical grounds that it
infringes on the patient's autonomy to be responsible for his or her own
care (Annas, 1993). Moreover, by focusing on treatment supervision,
the implementation of a universal DOTS strategy can result in a relative
neglect of problems related to the behaviour of providers, management
shortcomings in the health services and the specific problems of integrating tuberculosis services into primary care systems undergoing decentralisation and health reforms (Dujardin *et al.*, 1997, Chaulet, 1998).

Two reviews of the literature on interventions to improve adherence to tuberculosis treatment have been published recently. The first was restricted to published randomised controlled trials of interventions to promote adherence to curative or preventive treatment for tuberculosis (Volmink and Garner, 1997). Perhaps the most remarkable finding of this review was how few reported studies there are which have used a randomised controlled trial design to test interventions to improve tuberculosis treatment adherence, despite an extensive research literature on compliance to tuberculosis treatment (Sumartojo, 1993; Cohen, 1997). Of the five studies identified in the literature search, which included a review of the Medline database from 1966, only two included patients with active tuberculosis and the others looked at interventions to improve adherence with preventive therapy. Perhaps not surprisingly in published studies, all strategies to improve treatment adherence had a positive impact, whether the intervention was directed at patients or providers.

The review identified no published report of a randomised controlled trial evaluating DOT, despite its aggressive promotion by international agencies. This may be partly explained by historical and methodological factors. Interventions to improve adherence in a particular treatment setting are usually developed in response to perceived problems in service delivery, are implemented incrementally, adjusted in response to experience and validated by improvements in outcomes. It took almost a decade to develop and evaluate the IUATLD model for tuberculosis control in low-income countries. That model was based on a fully supervised intensive phase including injectable streptomycin delivered as in-patient treatment for the majority of patients, at least in sub-Saharan Africa. Other early examples of successful programmes based on intensive treatment supervision, such as in Madras and Hong Kong, were also developed gradually, reflecting the specific institutional and cultural characteristics of those settings. Evaluating one component of a complex context-specific service delivery model under routine conditions is not comparable, for instance, to a drug efficacy trial where the disruption of programme conditions through the application of eligibility criteria, blinding, and random allocation are necessary and acceptable. Randomised controlled trials to test the independent effects of a DOT strategy to enhance adherence under routine programme conditions are therefore only possible in certain settings where community randomisation is feasible or where patients allocated to different arms are treated by different providers — methodological requirements difficult to meet in field settings in developing countries (Gordis, 1979; Youngleson, 1988). Despite methodological constraints, randomised controlled trials of DOT service models in a particular setting are required to provide robust evidence to justify the investment costs of large-scale interventions.

The structured review of the literature on the relative effectiveness of programmes using DOT in achieving treatment completion for pulmonary tuberculosis carried out by the Public Health Tuberculosis Guidelines Panel provides a helpful guide to the diversity of DOT-based service models and the role of DOT among other interventions to improve treatment completion (Chaulk and Kazandjian, 1998). The panel reviewed 27 studies with treatment completion for pulmonary tuberculosis as an outcome, examined the intensity of DOT and evaluated the addition of other strategies designed around a patient's lifestyle, social and economic enablers and incentives, and culturally appropriate outreach and tracing. Studies from different settings in developing and developed countries were included in the review. In order to draw closer associations between the wide range of treatment outcomes and the diversity of DOT programmes, the panel grouped the studies into those using DOT with multiple incentives and enablers, those using DOT without multiple incentives and enablers, and those with a modified approach to DOT. Reports of treatment programmes without strategies of supervision were also reviewed for comparison.

The panel's recommendations and comments are worth reviewing in detail. As might be expected, it was found that the more actions taken to enable tuberculosis patients to take their medications, the more likely they were to complete treatment. Treatment organised around a patient's lifestyle was more acceptable and effective in terms of treatment completion. The panel's review defined an enabler-based or incentive-based model of DOT in which high rates of treatment completion had been replicated across time, geography and social infrastructure. The panel recommended that "a patient-centred strategy based on DOT... [that] should include appropriate incentives and enablers based on the individual needs of the patient, including transportation, outreach, financial and social incentives, reminder systems, and tracking for failed appointments". Further research on the effectiveness of various incentives and enablers among different populations is needed for the design of cost-effective service models in different settings.

Implementing DOT in a way which is acceptable to both providers and patients is a particular challenge where resources are limited and where traditional relationships between patient and health workers are not conducive to a patient-centred approach. The implementation of DOT in many countries is still viewed as a response to poor patient compliance attributed to certain demographic characteristics, beliefs and attitudes of the patients; general failings in the health system and provider attitudes are underrated and therefore not addressed (Farmer, 1996; 1997). The adoption of a DOT policy in the Western Cape province of South Africa did not change the rigid task-oriented manner in which patients were processed by clinic staff. Compliance was still viewed by many nurses as the patient's duty and non-adherence seen as 'irresponsible' (Dick *et al.* 1996a). In another study in the Western Cape, in which routine interviews between clinic nurses and tuberculosis patients were video-recorded, interactions were shown to be essentially nurse-centred with an unequal distribution of control and poor receptivity to or confirmation of the patient's perspective (Steyn *et al.*, 1997). In many developing countries there is also a perception that the education of patients and communities is secondary to the provision of services, whereas effective education and community participation are prerequisites to wider utilisation of appropriate services and improved treatment adherence (Dick and Lombard, 1997; see Chapters 11 and 21).

From the perspective of patients, the question remains open whether the implementation of a DOT strategy in a particular setting will reinforce the perception of a system unresponsive to their needs or result in more effective patient-oriented service. The success of direct observation as a strategy will depend on how attractive it is to both the patient and the treatment observer (Squire and Wilkinson, 1997), and incentives and enablers will be as important in developing or middle-income countries as they are in the US setting (Chaulk and Kazandjian, 1998). Financial incentives to village doctors in China (China Tuberculosis Control Collaboration, 1996) and a bond partly repayable upon treatment completion in Bangladesh (Chowdhury et al., 1997; see Chapter 16) are two examples.

The direct and opportunity costs of attending a clinic for supervised therapy can be high when transportation costs, or walking time, and clinic waiting time are taken into account. Patients will inevitably weigh up the opportunity cost of complying with treatment against their duties in the home, the farm or the workplace. In Islamic societies, there may be the additional time required for a person to accompany a woman to the clinic to consider. Though daily regimens are attractive because of their familiarity, when compared to intermittent therapy, the direct and indirect financial burden on the patient is doubled.

Flexibility in adapting a DOT-based programme to local health services and the social and cultural environment is of crucial importance. Recent WHO guidelines cite several examples in different settings, including 'manyattas' or temporary villages for rural nomads in northeastern Kenya, community supervisors in rural South Africa and extended family members in urban Guinea (World Health Organization, 1997b). More attention is now being focused on the characteristics and role of the treatment supervisor who can be an advocate for the patient within the family and community (Dick et al., 1996b; Dick and Schoeman, 1996). To be effective in that role, the DOT supervisor must be concerned about the welfare of the patient, have an influence on the patient's behaviour, and on some level be accountable to the health system. The nature of the 'social contract' between patient and supervisor has been little studied, but is important for developing realistic implementation guidelines to assist those organising DOT-based services.

Experience in most developing countries with DOT is, however, still limited and the success of alternatives to supervision of treatment by health workers is largely unknown. Community-based supervision by non-health workers in the Hlabisa district, South Africa, has achieved good treatment completion rates by a simplified case management approach (Wilkinson and Davies, 1997; Floyd *et al.*, 1997). Family member observation is another option, especially for patients with poor access to health services, or in Muslim societies where women's freedom of movement may be limited. Observational studies in Thailand and Malawi, where DOT by family members has been implemented, have shown high treatment completion rates (Ian Smith and Dermot Maher, personal communications).

Insufficient attention has also been paid to the distribution of medications to hospitalised patients. The assumption that inpatients, by virtue of being incarcerated, take all the pills they are given has not been borne by the evidence (Burkhardt and Nel, 1980). Even an official policy of DOT for hospitalised patients is not a guarantee of compliance. In a hospital serving a workforce of miners in South Africa with a high incidence of tuberculosis, the introduction of individualised dosage cards signed by both patient and treatment supervisor, thereby reinforcing the concept of a treatment contract with dual responsibilities, improved compliance as measured by urine monitoring for isoniazid and rifampicin from 62% to about 90% (Sonnenberg *et al.*, 1998).

It is unfortunate that the single-minded drive for DOT implementation has sidelined the often valuable experience of programmes that have been effective through other strategies. In India and Nepal, for instance, some non-governmental programmes serving hard to reach populations have achieved good cure rates through a mix of strategies, yet their results are often considered unsuitable for wider application or they feel pressured to change to DOT, even though appropriate service models for populations with poor access to health services have not been evaluated in these countries (Uplekar and Rangan, 1995; Jochem *et al.*, 1997).

Of special concern are the results of operational research studies carried out at urban DOT project areas in India under the World

Bank-sponsored revised National Tuberculosis Programme, showing that some health workers at DOT treatment sites deny certain patients access to such management, in some cases motivated by the perceived demands of their supervisors to demonstrate high adherence rates. In a perverse application of a universal DOT strategy, which is promoted precisely because it is impossible to predict which patients will not adhere to therapy, only 37 and 49% of patients, respectively, in two urban areas in Delhi demonstration sites were actually started on a supervised regimen over a three-month period of observation. Some patients refused such regimens because they could not meet requirements for attendance at the clinic during inflexible hours or were initially too ill to make regular visits. A larger number of patients were put on unsupervised regimens, however, because they could not pass the hurdles of the registration process, or were judged by the health worker to be likely not to adhere to it (Jain *et al.*, 1998).

The success of DOT depends on patient acceptance. It will repel patients if is perceived as punitive or inconvenient, even though medication costs may be subsidised, and they will turn to the private sector. A decision and sensitivity analysis on the potential negative effect of a universal DOT policy in the USA formally demonstrated what has always been understood: that if DOT discourages sufficient numbers of patients from accessing public services it can compromise the overall effectiveness of the programme (Heymann *et al.*, 1998). This observation is probably of more relevance in developing countries such as India, where a large proportion of patients already access private sector providers who are more responsive to patient's perceived needs and, by not participating in nominal reporting systems, do not expose patients to the consequences of the stigma associated with tuberculosis (Pathania *et al.*, 1997; Uplekar *et al.*, 1998).

Taking the implementation of DOTS as a marker for commitment to more effective tuberculosis programmes, WHO surveys in 1998 identified 96 countries where greater than 10% of the population has access to DOTS compared to only 19 in 1993 (World Health Organization, 1998). However, countries reporting treatment success over 70% as well as estimated case-detection rates of over 50% include only eight countries in sub-Saharan Africa, three in Latin America and one in South-East Asia. The challenge for tuberculosis programmes is great but the lessons of success point to greater community involvement. At the same time, the community cannot be viewed as a limitless resource (Squire and Wilkinson, 1997; Standing, 1997), in particular where the traditional care givers, women and girls, are already penalised by social codes and health systems unresponsive to their needs.

The complex issues surrounding the advocating of tuberculosis control strategies based on direct observation of therapy are further analysed in Chapter 9.

Community-based services for HIV-related tuberculosis

The development of community-based HIV-related tuberculosis care is a high priority, due to resource constraints limiting the increase in health facility provision in line with the increased caseload. Surprisingly, the huge increases in caseloads have had little impact on practices. In much of Africa the existing diagnostic, treatment and follow up procedures remain as they were before the HIV epidemic. Often where changes have been made, they are *ad hoc* responses, such as early unplanned hospital discharge, rather than the result of a considered strategy. While tuberculosis services are being strengthened in many countries where the WHO's DOTS strategy is being implemented, there has often been little progress in the provision of community-based tuberculosis care. An exception to this is the simplified and community-based approach in Hlabisa district, South Africa (Floyd *et al.*, 1997). In Hlabisa a number of simplifications have been introduced: reduced duration of hospital stay, planned discharge to community DOT supervisors supported by field workers, a biweekly treatment regimen after discharge and no sputum examinations subsequent to diagnosis. In the face of rapid increases in HIV-related tuberculosis, similar models need to be implemented elsewhere in order to cope with rising caseloads (De Cock, 1996; De Cock *et al.*, 1996; Wilkinson and Davies, 1997).

Planned change is required to cope with the increased burden of disease to mitigate the already common 'discharge to neglect' situation. There is a need for tuberculosis programmes, as well as for HIV/AIDS programmes, to work towards provision of 'comprehensive care across the continuum' (World Health Organization, 1994b). Comprehensive care includes clinical management, nursing care, counselling, voluntary HIV testing and social support. A care continuum includes discharge planning, referral networks, and links between government services, non-governmental organisations and community support groups for people with AIDS and their caregivers. Tuberculosis Services need to be integrated with existing inpatient and outpatient services, general health centres as well as with dedicated services for sexually-transmitted diseases and mother and child care. Prevention interventions as part of the overall care should include counselling of partners, supplying condoms, educating family members, using people with AIDS as peer educators and stimulating the formation of AIDS support groups. Such a comprehensive care system is not known to exist anywhere although some elements are provided by general health services, some by home care mobile services, and some by dedicated AIDS service organisations.

Home-based care through mobile services is another response to the problem of HIV-related tuberculosis and such a model was first developed at Chikankata Hospital in rural Zambia. A mobile team delivers the patient from hospital to home and provides continuing support through home visits. The mobile approach has been replicated by non-governmental organisations elsewhere in Africa although a recent WHO review of tuberculosis activities by home care organisations in Africa has revealed serious deficiencies in patient management (Maher *et al.*, 1997). The 'continuum of care' concept acknowledges the necessity of linking public and private health services. In many public health programmes, community health workers play this pivotal role, sometimes leading to heavy demands on their time as the burden shifts to community care, a consequence that must be addressed in planning.

Conclusion

This chapter has taken a traditional disease control perspective and grouped problems of service delivery in terms of case-detection and treatment. However, framing the failure of tuberculosis control in terms of technological constraints, poor quality of general health services and the failure to adopt a standard control strategy does not make explicit the association of tuberculosis with poverty and social marginalisation, the reality of stigma in many societies and the differential impact of this stigma on women. While the HIV pandemic has prompted a shift in the orientation of the international public health community towards infectious disease policies that relate health to social interventions, the rhetoric of tuberculosis control is still largely framed by a biomedical perspective that minimises the reality of tuberculosis as a social disease and is thus unable to add its voice to the need for broader social mobilisation through health professionals, organisations promoting social justice and communities themselves. These issues are taken up in later chapters.

References

Aber, V. R., Allen, B. W., Mitchison, D. A., Ayuma, P., Edwards, E. A. and Keyes, A. B. (1980) Quality control in tuberculosis bacteriology. 1. Laboratory studies on isolated postive cultures and the efficiency of direct smear examination. *Tubercle* **61**, 123–133.

Adeiga, A. A., Akinosho, R. O. and Onyewuche, J. (1994) Evaluation of immune responses in infants with different nutritional status: Vaccinated against tuberculosis, measles and poliomyelitis. *J. Trop. Pediatr.* **40**, 345–350.

Aisu, T., *et al.* (1995) Preventive chemotherapy for HIV-associated tuberculosis in Uganda: An operational assessment at a voluntary counselling and testing centre. *AIDS* **9**, 267–273.

Altare, F., *et al.* (1998) Impairment of mycobacterial immunity in human interleukin-12 receptor deficiency. *Science* **280**, 1432–1435.

156   *K. Jochem and J. Walley*

Aluoch, J. A., Edwards, E. A., Stott, H., Fox, W. and Sutherland, I. (1982) A fourth study of case-finding methods for pulmonary tuberculosis in Kenya. *Trans. R. Soc. Trop. Med. Hyg.* **79**, 679–691.

American Thoracic Society 1980. Guidelines for short-course tuberculosis chemotherapy. *Am. Rev. Resp. Dis.* **212**, 611–614.

American Thoracic Society/Medical Section of the American Lung Association. 1994. Treatment of tuberculosis and tuberculosis infection in adults and children. *Am. J. Resp. Crit. Care Med.* **149**, 1359–1374.

Andrews, R. and Radhakrishna, S. (1959) A comparison of two methods of sputum collection in the diagnosis of pulmonary tuberculosis. *Tubercle* **40**, 155–162.

Annas, G. (1993) Control of tuberculosis: The law and the public health. *N. Engl. J. Med.* **328**, 585–588.

Banerji, D. and Andersen, S. (1963) A sociological study of awareness of symptoms among persons with pulmonary tuberculosis. *Bull. Wld. Hlth. Orgn.* **29**, 665–683.

Barnes, P. F., Bloch, A. B., Davidson, P. T. and Snider, D. E. (1991) Tuberculosis in patients with human immunodeficiency virus infection. *N. Engl. J. Med.* **324**, 1644–1650.

Barnett, G. D. and Styblo, K. (1977) Bacteriological and X-ray status of tuberculosis following primary infection acquired in adolescence or later. *Bull. Int. Union Tuberc.* **52**, 5–16.

Bayer, R. and Wilkinson, D. (1995) Directly observed therapy for tuberculosis: History of an idea. *Lancet* **345**, 1545–1548.

Behr, M. and Small, P. (1997) Has BCG attenuated to impotence? *Nature* **389**, 133–134.

Blair, E. B., Brown, G. L. and Tull, A. H. (1976) Computer files and analyses of laboratory data from tuberculosis patients: II. Analyses of six years' data on sputum specimens. *Am. Rev. Resp. Dis.* **113**, 427–432.

Bloom, B. R. and Fine, P. E. M. (1994) The BCG experience: implications for future vaccines against tuberculosis. In: Bloom B., ed. *Tuberculosis — Pathogenesis, Protection and Control.* Washington DC: ASM Press, pp. 531–557.

Braun, M. J., *et al.* (1992) HIV infection and primary resistance to antituberculosis drugs in Abidjan, Côte d'Ivoire. *AIDS* **6**, 1327–1330.

Burkhardt, K. and Nel, E. (1980) Monitoring regularity of drug intake in tuberculous patients by means of simple urine tests. *S. Afr. Med. J.* **57**, 981–985.

Centers for Disease Control. (1986) Diagnosis and management of mycobacterial infection and disease in persons with human T-lymphotropic viurs type III/lymphoadenopathy-associated virus infection. *Morb. Mortal. Wkly. Rep.* **35**, 448–452.

Centers for Disease Control. (1991) Purified protein derivative (PPD) tuberculin anergy and HIV infection: Guidelines for anergy testing and management of anergic persons at risk of tuberculosis. *Morb. Mortal. Wkly. Rep.* **40** (RR-5), 27–32.

Centers for Disease Control. (1993) Initial therapy for tuberculosis in the era of multidrug resistance: Recommendations of the Advisory Council for the elimination of tuberculosis. *Morb. Mortal. Wkly. Rep.* **42**, 1–8.

Centers for Disease Control. (1994) Improving patient adherence to tuberculosis treatment. Atlanta, Georgia: US Department of Health and Human Services.

Chaisson, R. (1996) Potential role of rifabutin in prophylaxis for tuberculosis and infections due to multiple opportunistic pathogens. *Clin. Infect. Dis.* **22** (Suppl. 1): S61–66; discussion S66–69.

Chakraborty, A. K. R., *et al.* (1994) Prevalence of pulmonary tuberculosis in a peri-urban community of Bangalore under various methods of population screening. *Ind. J. Tuberc.* **41**, 17.

Chakraborty, A. K. R. (1996) Prevalence and incidence of tuberculosis infection and disease in India: A comprehensive review. New Delhi: World Health Organization SEARO.

Chaulet, P. (1987) Compliance with anti-tuberculosis chemotherapy in developing countries. *Tubercle* **68** (supplement): 19–24.

Chaulet, P. (1998) After health sector reform, whither lung health? *Int. J. Tuberc. Lung Dis.* **2**, 349–359.

Chaulet, P. and Zidouni, N. (1993) Evaluation of applied strategies of tuberculosis control in the developing world. In: Reichman LB, Hershfield ES, eds. *Tuberculosis: A Comprehensive International Approach*. New York, Marcel Dekker: pp. 601–627.

Chaulk, C. P., Moore-Rice, K., Rizzi, R. and Chaison, R. E. (1995) Eleven years of community-based directly observed therapy for tuberculosis. *J. J. Am. Med. Assoc.* **274**, 945–951.

Chaulk, C. P. and Kazandjian, V. (1998) Directly observed therapy for treatment completion of pulmonary tuberculosis: Consensus statement of the Public Health Tuberculosis Guidelines Panel. *J. Am. Med. Assoc.* **27**, 943–948.

China Tuberculosis Control Collaboration (1996) Results of directly observed short-course chemotherapy in 112, 842 Chinese patients with smear-positive tuberculosis. *Lancet* **347**, 358–362.

Chowdhury, A. M. R., Chowdhury, S. A., Islam, M. N., Islam, A. and Vaughan, J. P. (1997) Control of tuberculosis through community health workers in Bangladesh. *Lancet* **350**, 160–172.

Cocito, C. and Maes, H. (1998) Immunological relatedness of the protective mechanisms against tuberculosis and cancer. *Euro. J. Clin. Invest.* **28**, 1–12.

Cohen, F. (1997) Adherence to therapy in tuberculosis. *Annu. Rev. Nurs. Res.* **15**, 153–84.

Cohn, D., Bustreo, F. and Raviglione, M. C. (1997) Drug resistance in tuberculosis: Review of the worldwide situation and the World Health Organization/IUATLD global surveillance project. *Clin. Infect. Dis.* **24** (Suppl. 1): S121–S130.

Colditz, G. A., Brewer, T., Berkey, C., Wilson, M., Burdick, E., Fineberg, H. and Mosterller, F. (1995) The efficacy of bacillus Calmette-Guerin vaccination of newborns and infants in the prevention of tuberculosis: Meta-analyses of the published literature. *Pediatrics* **96**, 29–35.

Collins, C. H., Grange, J. M. and Yates, M. D. (1997) *Tuberculosis Bacteriology Organization and Practice*. 2nd edn. Oxford: Butterworth Heinemann.

Comstock, G., *et al.* (1967) A controlled trial of of community-wide isoniazid prophylaxis in Alaska. *Am. Rev. Resp. Dis.* **95**, 935–943.

Comstock, G. W., Baum, C. and Snider, D. E. (1979) Isoniazid prophylaxis among Alaskan Eskimos: A final report of the Bethel isoniazid studies. *Am. Rev. Resp. Dis.* **119**, 827–830.

Corlan, E., Marica, C., Macavei, C., Stanford, J. L. and Stanford, C. A. (1997a) Immunotherapy with *Mycobacterium vaccae* in the treatment of tuberculosis in Romania. 1. Newly-diagnosed pulmonary disease. *Resp. Med.* **91**, 13–19.

Corlan, E., Marica, C., Macavei, C., Stanford, J. L. and Stanford, C. A. (1997b) Immunotherapy with *Mycobacterium vaccae* in the treatment of tuberculosis in Romania. 2. Chronic or relapsed disease. *Resp. Med.* **91**, 21–29.

Crofton, J. (1962) The contribution of treatment to the prevention of tuberculosis. *Bull. Int. Union. Tuberc.* **32**, 643–653.

Cruz, J. R., Heldal, E., Arnidottir, T., Juarez, I. and Enarson, D. A. (1994) Tuberculosis case-finding in Nicaragua: Evaluation of routine activities in the control programme. *Tubercle Lung Dis.* **75**, 417–422.

De Cock, K. M. (1996) Tuberculosis control in resource-poor settings with high rates of HIV infection (editorial). *Am. J. Publ. Hlth.* **86**, 1071–1073.

De Cock, K. M., Binkin, N. J., Zuber, P. L., Tappero, J. W. and Castro, K. G. (1996) Research issues involving HIV associated tuberculosis in resource poor countries. *J. Am. Med. Assoc.* **276**, 1502–1507.

Desormeaux, J., *et al.* (1996) Widespread HIV counseling and testing linked to a community-based tuberculosis control program in a high-risk population. *Bull. Pan. Am. Hlth. Orgn.* **30**, 1–8.

Dick, J. and Schoeman, H. (1996) Tuberculosis in the community: 2. The perceptions of members of a tuberculosis health team towards a voluntary health worker programme. *Tubercle Lung Dis.* **77**, 380–383.

Dick, J., van der Walt, H., Hoogendoorn, L. and Tobias, B. (1996a) Development of a health education booklet to enhance adherence to tuberculosis treatment. *Tubercle Lung Dis.* **77**, 173–177.

Dick, J., Schoeman, J. H., Mohaammed, A. and Lombard, C. (1996b) Tuberculosis in the community: 1. Evaluation of a volunteer health worker programme to enhance adherence to anti-tuberculosis treatment. *Tubercle Lung Dis.* **77**, 274–279.

Dick, J. and Lombard, C. (1997) Shared vision — A health education project designed to enhance adherence to anti-tuberculosis treatment. *Int. J. Tuberc Lung Dis.* **1**, 181–186.

Dujardin, B., Kegels, B., Buve, A. and Mercenier, P. (1997) Tuberculosis control: Did the programme fail or did we fail the programme? (Editorial). *Trop. Med. Int. Hlth.* **2**, 715–718.

Elink Schuurman, M. W., Srisaenpang, S., Pinitsoontorn, S., Bijleveld, I., Vaeteewoothacharn, K. and Methapat, C. (1996) The rapid village survey in tuberculosis control. *Tubercle Lung Dis.* **77**, 549–554.

Enarson, D. (1991) Principles of IUALTD collaborative tuberculosis programmes. *Bull. Int. Union Tuberc.* **66**, 195–200.

Enarson, D. A., Rieder, H. L., Arnadottir, T. and Trébucq, A. (1996) *Tuberculosis Guide for Low Income Countries.* Frankfurt am Main: PMI Verlagsgruppe.

Etkind, S. C. (1993) The role of the public health department in tuberculosis. *Med. Clin. North Am.* **77**, 1303–1314.

Farmer, P. (1996) Social inequalities and emerging infectious diseases. *Emerg. Infect. Dis.* **2**, 259–269.

Farmer, P. (1997) Social scientists and the new tuberculosis. *Soc. Sci. Med.* **44**, 347–358.

Ferebee, S. (1969) Controlled chemoprophylaxis trials in tuberculosis: A general review. *Adv. Tuberc. Res.* **17**, 28–106.

Fine, P. E. M. (1995) Variation in protection by BCG: Implications of and for heterologous immunity. *Lancet* **346**, 1339–1345.

Floyd, K., Wilkinson, D. and Gilks, C. F. (1997) Comparison of cost effectiveness of directly observed treatment (DOT) and conventionally delivered treatment for tuberculosis: Experience from rural South Africa. *Br. Med. J.* **315**, 1407–1411.

Fox, W. (1958) The problem of self administration of drugs with particular reference to pulmonary tuberculosis. *Tubercle* **39**, 269–274.

Fox, W. (1961) Self-administration of medicaments. A review of published work and a study of the problems. *Bull. Int. Union Tuberc.* **31**, 307–331.

Fox, W. (1981) Whither short-course chemotherapy? *Br. J. Dis. Chest* **75**, 331–357.

Frieden, T. R., Sterling, T., Pablos-mendez, A., Kilburn, J. O., Cauthen, G. M. and Dooley, S. W. (1995) Tuberculosis in New York City — Turning the tide. *N. Engl. J. Med.* **333**, 229–233.

Galtung Hansen, O. (1955) *Tuberculosis Mortality and Morbidity and Tuberculin Sensitivity in Norway.* Geneva: World Health Organization (EURO-84-15).

Gebre, N., Karlsson, U., Jonsson, G., Macaden, R., Wolder, A., Assefa, A. and Miorner, V. (1995) Improved microscopical diagnosis of pulmonary tuberculosis in developing countries. *Trans. R. Soc. Trop. Med. Hyg.* **89**, 191–193.

Gonzalez, E., Armas, L. and Alonso, A. (1994) Tuberculosis in the Republic of Cuba: Its possible elimination. *Tubercle Lung Dis.* **75**, 188–194.

Gordis, L. (1979) Methodologic issues in the measurement of patient compliance. In: Haynes, B., Tayler, D., Sackett, D., eds. *Compliance in Health Care.* Baltimore: The Johns Hopkins University Press, pp. 51–65.

Grange, J. M. (1997) Vaccination against tuberculosis: Past problems and future hopes. *Semin. Resp. Crit. Care Med.* **18**, 459–470.

Grange, J. M., Stanford, J. L. and Rook, G. A. W. (1995) Tuberculosis and cancer: Parallels in host responses and therapeutic approaches? *Lancet* **345**, 1350–1352.

Greenberg, S. D., Frager, D., Suster, B., Walker, S., Stavropoulos, C. and Rothpearl, A. (1994) Active pulmonary tuberculosis in patints with AIDS: Spectrum of radiographic findings (including a normal appearance). *Radiology* **193**, 115–119.

Grzybowski, S., Barnett, G. D. and Styblo, K. (1975) Contacts of cases of active pulmonary tuberculosis. *Bull. Int. Union Tuberc.* **50**, 90–106.

Halsey, N., *et al.* (1998) Randomised trial of isoniazid versus rifampicin and pyrazinamide for prevention of tuberculosis in HIV-1 infection. *Lancet* **351**, 786–792.

Harries, A. D., Maher, D., Mvula, B. and Nyangulu, D. S. (1995) An audit of HIV testing and HIV serostatus in tuberculosis patient, Blantyre, Malawi. *Tubercle Lung Dis.* **76**, 413–417.

Harries, A. D., Kamenya, A., Subramanyam, V. R., Salanponi, F. M. and Nyangulu, D. S. (1996) Sputum smears for diagnosis of smear-positive pulmonary tuberculosis. *Lancet* **347**, 834–835.

Harries, A. D., *et al.* (1997a) The pattern of tuberculosis in Queen Elizabeth Central Hospital, Blantyre, Malawi: 1986–1995. *Int. J. Tuberc. Lung Dis.* **1**, 346–351.

Harries, A. D., *et al.* (1997b) Screening pulmonary tuberculosis suspects in Malawi: Testing different strategies. *Trans. R. Soc. Trop. Med. Hyg.* **91**, 416–419.

Haynes, R. B., Taylor, D. W. and Sackett, D. L. (1979) *Compliance in Health Care.* Baltimore: The Johns Hopkins University Press.

Haynes, R. B. (1979) Determinants of compliance: The disease and mechanics of treatment. In: Haynes, R. B., Taylor, D. W., Sackett, D. L., eds. *Compliance in Health Care.* Baltimore: The Johns Hopkins University Press.

Haynes, R. B., McKibbon, K. A. and Kanani, R. (1996) Systematic review of randomised trials to assist patients to follow prescriptions for medications. *Lancet* **348**, 383–386.

Heymann, S. J. (1993) Modelling the efficacy of prophylactic and curative therapies for preventing the spread of tuberculosis in Africa. *Trans. R. Soc. Trop. Med. Hyg.* **87**, 406–411.

Heymann, S. J., Serll, R. and Brewer, T. F. (1998) The influence of program acceptability on the effectiveness of public health policy: A study of directly observed therapy for tuberculosis. *Am. J. Publ. Hlh.* **88**, 442–445.

Hong Kong Chest Service/British Medical Research Council. (1984) Study of a fully supervised programme of chemotherapy for pulmonary tuberculosis given once weekly in the continuation phase in rural areas of Hong Kong. *Tubercle* **65**, 5–15.

Hong Kong Chest Service/British Medical Research Council. (1987) Five-year follow-up of a controlled trial of five six-month regimens of chemotherapy for pulmonary tuberculosis. *Am. Rev. Resp. Dis.* **136**, 1339–1342.

Hong Kong Chest Service/British Medical Research Council. (1992) A double-blind placebo-controlled clinical trial of three antituberculosis chemoprophylaxis regimens in patients with silicosis in Hong Kong. *Am. Rev. Resp. Dis.* 145, 36–41.

International Union Against Tuberculosis Committee on Prophylaxis. 1982. Efficacy of various durations of isoniazid preventive therapy for tuberculosis: Five years of follow-up in the IUAT trial. *Bull. Wld. Hlth. Orgn.* 60, 555–564.

Ipuge, Y., Rieder, H. L. and Enarson, D. A. (1996) The yield of acid-fast bacilli from serial smears in routine microscopy laboratories in rural Tanzania. *Trans. R. Soc. Trop. Med. Hyg.* 90, 258–261.

Iseman, M. and Sbarbaro, J. (1987) Short-course chemotherapy of tuberculosis: Hail Britannia (and friends)! *Am. Rev. Resp. Dis.* 136, 697–698.

Jain, R., *et al.* (1998) Operations research to assess needs and perspectives of tuberculosis patients and providers of tuberculosis care in Nehru Nagar and Moti Nagar chest clinic areas of Delhi. Interim Report. Delhi and London: Lala Ram Swarup Institute for Tuberculosis and Allied Diseases/London School of Hygiene and Tropical Medicine.

Jochem, K., Fryatt, R. J., Harper, I., White, A., Luitel, H. and Dahal, R. (1997) Tuberculosis control in remote districts of Nepal comparing patient-responsible short-course chemotherapy with long-course treatment. *Int. J. Tuberc. Lung Dis.* 1, 502–508.

Johnson, B. J., *et al.* (1995). Clinical and immune responses ot tuberculosis patients treated with low-dose IL-2 and multidrug therapy. *Cytokines Mol. Ther.* 1, 185–196.

Johnson, B. J., Estrada, I., Shen, Z., Ress, S., Wilcox, P., Colston, M. J. and Kaplan, G. (1998) Differential gene expression in response to adjunctive recombinant human interleukin-2 immunotherapy in multidrug-resistant tuberculosis patients. *Infect. Immun.* 66, 2426–2433.

Karonga Prevention Trial Group. 1996. Randomised controlled trial of single BCG, repeated BCG, or combined BCG and killed *Mycobacterium leprae* vaccine for prevention of leprosy and tuberculosis in Malawi. *Lancet* 348, 17–24.

Klein, N., Duncanson, F. P., Lenox, T. H., Pitta, A., Cohen, S. C. and Wormser, G. P. (1989) Use of mycobacterial smears in the diagnosis of pulmonary tuberculosis in AIDS/ARC patients. *Chest* 95, 1190–1192.

Kochi, A. (1991) The global tuberculosis situation and the new control strategy of the World Health Organization. *Tubercle* 72, 1–6.

Liefooghe, R., Baliddawa, J. B., Kipruto, E. M., Vermiere, C. and De Myunck, A. O. (1997) From their own perspective. A Kenyan community's perception of tuberculosis. *Trop. Med. Int. Hlth.* 2, 809–821.

Madico, G., *et al.* (1995) Community infection ratio as an indicator for tuberculosis control. *Lancet* 345, 416–419.

Maher, D., Hausler, H. P., Raviglione, M. C., Kaleeba, N., Aisu, T., Fourie, B. and Nunn, P. (1997) Tuberculosis care in community care organizations in sub-Saharan Africa: Practice and potential. *Int. J. Tuberc. Lung Dis.* 1, 276–283.

162 K. Jochem and J. Walley

McDonald, R. J., Memon, A. M. and Reichman, L. B. (1982) Successful supervised ambulatory management of tuberculosis treatment failures. *Annu. Int. Med.* **96**, 297–302.

Miles, S. H. and Maat, R. B. (1984) A successful supervised outpatient short-course tuberculosis treatment program in an open refugee camp on the Thai-Cambodian border. *Am. Rev. Resp. Dis.* **130**, 827–830.

Ministry of Public Health of the People's Republic of China. 1992. Nationwide random survey for the epidemiology of tuberculosis in 1990. Beijing: Ministry of Public Health.

Moodie, A. (1967) Mass ambulatory chemotherapy in the treatment of tuberculosis in a predominantly urban community. *Am. Rev. Resp. Dis.* **95**, 384–397.

Murray, C. J., Styblo, K. and Rouillon, A. (1990) Tuberculosis in developing countries: Burden, intervention and cost. *Bull. Int. Union Tuberc. Lung Dis.* **65**, 6–24.

Murray, C. J., DeJonghe, E., Chum, H. J., Nyangulu, D. S., Salomao, A. and Styblo, K. (1991) Cost-effectiveness of chemotherapy for pulmonary tuberculosis in three sub-Saharan African countries. *Lancet* **338**, 1305–1308.

Murray, C. J., *et al.* (1993). Tuberculosis. In: Jamison, D. T., Mosley, W. H., Measham, A. R., J. Bobadilla, J., eds. *Disease Control Priorities in Developing Countries*. New York: Oxford University Press, pp. 233–259.

Nichter, M. (1994). Illness semantics and international health: The weak lungs/tuberculosis complex in the Philippines. *Soc. Sci. Med.* **38**, 649–663.

O'Brien, R. J. and Perriëns, J. H. (1995) Preventive therapy for tuberculosis in HIV infection: The promise and the reality (editorial). *AIDS* **9**, 665–673.

Onyebujoh, P., Abdulmumini, T., Robinson, S., Rook, G. A. W. and Stanford, J. L. (1995) Immunotherapy with *Mycobacterium vaccae* as an addition to chemotherapy for the treatment of pulmonary tuberculosis under difficult conditions in Africa. *Resp. Med.* **89**, 199–207.

Orme, I. M. (1997) Progress in the development of new vaccines against tuberculosis. *Int. J. Tuberc. Lung Dis.* **1**, 95–100.

Pathania, V., Almeida, J. and Kochi, A. (1997) Tuberculosis patients and private for-profit health care providers in India. Geneva: World Health Organization/Global Tuberculosis Programme.

Pust, R. (1982) The risk factor approach to sputum-smear diagnosis. *Wld. Hlth. Forum* **3**, 78–80.

Raviglione, M. C., Dye, C., Schmidt, S. and Kochi, A. (1997) Assessment of worldwide tuberculosis control. *Lancet* **350**, 624–629.

Rieder, H. and Enarson, D. (1995) A computer-based ordering system for supplies in national tuberculosis programs. *Tubercle Lung Dis.* **76**, 450–454.

Rieder, H., *et al.* (1997) Evaluation of a standardized recording tool for sputum smear microscopy for acid-fast bacilli under routine conditions in low income countries. *Int. J. Tuberc. Lung Dis.* **1**, 339–345.

Rouillon, A., Perdrizet, S. and Parrot, R. (1976) Transmission of tubercle bacilli: The effects of chemotherapy. *Tubercle* **57**, 275–299.

Sbarbaro, J. A. (1980) Public health aspects of tuberculosis: Supervision of therapy. *Clin. Chest Med.* **1**, 253–263.

Sbarbaro, J. A. (1988) All patients should receive directly observed therapy in tuberculosis. *Am. Rev. Resp. Dis.* **138**, 1075–1076.

Simooya, O. O., Maboshe, M. N., Kaoma, R. B., Chimfwembe, E. C., Thur air ajah, A. and Mukunyandekla, M. (1991) HIV infection in newly diagnosed tuberculosis patients in Ndola, Zambia. *Centr. Afr. J. Med.* **37**, 4–7.

Singapore Tuberculosis Service/British Medical Research Council. 1988. Five-year follow-up of a clinical trial of three six-month regimens of chemotherapy given intermittently in the continuation phase in the treatment of pulmonary tuberculosis. *Am. Rev. Resp. Dis.* **137**, 1147–1150.

Skinner, M. A., Yuan, S., Prestidge, R., Chuk, D., Watson, J. D. and Tan, P. L. (1997) Immunization with heat-killed *Mycobacterium vaccae* stimulated CD8+ cytotoxic T cells specific for macrophages infected with *Mycobacterium tuberculosis. Infect. Immun.* **65**, 4525–4530.

Sonnenberg, P., Ross, M. H., Shearer, S. C. P. M. and Murray, J. (1998) The effect of dosage card on compliance with directly observed tuberculosis therapy in hospital. *Int. J. Tuberc. Lung Dis.* **2**, 168–171.

Squire, S. B. and Wilkinson, S. (1997) Strengthening DOTS through community care for tuberculosis: Observation alone isn't the key. *Br. Med. J.* **315**, 1395–1396.

Standing, H. (1997) Gender and equity in health reform programmes: A review. *Hlth. Pol. Plann.* **12**, 1–18.

Sterne, J. A. C., Rodrigues, L. C. and Guedes, I. N. (1998) Does the efficacy of BCG decline with time since vaccination? *Int. J. Tuberc. Lung Dis.* **2**, 200–207.

Steyn, M., van der Merwe, N., Dick, J., Borcherds, R. and Wilding, R. J. (1997) Communication with tuberculosis patients; a neglected dimension of effective treatment? *Curationis* **20**, 53–56.

Styblo, K. (1985). The relationship between the risk of tuberculous infection and the risk of developing infectious tuberculosis. *Bull. Int. Union Tuberc.* **60**, 117–119.

Styblo, K. (1991) *Epidemiology of Tuberculosis.* The Hague: Royal Netherlands Tuberculosis Association.

Styblo, K. and Meijer, J. (1976) Impact of BCG vaccination programmes in children and young adults on the tuberculosis problem. *Tubercle* **57**, 17–43.

Styblo, K. and Salomao, M. A. (1993) National tuberculosis control programs. In. Reichman LB, Hershfield ES, eds. *Tuberculosis: A Comprehensive International Approach.* New York: Marcel Dekker, pp. 573–600.

Sumartojo, E. (1993) When tuberculosis treatment fails. A social behavioral account of patient adherence. *Am. Rev. Resp. Dis.* **147**, 1311–1320.

Ten Dam, H. G. and Pio, A. (1982). Pathogenesis of tuberculosis and effectiveness of BCG vaccination. *Tubercle* **63**, 225–233.

164 K. Jochem and J. Walley

Theuer, C. P., Hopewell, P. C., Elias, D., Schecter, G. F., Rutherford, G. W. and Chaisson, R. E. (1990) Human immunodeficiency virus infection in tuberculosis patients. *J. Infect. Dis.* **162**, 8–12.

Toman, K. (1979) *Tuberculosis Case-Finding and Chemotherapy: Questions and Answers.* Geneva: World Health Organization.

Tuberculosis Chemotherapy Centre Madras. (1964) A concurrent comparison of intermittent (twice-weekly) isoniazid plus streptomycin and daily isoniazid plus PAS in the domiciliary treatment of pulmonary tuberculosis. *Bull. Wld. Hlth. Orgn.* **31**, 247–271.

Uplekar, M. and Rangan, S. (1995) Alternative approaches to improve treatment adherence in tuberculosis control programme. *Ind. J. Tuberc.* **42**, 67–74.

Uplekar, M., Juvekar, S., Morankar, S., Rangan, S. and Nunn, P. (1998) Tuberculosis patients and practitioners in private clinics in India. *Int. J. Tuberc. Lung Dis.* **2**, 324–329.

Van Deun, A. and Portaels, F. (1998) Limitation and requirements for quality control of sputum smear microscopy for acid-fast bacilli. *Int. J. Tuberc. Lung Dis.* **2**, 756–765.

Volmink, J. and Garner, P. (1997) Systematic review of randomised controlled trials of strategies to promote adherence to tuberculosis treatment (paper). *Br. Med. J.* **315**, 1403–1406.

Vynnyky, E. and Fine, P. E. M. (1997) The annual risk of infection with *Mycobacterium tuberculosis* in England and Wales since 1901. *Int. J. Tuberc. Lung Dis.* **1**, 389–396.

Weis, S. P., et al. (1994) The effect of directly observed therapy on the rates of drug resistance and relapse in tuberculosis. *N. Engl. J. Med.* **330**, 1179–1184.

Whalen, C. C., et al. (1997) A trial of three regimens to prevent tuberculosis in Ugandan adults infected with the human immunodeficiency virus. *N. Engl. J. Med.* **337**, 801–808.

Wilkinson, D. and Davies, G. (1997) Coping with Africa's increasing tuberculosis burden: Are community supervisors an essential component of the DOT strategy? *Trop. Med. Int. Health* **2**, 700–704.

World Health Organization (1994a) *World Health Organization Tuberculosis Programme: Framework for Effective Tuberculosis Control.* Geneva: World Health Organization. (WHO/TB/94.179)

World Health Organization (1994b) Comprehensive Care Across the Continuum: Aide-Memoire for National AIDS Programme Planners and Reviewers. Geneva: World Health Organization/GPA.

World Health Organization (1996) *Groups at Risk: World Health Organization Report on the Tuberculosis Epidemic 1996.* Geneva, World Health Organization.

World Health Organization (1997a) *Report on the Tuberculosis Epidemic, 1997.* Geneva: World Health Organization Global Tuberculosis Programme.

World Health Organization (1997b) *Treatment of Tuberculosis: Guidelines for National Programmes.* 2nd edition. Geneva: World Health Organization.

World Health Organization (1997c) *Anti-Tuberculosis Drug resistance in the World. Report of the World Health Organization/IUATLD Global Project on Anti-tuberculosis Drug Resistance Surveillance, 1994–1997.* Geneva: World Health Organization Global Tuberculosis Programme.

World Health Organization (1998) *Global Tuberculosis Control 1998.* Geneva: World Health Organization.

World Health Organization/IUATLD. (1993) Tuberculosis preventive therapy in HIV-infected individuals: A joint statement of the World Health Organization Tuberculosis Programme and the Global Programme on AIDS, and the International Union Against Tuberculosis and Lung Disease (IUATLD). *Wkly. Epidemiol. Rec.* **68**, 361–368.

World Bank (1993) *World Development Report 1993: Investing in Health.* New York: Oxford University Press.

Yanai, H., Uthaivoravit, W., Mastro, T. D., Limpakarnjanarat, K., Sawanpanyalert, P., Morrow, R. H. and Nieburg, P. (1997) Utility of tuberculin and anergy skin testing in predicting tuberculosis infection in human immunodeficiency virus-infected persons in Thailand. *Int. J. Tuberc. Lung Dis.* **1**, 427–434.

Youngleson, S. (1988) Measuring patient compliance in the treatment of pulmonary tuberculosis in Cape Town — Pitfalls in study design. *S. Afr. Med. J.* **7**, 28–30.

Zhang, L. and Kan, G. (1992) Tuberculosis control programme in Beijing. *Tubercle Lung Dis.* **73**, 162–166.

CHAPTER 7

TUBERCULOSIS TREATMENT IN THE PUBLIC AND PRIVATE SECTORS — POTENTIAL FOR COLLABORATION

Ruairí Brugha and Anthony B. Zwi

Introduction

In this chapter, we explore some of the features of tuberculosis which have contributed to its resurgence over the last decade, and the particular contribution of the for-profit private sector in its control in low- and middle-income countries is examined. The comparative advantages and disadvantages of private providers are described, and reasons why both public and private providers frequently fail to address the needs of patients, families and communities are suggested. The complex and interacting range of factors that influence the behaviour of private providers, and the responses of patients to the services available to them, are outlined, thereby enabling opportunities for National Tuberculosis Programmes to work with different types of providers, patients and their families to be identified. Some important lessons emerge from this analysis: tuberculosis is a complex problem which, in the absence of treatment which is rapidly and completely effective or a novel vaccine, will continue to remain refractory to simple, single-faceted technical solutions. Effective and sustainable tuberculosis control programmes need to be based on an understanding of the rationales underlying patient and provider behaviours in the social and economic contexts in which they live, and must satisfy the needs of each. Current health sector reforms (see Chapter 18) may provide opportunities for forging partnerships at the local level, involving private providers, public sector programmes and other stakeholders who play a role in responding to the health and social burdens posed by tuberculosis, although such innovations are likely to be contested by at least some of the key stakeholders.

A Private Disease of Public Health Importance

Tuberculosis, like other diseases of major public health importance such as sexually transmitted diseases and malaria, is more frequently managed in the private than in the public health care sector in many low- and middle-income countries (Uplekar and Rangan, 1993; Adu-Sarkodie, 1997; McCombie, 1996). These diseases share a number of characteristics: they disproportionately affect the poor; people who are ill with these diseases often seek, or are provided with, symptomatic treatment which does not result in cure; and effective treatment is a 'mixed public-private good with positive externalities' (Bennett, 1991), i.e. a failure to manage them effectively is detrimental not only to the infected individual but also to society at large. In relation to tuberculosis, the private sector is especially important in Asian countries; in Africa tuberculosis care is mainly provided through the public sector, albeit often with some support from non-governmental organisations.

A diagnosis of tuberculosis, like that of a sexually transmitted disease, carries high social costs: the diagnosis itself may be stigmatising due to its implications for one's family and community relationships (Hudelson, 1996; see Chapter 14). Tuberculosis also carries high economic costs which can impoverish families as well as individuals through loss of employment and the cost of obtaining treatment (Uplekar and Rangan, 1996). The social and economic costs of tuberculosis impinge particularly on those in dependent relationships, such as women, leading them to hide the nature of their illness and adopt ineffective strategies to deal with the disease (Hudelson, 1996; Nair *et al.*, 1997). A unique feature of mycobacterial infections (tuberculosis and leprosy), among the diseases of major public health importance, is that they require uninterrupted treatment for many months for a complete cure. A perception that being diagnosed as having tuberculosis is akin to a death sentence (see, for example, Sontag, 1979) may bring with it a denial that the disease is present at all.

These factors have contributed to the emergence of the private sector as a major provider of tuberculosis-related health care in countries where private providers play a dominant role; their involvement in the development of appropriate national strategies is therefore likely to be crucial to the successful control of tuberculosis in such countries. While we argue that the role of private providers needs to be recognised and incorporated into disease control strategies, we realise that this has to take place within a broader context of increasing choice, assuring quality, and guaranteeing that the poor have access to effective services. Every health policy innovation deserves, and indeed demands, to be critically assessed in terms of its anticipated and unanticipated benefits and harms; policies which are widely promoted need to be able to demonstrate that they do more good than harm (Irwig *et al.*, 1998). The strategies for public-private sector collaboration highlighted here need to be rigorously scrutinised and assessed. It is, however, only by recognising the problems and opportunities, and by thoroughly assessing such innovations, that evidence-based policy will be formulated and more widely promoted.

Private or Public Sector Care?

The importance of private providers — including medical practitioners qualified in Western-style medicine, those qualified in other systems of medicine, and unqualified providers — in terms of the proportion of the population that they serve in many low- and middle-income countries, is increasingly being recognised (Bhat, 1993; Aljunid, 1995; Pathania et al., 1997; Swan and Zwi, 1997). In sub-Saharan Africa, private drug retail outlets are the main source of Western-style (allopathic) drugs, mostly inappropriately dispensed (Ross-Degnan et al., 1992; Trostle, 1996). In the Indian Subcontinent, unqualified private providers who dispense allopathic medicines with little or no formal training are often the only accessible or affordable providers in rural areas (Rohde and Visnwanathan, 1995) and urban slums (Garner and Thaver, 1993). Elsewhere in urban areas, a range of private medical practitioners provide the bulk of care, with anti-tuberculosis and other allopathic drugs inappropriately prescribed or dispensed by most private providers. In India, this complexity is deepened further by an additional range of non-allopathic providers, many of whom play some role in dispensing pharmaceuticals, despite a lack of training in how to do so.

In India, it is estimated that at least 60% of tuberculosis patients initially seek care in private clinics (Uplekar and Rangan, 1996). In two studies from Pakistan, two-thirds of tuberculosis patients (Association for Social Development, 1996) and 80% of 152 hospitalised cases (Marsh et al., 1996) reported seeking care initially from a private medical practitioner. Frequent movement of patients between the private and public sectors has been reported for India (Rangan, 1995; Uplekar and Rangan, 1996) and Nepal (Durkin-Longley, 1984). Inability to bear the expense of treatment in the private sector is a principal reason for patients shifting to government services (Uplekar and Rangan, 1996, Nair et al., 1997). However, having commenced treatment in the private sector, two-thirds of patients remain there (Uplekar et al., 1996).

Important shortcomings in the diagnosis and case-management of tuberculosis by private providers have been reported, including failure to confirm the diagnosis with laboratory tests, reliance on radiological diagnosis alone, inappropriate treatment regimens, failure to educate patients and poor case holding (Uplekar and Shepard, 1991; Marsh et al., 1996). Among the negative effects attributable to these shortcomings are the emergence of multidrug-resistant tuberculosis, high costs and high transmission rates. Private providers are unlikely to play a substantive role in relation to other public health aspects of tuberculosis control such as community education, health promotion and contact tracing, given that they typically restrict their role to individual-oriented curative care (Swan and Zwi, 1997). Assertions about the comparative technical superiority of private or public sector care are, however, of limited value outside of the particular context in which the care is delivered, and without regard to the factors that determine quality of care in both sectors. The limited available evidence indicates that the preferential use by patients of technically low-quality private sector services is because public sector services are performing at least as badly (Uplekar and Rangan, 1996), or are considered to be substantially less satisfactory by service users. We have, however, located no published studies which systematically compare the quality of care offered in the public and private sectors in particular countries: this is in itself an indication of how the two health care sectors have, until relatively recently, been compartmentalised and separated from one another by, amongst others, many analysts.

The comparative advantages of attending a private practitioner for a variety of conditions from the service users point of view are increasingly recognised from household and other surveys (Duggal and Amin, 1989; Yesudian, 1991; World Bank, 1993; Uplekar and Rangan, 1996; Nair *et al.*, 1997; Swan and Zwi, 1997): easier accessibility (and therefore shorter travelling time and costs), shorter waiting periods, availability of doctors and drugs, considerate staff attitudes, continuity of care in a stable doctor-patient relationship, and sometimes credit or payment in instalments. Of particular importance for tuberculosis patients is the perception of a greater degree of confidentiality of care in the private sector — a feature which may be more difficult to achieve in a designated public clinic.

It is commonly assumed that the private sector is mainly utilised by wealthier patients; McPake (1997) shows, however, that the pattern of access to private health care differs for people of different socio-economic status, but even the poorest may access private health care, for example, through purchasing drugs from market traders in order to self-treat.

Furthermore, private health care expenditure has been found to be considerable in low-income groups in Africa, Asia and Latin America, in part because of the wide variety of accessible and affordable trained and untrained private providers (Hanson, 1993; Aljunid, 1995; Yesudian, 1994). Health care expenditure, whether private or public, probably accounts for a higher proportion of total expenditure among poorer than wealthier persons (Pannarunothai and Mills, 1997).

In general, being on treatment for tuberculosis poses a significant financial burden on those affected, many of whom are least capable of bearing these costs. In Pune, India, it was estimated that, on average, patients spent almost half their monthly income on tuberculosis treatment, and that one third of the patients were indebted due to the cost of treatment (Uplekar and Rangan, 1996). A study conducted in Bombay in 1992 showed that a third of the tuberculosis patients interviewed spent 9% of their income solely on travel to the clinic to collect drugs (Rangan, 1995). In a Ugandan study it was estimated that approximately 70% of the total cost of tuberculosis treatment was borne by the patient (Saunderson, 1995). Private care may also be cheaper than public sector treatment in economic terms, especially if the latter involves unofficial and illicit charges (Asiimwe *et al.*, 1997), wasted trips to public facilities due to irregular drug supplies (Uplekar and Rangan, 1996) and greater opportunity costs through lost earnings as a result of attending for care. Daily or twice weekly directly observed treatment, for which patients are required to travel some distance regularly to public clinics for the supervision of treatment, may impose high costs on patients in some settings. Failure to recognise these costs, which are often hidden, contributes to the inability of many public sector policy makers and programme managers to understand why those with tuberculosis seek care in the private sector, and to the failure to recognise a potential role for these providers in the development of national tuberculosis control programmes.

A More Informed Approach to Private Sector Tuberculosis Control

Much of the failure of national tuberculosis control programmes in the past can be ascribed to a lack of commitment of resources, especially to ensuring a regular and easily-accessible drug supply to patients (Nagpaul, 1982). The renewed international concern with tuberculosis (see, for example, World Bank, 1993; World Health Organization, 1996) and calls to mobilise greater resources for global tuberculosis control present opportunities to rethink how best to respond to tuberculosis. This could be both upstream, in terms of prevention (outside the scope of this chapter, but see Chapter 20), and downstream, in terms of control, where increasing coverage of diagnostic and treatment services, and improving the quality of care delivered to those with tuberculosis would bring needed benefits. More efficient and rational utilisation of available health care resources, and greater recognition of the complementary strengths of public and private providers, is an important part of such an agenda. A number of commentators on the World Health Organization's (WHO) campaign based on directly observed therapy have highlighted the need to devote greater attention to recognising and working with the private sector (Bam, 1997; Lieberman, 1997).

Health care providers, like patients, act in rational ways, influenced by a variety of factors, including their professional characteristics (knowledge, skills, access to essential supports and resources), personal aspirations (for income and for respect and recognition from patients, their families, communities and colleagues, including public sector colleagues), the perceived needs of their clients (demands of patients or their families for particular forms of treatment), and health system characteristics (competition and perceptions of how other providers are acting, the relationship between public and private sectors, and the organisation of national disease control programmes) (Brugha and Zwi, 1998). Multi-faceted strategies which are based on an understanding of the complex influences which determine provider behaviour, in the social and professional contexts in which they operate, are more likely to be effective than approaches based on a simplistic cause-and-effect model which assumes that profit-maximisation is the sole influence on private practitioner behaviours (Brugha and Zwi, 1998). Understanding the complexity of factors influencing provider practices may help to uncover a range of potential levers which could be used to support a shift towards improving the quality of care provided.

While there has been some research to assess the quality of tuberculosis care in the private sector, little has been done to explain the reasons for provider behaviour. The research by Uplekar and his colleagues in India suggests a provider knowledge deficit, in view of the many different and inappropriate treatment regimens used and the high proportion of private providers who were unaware of the existence of the National Tuberculosis Programme, let alone guidelines on tuberculosis management (Uplekar and Shepard, 1991; Uplekar *et al.*, 1996). Our ongoing research on the role of private providers in malaria control in an urban area of India reveals a high level of interest and commitment to regular continuing medical education among those trained in Western-style medicine (general practitioners, specialists and chemists) and those trained in other systems of medicine (such as Ayurveda and homoeopathy), with little or no input and no guidelines disseminated by municipal or national programmes (unpublished data). In other countries, where national programme managers organised continuing medical education seminars for private providers on appropriate tuberculosis case management, they proved to be popular (Berman *et al.*, 1995).

Primary care providers in low- and middle-income countries, as in high-income countries, depend on a fast turnover of patients and lack the time and often the skills to educate, counsel and reassure suspected or diagnosed tuberculosis patients. Private providers live and work in an environment where tuberculosis and its care are socially stigmatised, and they often reinforce the stigma by avoiding or concealing the diagnosis of tuberculosis from patients (Uplekar *et al.*, 1996). Private providers may fear that an unwelcome sputum investigation or diagnosis, hurriedly given to a patient, will result in the patient deserting them for a competitor; or that they may gain a reputation as a 'tuberculosis doctor', thereby deterring other patients. A sputum investigation may require a number of patient visits to a public sector laboratory, staffed by poorly-motivated personnel, and thereby incurring greater opportunity costs for patients. More than with a chest radiograph, a sputum examination already carries the implication of tuberculosis and may be less attractive to providers and be feared by patients. The economic demands of treatment adherence may be considerable and symptomatic relief may result in patients stopping treatment. The lack of support to counsel patients and to promote treatment adherence may be outweighed by the costs and expectation of failure. In addition, successful tuberculosis management and high cure rates may not be valued or esteemed by most of one's public and private sector colleagues.

Successful tuberculosis control, especially in those resource-poor settings where private providers have a dominant role, needs to be based on an evaluation of the quality of care supplied by public and private providers, the professional, social and economic factors and contexts which influence provider practices, and the realisation of the need for a profound change in the perceptions, attitudes and cultures in which the different players operate: programme managers, public and private providers, employers, communities, families and patients. As Donovan and Blake (1992) remark: "In effect, patients carry out their own cost-benefit analysis for each treatment they are offered". The benefits patients receive, whether in the public or private sectors, relative to the costs they, their families and their communities, incur, need to be greatly increased if tuberculosis is to be more effectively controlled.

Strategies for Promoting Improved Private Sector Tuberculosis Control

A combination of different strategies needs to be considered for promoting quality of care in the private sector, taking into account the complexities identified above. Many of these strategies, listed in Table 1,

Table 1. Examples of potential interventions to improve private sector delivery of tuberculosis care

Initiatives directed at or through **provider organisations**:
• Developing local organisational networks and links.
• Enhancing provider skills and knowledge through a variety of mechanisms (e.g. training, dissemination of guidelines, audit systems and use of local opinion leaders).
• Offering incentives and support to providers who deliver services of a specified, agreed standard.
• Accreditation of providers as an incentive to good practice.

Initiatives directed at **service users**:
• Enhancing knowledge and power of service users in order that they demand high-quality services.
• Developing or supporting consumer/service user representative groups to enable them to monitor provider practices and serve as advocates for patients.
• Developing partnerships between consumer groups and professional bodies.

Initiatives directed more broadly at **health systems**:
• Enhancing/developing monitoring and quality control systems which are feasible and acceptable to private providers and public sector programme managers.
• Maintaining a regulatory framework to underpin and support good private provider practices.
• Providing access to essential resources (drugs, diagnostic services, administrative support), subject to evidence of adherence to agreed standards.
• Enhancing the skills of public sector managers for working with the different interest groups (private providers, patients and community) in order to develop common strategies.

are interdependent and potentially synergistic, but for clarity they are discussed separately.

Provider Organisational Initiatives

The development and successful implementation of strategies for modifying provider practices require a comprehensive identification of existing provider organisations and networks or, in the absence of such formal structures, the identification of any informal networks and potential opinion leaders among the provider target group. Where such networks exist, the potential to enter into dialogue and establish links, both with and between the different stakeholders, with a view to reaching consensus on how to move forward, is greatly enhanced. In many countries, those formally trained in Western-style medicine and, in a few countries such as India, those trained in other medical systems, are well organised through representative bodies with elected office-holders and formal constitutions. These bodies represent their members' interests in negotiations with other bodies, organise regular and well-attended continuing medical education sessions, and co-ordinate members' involvement in special health programmes. Such bodies may provide channels which can be used to improve and extend services offered.

A prerequisite for change is that those who need to be involved in changing practice perceive that a problem exists, and have a shared perception of the problem (Williamson, 1992). The degree to which private providers are organised in representative bodies, and are open to the influence of their peers, will determine what approaches should be taken. Lessons learned from the implementation of clinical guidelines in pilot sites within the National Health Service of the United Kingdom include the need to involve key stakeholders from an early stage in agreeing the need, and identifying priority areas, for change; the central role of clinicians as motivators and agents of change; the importance of utilising existing professional networks in the adaptation and dissemination of guidelines, and the linkage of this process to clinical audit and quality assurance processes (Humphris and Littlejohns, 1996). By the use of methods such as stakeholder analysis (Overseas Development Administration, 1995) and political mapping (Reich, 1994), it may be possible to assess the relative importance of different groups and organisations to the success of practice-modifying initiatives; and through consensus building techniques, such as Delphi methods, identify which kinds of strategies are likely to win the active support of the different stakeholders, including private providers, and how such strategies should be designed so as to gain maximum support (Brugha and Zwi, 1998).

Provider Skills and Knowledge

Evidence from high-income countries suggests that improvements in patient care require more than the dissemination of evidence-based guidelines through continuing medical education and other training strategies (Oxman et al., 1995). Interventions may result in increased levels of knowledge, unaccompanied by improvements in practice. A review of 91 studies, in which the effectiveness of clinical guidelines in changing the practices of health professionals was rigorously evaluated, led to the conclusion that the key features of successfully implemented interventions were "active professional participation and implementation strategies that are closely related to decision making" (Grimshaw et al., 1995). Guidelines, if they are to be effective, have to be carefully developed through an inclusive process and need to be appropriately directed and disseminated at the right target groups (Thomson et al., 1995). A prerequisite to applying the lessons learned from research in health care practice is an understanding of how knowledge is interpreted locally and of the connection between what is advocated globally and their own local situation (Ferlie et al., 1996), and of the beliefs of practitioners (Graham, 1996).

In low- and middle-income countries, a range of different categories of private practitioner may be involved, in one way or another, in delivering (or failing to deliver) tuberculosis control services. Continuing medical education strategies need to take into account the time constraints and practice hours of private providers, use strategies which are tailored to the particular target group, and utilise different strategies for reaching the variety of relevant providers. Local opinion leaders need to be involved in designing and supporting continuing medical education messages and strategies. The existence of referral linkages, formal or informal, between different private providers may provide opportunities for reinforcing continuing medical education and providing audit and feedback to the referring provider on case management. Our ongoing research in India demonstrates that such informal (and often personal and/or financial) linkages between specialists privately practising Western-style medicine and a variety of different types of private primary care providers are common (unpublished data).

Provider Incentives and Supports

Improving provider knowledge, though essential, is not a sufficient measure for improving quality of care in the private sector and other ways of influencing their practice need to be considered. Private providers are usually more aware or concerned than public sector workers about the ability of their patients to pay for laboratory investigations and lengthy courses of treatment, as these may influence the loyalty of clients to the provider. In India, private providers prefer to use private rather than public laboratories because these are able to provide results more rapidly and are perceived to be more reliable (unpublished data). Financial incentives or subsidies could be considered for supporting private sector care but may create the potential for abuse by private providers. The supply of drugs or the direct reimbursement of private providers by public sector programmes may, for example, promote the diversion or misuse of resources, or the creation of phantom patients. The use of voucher systems or the reimbursement of diagnosed patients, who utilise designated and accredited private laboratories and drug retail outlets, warrants consideration although they may also not be immune to abuse and would need to be closely monitored. Such systems would, however, place the control more in the hands of patients who would have the greatest interest in ensuring the success of such systems. Counselling supports to private providers (see *A role for service users*, below) are much less likely to be abused.

Any form of public financing of privately-provided services, such as the contracting out or franchising of tuberculosis control services to private organisations, would require the capacity and resources in the public sector, or at least financed by the public sector, to monitor their effects. International agencies are increasingly advocating a change in the role of governments in low- and middle-income countries away from provision towards the financing and regulation of health services (World Bank, 1997).

Monitoring and Quality Control

The identification of mechanisms for the monitoring and quality control of services of public health importance, in the public as well as the private sector, is increasingly recognised as a priority for governments. There has, however, been little research on identifying effective quality assurance systems (Heiby, 1996), or on the development and evaluation of acceptable, feasible and efficient mechanisms for monitoring service quality (Cibulskis and Izard, 1996), which are necessary for the efficient use of regulatory controls and incentives for influencing provider practices. Routine passive data return systems involve significant transaction and opportunity costs for busy private providers. Their validity and reliability are often uncertain, and busy private providers are unlikely to participate in such systems unless they perceive some benefits. Active surveillance systems, where health authorities send trained personnel to collect data on a range of diseases and control programmes of public health importance, may be more costly but the advantages for public health managers and health service planners may outweigh the costs. The co-operation of private providers in such systems is more likely if a consultative stakeholder approach is utilised, as recommended above (see *Provider organisational initiatives*, above), and if it is combined with some form of provider accreditation (see below).

Patients and their families may be best placed to monitor and report on the care received from providers. They could be enabled to do this by the implementation of shared care arrangements under which tuberculosis patients attending private providers register initially with a public sector programme, and subsequently attend the public sector to establish that sputum conversion has occurred and, later, to confirm that they have been cured. Patient-held case records, supported by an in-depth interview by a public sector health worker, clinical examination and sputum tests would help determine the outcome of treatment. Service users have been clearly shown to be reliable at maintaining their own health records (Brugha and Kevany, 1995). Private providers would, however, need to see clear advantages for themselves in participating in such arrangements.

Regulation and Accreditation

"Regulation has been defined as government 'action to manipulate prices, quantities [and distribution], and quality of products'" (Maynard, 1992, cited by Kumaranayake, 1997). Those who may be involved in the regulatory process include governmental and non-governmental agencies, health care professionals, commercial interests, community and consumer groups (Kumaranayake, 1997). In the case of tuberculosis control, regulation is or should be concerned with the management of individual patients, and the exclusive and appropriate use of anti-tuberculosis drugs for tuberculosis control. In many low- and middle-income countries there exists a lack of governmental capacity for regulatory enforcement, high transaction and administrative costs, an undermining of governmental efforts as a result of corruption, and an unwillingness of professional organisations (medical registration councils and representative associations) to become involved. In addition, the profit-maximising activities of many national and international pharmaceutical distributors may promote inappropriate prescribing of drugs (Kamat and Nichter, 1997).

Despite the many failures there have been some notable successes: in India, the 1986 Consumer Protection Act (COPRA) has been used to protect patients' rights through enforcing norms designed to protect consumers' rights, where these had been historically neglected by the

Indian Medical Association and Indian Medical Council (Bhat, 1996). The effects of such alternative consumer-oriented approaches are still unclear, as judicial decisions may not be underpinned by adequate professional knowledge and unwelcome outcomes could include litigiously defensive practices, such as inappropriately excessive levels of clinical investigation (Bhat, 1996). Our own ongoing research in India confirms a significant level of awareness of the COPRA among private practitioner representatives and a belief in many quarters that it will, and already does, influence provider behaviour. Kumaranayake (1997) suggests that a basic legislative regulatory framework is essential, even where enforcement capacity is low, especially for those low- and middle-income countries in which the private sector is rapidly growing.

Regulatory mechanisms include controls and incentives. As regulatory controls are either used to address blatant medical negligence rather than to improve the quality of medical care, or are left to gather dust, there is increasing interest in the potential of incentives for shifting provider behaviour in low- and middle-income countries (Bennett et al., 1994). The resources and support systems which enable private practitioners to provide effective and affordable tuberculosis care include access to diagnostic services, regular supplies of anti-tuberculosis drugs, and support in providing patient counselling and education.

Interest has recently been expressed in exploring the utility of other more generic and multi-faceted types of incentives such as provider accreditation (World Bank, 1997). Accreditation has been defined by Scrivens (1996) as "the procedure by which an authoritative body gives formal recognition that a body or a person is competent to carry out specific tasks". It is concerned with "assessing quality of organisational processes and performance using agreed upon standards, compliance with which is assessed by surveyors" (Scrivens, 1995). An additional feature of accreditation is that it is frequently linked to initiatives for promoting better clinical practice and therefore requires the co-operation and participation of health professionals in the process. Accreditation is usually awarded to providers for time-limited periods, thus maintaining pressure upon them to continue to assure high standards of service provision.

In low- and middle-income country settings, where all the players including private providers recognise the inability of external regulatory controls to substantially shift provider behaviour, participatory strategies such as accreditation, introduced through agreement and consensus, are more likely than punitive controls to result in sustainable improvements in provider behaviour at the population level. The aim of accreditation is to raise the standard of care of all accredited providers, rather than to identify and punish the poorest or most dangerous outliers, based on the principle that "a rising tide raises all boats" (Brugha, Kumaranayake and Zwi, unpublished data). Nevertheless, an effective accreditation system, with high levels of consumer education, would aim to reduce reliance on services which are of recognisably poor quality. Incentives need to be built into accreditation systems to make them attractive to private providers: underpinning them with community education programmes and extensive media coverage to promote the accredited providers would reward such providers while at the same time promoting use of the higher quality services on offer. Logos which identify accredited providers could be promoted through local community and media campaigns while other mechanisms, such as child-to-family campaigns and social marketing, could also be utilised.

As with other incentive-based strategies, accreditation could be open to abuse. Mechanisms for monitoring and evaluating accreditation systems, and the quality of care patients receive from accredited providers, need to be agreed between the different stakeholders involved. In high-income countries, monitoring involves the submission to the accrediting body of complex data sets which describe a range of process activities undertaken by the provider (organisation). More appropriate and affordable monitoring systems could be piloted in resource-poor settings, including regular examinations to test provider knowledge of national programme guidelines, surprise practice visits by teams which include members of the provider's own representative body, reports of patients and other key informants, and the use of simulated client visits to providers' practices (Madden et al., 1997). Accredited providers could be required to demonstrate that they participate, at regular intervals, in programmes of continuing professional development.

A Role for Service Users

Economic status and literacy or educational level have long been recognised as highly influential determinants of health, access to health care and health service utilisation. In the presence of 'free' public sector tuberculosis services it is often assumed that lack of adherence to treatment is due to patient ignorance and lack of motivation, and can simply be addressed through health education. Case studies, as reported by Uplekar (1996) and Farmer (1997), demonstrate that patients often make considerable efforts and sacrifices to adhere to treatment regimens, at great economic cost, but are let down by the shortcomings of the available tuberculosis services and encounter barriers when attempting to access them. As Farmer (1997) states, such settings "are crying out for measures to improve the quality of care, not the quality of patients". In a review of the issues related to adherence to tuberculosis treatment, Sumartojo (1993) highlighted the importance of improving the health system and the interface of the health service with its users, if treatment was to be more effective. The importance of addressing the key human and/or organisational failures of the health system rather than focusing simply on technical issues and human failures has also been highlighted (Dujardin et al., 1997).

Patient-pressure and the belief that patients will prefer to self-medicate or visit 'quack doctors' are frequently cited by public and private providers as reasons for adopting treatment practices which they apparently know to be harmful or ineffective (Ofori–Adjei and Arhinful, 1996; Santoso 1996; Nizami et al., 1996). Busy private providers, especially single-handed ones with high patient turnover rates, have insufficient time and often lack the skills to ensure that their patients have an understanding of optimal treatment-taking behaviour. Where doctors are organised in group practices (less common in low- and middle-income countries than in more developed ones), as reported by Uplekar in Bombay (Chapter 8), the assignment of publicly-funded counsellors to support private providers in the delivery of diseases of public health importance — tuberculosis, sexually transmitted diseases, family planning — would most likely be attractive to them. This would be even more so if such workers could also assist in carrying out other priority public health tasks such as patient registration, treatment documentation, and collation and return of data to public sector programme managers. Governments might also consider sub-contracting such activities to non-governmental organisations who specialise in tuberculosis control (Nair *et al.*, 1997). Single-handed general practitioners might be willing to refer patients who require initial education and counselling to designated public sector services, if they were reassured that client loyalty would be reinforced rather than undermined.

There is a need, however, for the focus to shift from the education of patients to education by patients. This requires a conceptual shift from seeing the patient as ignorant, passive and compliant to seeing the patient as a knowledgeable, rational and active agent who is in control of his or her treatment and can influence how that treatment is delivered (see also Ogden, Chapter 9). As Donovan and Blake (1992) conclude: "The key to improving rates of compliance (although effectively doing away with the concept), is the development of active, co-operative relationships between patients and doctors. For this to be successful, doctors will need to recognise patients' decision-making abilities, to try to understand patients' needs and constraints, and to work with patients in the development of treatment regimes." Tuberculosis patients and their families, who lie at the bottom of the chain of service delivery, are in the best position to identify and report health service barriers (as described above). The importance of client loyalty to private providers, and the evidence that many patients only utilise public sector services when their savings are exhausted, suggest a greater willingness and ability of private providers to overcome many of these barriers.

If the perspectives of patients and their families are to be incorporated into the design and delivery of tuberculosis programmes, the managers of the programmes need to find ways to include them, alongside the different health care providers, as equal partners. The use of the Consumer Protection Act in India to represent patients' interests indicates the emerging importance of consumer protection groups (Bhat, 1996). In the absence of consumer representative groups, programme managers should consider measures to foster the development of voluntary groups of tuberculosis patients, ex-patients and their families to participate in programme design. A cure rate of 81% has been achieved in a highly cost-effective public tuberculosis programme in South Africa where patients and their families were free to select treatment supervisors of their choice: 56% selected non-health workers (Floyd *et al.*, 1997).

Choice of provider is only meaningful for patients and their families where at least some high-quality alternatives are available, which is frequently not the case. Once quality of care is being effectively addressed in the public and private sectors, there may be a role for educating patients and communities on how to recognise and select those providers who offer a technically high-quality service, thereby ensuring that competition drives quality improvements (see sections on monitoring and quality control and regulation and accreditation). Community-wide education campaigns will only have a realistic chance of changing the culture of denial and social ostracism that understandably exists in many communities when effective, acceptable and affordable treatment options are made available to communities.

Tuberculosis Control in Reforming Health Systems

Affordable and accessible high-quality tuberculosis control services are a human right and ensuring their availability is the responsibility of the state. The major involvement of the for-profit private sector in the delivery of services of public health importance should not be seen by governments as a cause for complacency, inertia, or as an excuse for leaving the challenge of controlling tuberculosis to non-state agents and agencies. International policy makers envisage the limitation of the role of governments in the financing and regulation of health care in low- and middle-income countries in the future (World Bank, 1997). Governments must act as the guarantors for the availability of high-quality health care to the whole population. There are a variety of reasons for retaining a strong role for the government in delivering services of public health importance: the state should guarantee access to public health care, especially for the poor, and not leave it to the uncertainties of the market place; it should maintain a monitoring and regulatory role which is conditioned and refined by active involvement in service delivery; and it should maintain high-quality public sector care in order to promote high-quality care in the private sector through both competition and support.

An aspect of health sector reform which is at least as important to the health of populations as the strong and growing role of the private sector, and is impinging more immediately on how national control programmes such as National Tuberculosis Programmes are organised, is health service decentralisation (see also Chapter 18). The oscillation over the last 30 years between a selective, vertical programme approach to tuberculosis, malaria, family planning and immunisation services, and a horizontal, comprehensive primary health care approach to health service delivery (see Rifkin and Walt, 1986 and Chapter 4), is moving inexorably with current health sector reforms towards the latter through the devolution of power and resources to the district. Enhancing the role of local government in health service provision, at least in urban areas in low- and middle-income countries, will also provide opportunities for developing comprehensive, intersectoral care.

The World Health Organization's Global Tuberculosis Programme's struggle to convince low- and middle-income countries to adopt a uniform approach to tuberculosis control, through its 'Use DOTS More Widely' campaign, will increasingly be confronted by districts, municipalities and states where health service managers are being offered, or are demanding, greater freedom and flexibility to adopt case-holding strategies which may include directly observed therapy approaches, and which suit their particular professional and cultural contexts. Countries such as Ghana and Zambia, which have travelled further down the road of decentralisation than most sub-Saharan African countries, are struggling to maintain a balance between ensuring vertically driven, technically high-quality assurance systems, and local control of service delivery strategies.

Once the rapid pace of public sector health service decentralisation slows down, decentralisation will offer great opportunities for forging partnerships between public sector health service managers and the range of different private providers, non-governmental organisations and community groups which are operating in each local context. Many of the strategies and approaches we have outlined in this chapter — developing local organisational networks and links, provider training and in-service training, optimising use of all available human and financial resources at the local level, promoting and rewarding private (and public) providers who offer high-quality care, and empowering communities to demand and obtain affordable high quality care — may thrive in such an environment. Other fundamental challenges, such as shifting the focus of tuberculosis from downstream care to upstream prevention (see Chapter 20), protecting the health of the poor, and promoting equity, remain. Directing the attention of governments and international policy makers to these issues merits ongoing analysis and advocacy.

References

Adu-Sarkodie, Y. A. (1997) Antimicrobial self medication in patients attending a sexually transmitted diseases clinic. *Int. J. Sexually Transmitted Disease and AIDS* **8**, 456–458.

Aljunid, S. (1995) The role of private medical practitioners and their interactions with public health services in Asian countries. *Hlth. Pol. Plann.* **10**, 333–349.

Asiimwe, D. *et al.* (1997) The private-sector activities of public sector workers in Uganda. In: Bennett, S., McPake, B., Mills, A. eds. *Private Health Providers in Developing Countries*. London: Zed Books. Chapter 5.

Association for Social Development. (1996) *Qualitative Study on Tuberculosis Patients at the Tuberculosis Centre, Rawalpindi.* Islamabad: Association for Social Development.

Bam, D. S. (1997) In Nepal it is the breakthrough of the decade. *World Health Forum* **18**, 236–238.

Bennett, S. (1991) *The Mystique of Markets: Public and Private Health Care in Developing Countries.* Department of Public Health and Policy, PHP Departmental Publication No. 4 London School of Hygiene and Tropical Medicine.

Bennett, S. *et al.* (1994) Carrot and stick: State mechanisms to influence private provider behaviour. *Hlth. Pol. Plann.* **9**, 1–13.

Berman, P. *et al.* (1995) *Kenya: Non-Governmental Health Care Provision. Data for Decision Making Project.* Boston: Harvard University.

Bhat, R. (1993) The private/public mix of health care in India. *Hlth. Pol. Plann.* **8**, 43–56.

Bhat, R. (1996) Regulation of the private sector in India. *Int. J. Hlth. Plann. Management* **11**, 253–274.

Brugha, R. and Kevany, J. (1995) Immunisation determinants in the Eastern Region of Ghana. *Hlth. Pol. Plann.* **10**, 312–318.

Brugha, R. and Zwi, A. (1998) Improving the quality of privately provided public health services in low- and middle-income countries: Challenges and strategies. *Hlth. Pol. Plann.* **13**, 107–120.

Cibulskis, R. and Izard, J. (1996) Monitoring systems. In: Janovsky, K., ed. *Health Policy and Systems Development, An Agenda for Research.* Geneva: World Health Organization. Chapter 12, pp. 191–206.

Donovan, J. L. and Blake, D. R. (1992) Patient non-compliance: Deviance or reasoned decision-making? *Soc. Sci. Med.* **34**, 507–513.

Duggal, R. and Amin, S. (1989) *Cost of Health Care: A household Survey in An Average Indian District.* Bombay: The Foundation for Research in Community Health.

Dujardin, B., Kegels, G., Buve, A. and Mercenier, P. (1997) Tuberculosis control: Did the programme fail or did we fail the programme? *Trop. Med. Intl. Hlth.* **2**, 715–718.

Durkin-Longley, M. (1984) Multiple therapeutic use in urban Nepal. *Soc. Sci. Med.* **19**, 867–872.

Farmer, P. (1997) Social scientists and the new tuberculosis. *Soc. Sci. Med.* **44**, 347–358.

Ferlie, E., Fitzgerald, L. and Wood, M. (1996) *Achieving Change in Clinical (Communities of) Practice: Scientific, Organisational and Behavioural Processes.* University of Warwick, UK: Centre for Corporate Strategy and Change.

Floyd, K., Wilkinson, D. and Gilks, C. (1997) *Community-Based, Directly Observed Therapy for Tuberculosis: An Economic Analysis.* Tygerberg, South Africa: Medical Research Council.

Garner, P. and Thaver, I. (1993) Urban slums and primary health care. *Brit. Med. J.* **306**, 667–668.

Graham, I. (1996) I believe therefore I practise. *Lancet* **347**, 4–5.

Grimshaw, J., *et al.* (1995). Developing and implementing clinical practice guidelines. *Quality in Health Care* **4**, 55–64.

Hanson, K. (1993) *Non-Government Financing and Provision of Health Services in Africa, A Background Paper. Data for Decision Making Project.* Boston: Harvard University.

Heiby, J. (1996). Quality of health services. In: Janovsky, K., ed. *Health Policy and Systems Development, An Agenda for Research.* Geneva: World Health Organization. Chapter 11.

Hudelson, P. (1996) Gender differentials in tuberculosis: The role of socio-economic and cultural factors. *Tubercle. Lung Dis.* **77**, 391–400.

Humphris, D. and Littlejohns, P. (1996) Implementing clinical guidelines: Preparation and opportunism. *J. Clin. Effect* **1**, 5–10.

Irwig, L., Zwarenstein, M., Zwi, A. and Chalmers, I. (1998) A flow diagram to help select interventions and research for health care. *Bull. Wld. Hlth. Org.* **76**, 17–24.

Kamat, V. R. and Nichter, M. (1997) Monitoring product information: An ethnographic study of pharmaceutical sales representatives in Bombay, India. In: Bennett, S., McPake, B., Mills, A., eds. *Private Health Providers in Developing Countries.* London: Zed Books. Chapter 8

Kumaranayake, L. (1997) The role of regulation: Influencing private sector activity within health sector reform. *J. Int. Devl.* **9**, 641–649.

Lieberman, S. (1997) A good start. *World Health Forum* **18**, 239–241.

Madden, J. M., Quick, J. D., Ross-Degnan, D. and Kafle, K. K. (1997) Undercover careseekers: Simulated clients in the study of health provider behaviour in developing countries. *Soc. Sci. Med.* **45**, 1465–1482.

Marsh, D. R., *et al.* (1996) Front-line management of pulmonary tuberculosis; an analysis of tuberculosis and treatment practices in urban Sindh, Pakistan. *Tubercle Lung Dis.* **77**, 86–92.

McCombie, S. C. (1996) Treatment seeking for malaria: A review of recent research. *Soc. Sci. Med.* **43**, 933–945.

McPake, B. (1997) The role of the private sector in health service provision. In: Bennett, S., McPake, B., Mills, A., eds. *Private Health Providers in Developing Countries.* London: Zed Books. Chapter 2.

Nagpaul, D. R. (1982) Why integrated tuberculosis programmes have not succeeded as per expectations in many developing countries — A collection of observations. *Ind. J. Tuberc.* **29**, 149.

Nair, D. M., George, A. and Chacko, K. T. (1997) Tuberculosis in Bombay: New insights from poor urban patients. *Hlth. Pol. Plann.* **12**, 77–85.

Nizami, S. Q., Khan, I. A. and Bhutta, A. Z. (1996) Drug prescribing practices of general practitioners and paediatricians for childhood diarrhoea in Karachi, Pakistan. *Soc. Sci. Med.* **42**, 1133–1139.

Ofori-Adjei, D. and Arhinful, D. (1996) Effect of training on the clinical management by medical assistants in Ghana. *Soc. Sci. Med.* **42**, 1169–1176.

Overseas Development Administration. (1995) Guidelines for Stakeholder Analysis. London: Overseas Development Administration.

Oxman, A. D., Thomson, M. A., Davis, D. A. and Haynes, B. (1995) No magic bullets: A systematic review of 102 trials of interventions to improve professional practice. *Can. Med. Assoc. J.* **153**, 1423–1431.

Pannarunothai, S. and Mills, A. (1997) The poor pay more: Health-related inequality in Thailand. *Soc. Sci. Med.* **44**, 1781–1790.

Pathania, V., Almeida, J. and Kochi, A. (1997) *TB Patients and Private For-Profit Health Care Providers in India.* Geneva: World Health Organization Global Tuberculosis Programme.

Rangan, S. (1995) User perspective in urban tuberculosis control. In: Chakraborty, A. K., Rangan, S., Uplekar, M., eds. *Urban Tuberculosis Control: Problems and Prospects.* Bombay: The Foundation for Research in Community Health, pp. 97–106.

Reich, M. (1994) *Political Mapping of Health Policy, A Guide for Managing the Political Dimensions of Health Policy.* Boston, Massachusetts: Harvard School of Public Health.

Rifkin, S. B. and Walt, G. L. (1986) Why health improves: Defining the issues concerning 'comprehensive primary health care' and 'selective primary health care'. *Soc. Sci. Med.* **23**, 559–566.

Rohde, J. E. and Viswanathan, H. (1995) *The Rural Private Practitioner.* Delhi: Oxford University Press, pp. 108–121.

Ross-Degnan, D., Laing, R. and Quick, J. (1992) A strategy for promoting improved pharmaceutical use: the international network for rational use of drugs. *Soc. Sci. Med.* **35**, 1329–1341.

Santoso, B. (1996) Small group intervention vs. formal seminar for improving appropriate drug use. *Soc. Sci. Med.* **42**, 1185–1194.

Saunderson, P. R. (1995) An economic evaluation of alternative programme design for tuberculosis control in rural Uganda. *Soc. Sci. Med.* **40**, 1203–1212.

Scrivens, E. (1995) International trends in accreditation. *Int. J. Hlth. Plann. Management* **10**, 165–181.

Scrivens, E. (1996) Recent developments in accreditation. *Int. J. for Qual. in Hlth. Care* **7**, 427–433.

Sontag, S. (1979) *Illness as Metaphor.* New York: Vintage Books.

Sumartojo, E. (1993) When tuberculosis treatment fails: A social behavioural account of patient adherence. *Am. Rev. Resp. Dis.* **147**, 1311–1320.

Swan, M. and Zwi, A. (1997) *Private Practitioners and Public Health: Close the Gap or Increase the Distance.* Department of Public Health and Policy, PHP Departmental Publication No. 24. London: London School of Hygiene and Tropical Medicine.

Thomson, R., Lavender, M. and Madhok, R. (1995) How to ensure that guidelines are effective. *Brit. Med. J.* **311**, 237–242.

Trostle, J. (1996) Inappropriate distribution of medicines by professionals in developing countries. *Soc. Sci. Med.* **42**, 1117–1120.

Uplekar, M. W. and Shepard, D. S. (1991) Treatment of tuberculosis by private general practitioners in India. *Tubercle* **72**, 284–290.

Uplekar, M. W. and Rangan, S. (1993) Private doctors and tuberculosis control in India. *Tubercle Lung Dis.* **74**, 332–337.

Uplekar, M. W. and Rangan, S. (1996) *Tackling Tuberculosis: The Search for Solutions.* Bombay: The Foundation for Research in Community Health.

Uplekar, M. W., Juvekar, S. and Morankar, S. (1996) *Tuberculosis Patients and Practitioners in Private Clinics.* Bombay: The Foundation for Research in Community Health.

Williamson, P. (1992) Health Bulletin **50** (1), 78–86.

World Bank. (1993) *World Development Report 1993. Investing in Health.* Oxford: Oxford University Press for the World Bank.

World Bank. (1997) *Sector Strategy: Health, Nutrition and Population.* Washington DC: World Bank.

World Health Organization. (1996) *Investing in Health Research and Development.* Report of the *Ad Hoc* Committee on Health Research Relating to Future Intervention Options. Geneva: World Health Organization.

Yesudian, C. A. K. (1991) *Urban Health Services, Issues and Challenges — A Case Study of Bombay.* Paper presented at the World Health Organization study group meeting on primary health care in urban areas, Geneva. Geneva: World Health Organization.

Yesudian, C. A. K. (1994) Behaviour of the private health sector in the health market of Bombay. *Hlth. Pol. Plann.* **9**, 72–80.

CHAPTER 8

INVOLVING THE PRIVATE MEDICAL SECTOR IN TUBERCULOSIS CONTROL: PRACTICAL ASPECTS

Mukund Uplekar

Introduction

Throughout history, health care has been provided privately. In every society, certain individuals obtained skills in healing or drug preparation and made these available to their people. In exchange, communities took good care of these healers and respected them, offering financial reward that most could afford (Roth, 1987). In many African and South Asian countries, missionaries were responsible for introducing Western medicine while the state under colonial rule established facilities for essential workers, but it was only after independence that state provision of health care services became widespread (Bennett *et al.*, 1997). It was obvious that for health problems of major public importance, curative medical care centred on individuals formed only a small part of disease control measures and the states rather than private providers were in a better position to offer all the preventive, promotive and curative components of health care. Expansion of state-funded and organised health care services in poor countries occurred mostly during the 1960s and 1970s. The Alma-Ata Declaration (World Health Organization, 1979) reaffirmed the primary role of the state in the provision of equitable health care to the people. The response to this Declaration was, however, very short-lived and the period from 1978 to 1987 witnessed a gradual reversal of the theme of the primary role of government in health care. The rapid growth of the private health sector was prompted and promoted by several factors: the decline in state funding for health, the continuing training of medical personnel who could not find adequate employment in state institutions, and a growing middle class dissatisfied with the public sector and willing to pay for private health care (Prakash, 1996). Initiated by the World Bank and aided and abetted by bilateral donors such as the USAID, the policy agenda aimed at the diminution of the role of government involvement in health care and promotion of the private sector was clearly articulated for the first time in 1987 (World Bank, 1987). There has been much argument in favour of the private health sector ever since, despite a lack of firm knowledge on the effectiveness of private health care providers in poor countries.

Tuberculosis has always been a major public health problem in poor countries and the private sector has almost always played a key role in the provision of care for patients with this disease. With about 14 million prevalent cases, India alone bears a third of the world's burden of tuberculosis, and an estimated 60% of these cases in India are managed by the private practitioners (Uplekar and Rangan, 1993). Thus, over a sixth of the world's burden of tuberculosis is managed by the Indian private sector alone. The situation is not very different in other South-East Asian countries. Seventy per cent of health care provision in Pakistan is in the private sector and, in Africa, Kenya and Ghana are two countries which also have a significant presence of private practice (McPake, 1997). Yet, the private medical sector has never attracted as much attention as it is doing today. It seems that both tuberculosis and the private health sector owe the boost in the world-wide attention they have received to the World Bank's current policies and their pursuance by the World Health Organization (WHO) and the national governments (World Bank, 1993).

This chapter addresses the practical aspects of private sector involvement in tuberculosis control. While much is being discussed and written about the private sector and the public/private mix in health care, documented literature on practical efforts or experiments involving the private sector in poor countries is extremely scanty. The situation in affluent countries may not be very different (Reichman, 1997). The chapter draws heavily from the Indian setting, which not only has a National Tuberculosis Programme (NTP) which has been in place for over three decades, but also the largest private medical sector. The characteristics of the private medical sector are first described and its role in public health in general and tuberculosis control in particular are then discussed. Experiences in other countries, in dissimilar situations, are also cited. A few specific examples of private sector initiatives in tuberculosis control activities and their outcome are presented thereafter. The chapter ends with a discussion on possible practical steps that could be undertaken to evaluate and institute sustainable public-private collaboration for tuberculosis control.

The Private Medical Sector and Health Care

Health conditions around the world have improved more in the past 40 years than throughout all previous human history (World Bank, 1993). And there are strong correlations between the decline of mortality and the accelerated socio-economic improvement in the high-income countries and developing countries. What have been the role and contribution of the private medical sector in achieving these improvements in peoples' health world wide? There is little convincing evidence that the private medical sector has made a positive contribution to public health in general. Notwithstanding, it continues to enjoy power and patronage among both the common people and the policy makers. Privatisation in all the sectors including health care has become an integral part of the present wave of globalisation. Bennett (1992) emphasises that in those developing countries where the private sector is allowed, it tends to be far more active than in the industrialised world.

Several surveys in India have shown that people in rural areas prefer to pay unqualified quacks than to avail themselves of free medical care from qualified doctors staffing the public health facilities (Duggal *et al.*, 1995). The situation among urban populations is no different. This has also been reported in other countries including Pakistan, Mexico and the Philippines (Thavar and Harpham, 1997). There are several reasons why the private sector remains the preferred provider. Private providers take better care of the psychological needs of their patients since they have a relatively greater sense of responsibility towards them. They are more sympathetic and responsive, which helps them develop a closer relationship not only with the patients but also with their families and community. They provide service for a fee but usually offer flexibility of payment. Unlike public facilities, they are available at times that suit most of their clients and are willing to offer services at their own homes (Uplekar and George, 1993). While all this may, very often, be at the cost of the quality and content of their services, the lay people are generally not aware of this.

In India, the way that the private medical sector has been allowed to grow unchecked and develop totally by itself has helped it to evolve its present character. 80% of about a million registered doctors in India are in private practice. Formal courses are available in modern Western medicine, Ayurveda, Homoeopathy and Unani systems. Although the Western type of medicine does not necessarily form a part of the curricula in other courses, most of those trained in the colleges for alternative systems end up acquiring skills in Western medicine — sufficient to enable them to set up in general practice — by working in a hospital or with a senior practitioner. In addition, there are a large number of quacks — about 30,000 in Delhi alone — according to the estimates of the Quackery Eradication Committee of the Delhi Medical Association (India Today, 1997). The most important feature is that while about 75% of Indians live in villages, about 80% doctors are based in cities (Government of India, 1993). While the rural majority continues to have poor access to medical care which, when accessible, is often of very poor standard, the cities are over-saturated with medical establishments.

The public and the private sectors function as two parallel systems. Mandatory continuing medical education does not exist. The medical councils who give the license to practice do not have the wherewithal to regulate their own licentiates. The system of recertification is absent. Membership of professional organisations and associations is purely voluntary and only a fourth of those qualified in Western medicine are members of the Indian Medical Association, the largest representative organisation. Medical colleges, barring a few, are preoccupied with clinical and academic activities and are dominated, as elsewhere in the world, by clinicians. Neither they, nor their subdued counterparts in the departments of Preventive and Social Medicine, inculcate among the students even the basic minimum understanding of community health in clinical practice (Rangan and Uplekar, 1993). The obvious reason why private practice is attractive is the handsome monetary reward it offers. In the absence of any organised educational activity, a majority of the first-level private providers manage their clients by either copying consultants' prescriptions or through knowledge gained from the half-truths received from sales representatives of drug companies. Kapil (1988) compares the medical market in India today to that described for 19th century England, which was in transition from an agrarian to an industrial system.

The Private Medical Sector and Tuberculosis Control

High-quality care for tuberculosis control depends upon a diagnosis based on microscopic examination of three sputum smear samples, patients taking drugs under the supervision of a care-giver, a regular supply of good-quality drugs, and individual registration, monitoring and outcome evaluation (by sputum smear examination) of each initially smear-positive patient (World Health Organization, 1997). All that is expected of a private practitioner managing patients with pulmonary tuberculosis is to subject patients with long-standing cough to a sputum examination before diagnosis, prescribe approved drug regimens, supervise treatment to ensure regular drug consumption, and monitor and evaluate the outcome of treatment of individual patients while keeping a record of it. To what extent are these minimum expectations met by the private practitioners?

Our own studies in India (Uplekar and Rangan, 1993, 1996; Uplekar et al., 1998) revealed that patients with tuberculosis do shop around before they are diagnosed. Usually, they first seek help from a private practitioner and about half of them are diagnosed at the first source of help itself. Yet, on average, there is a time interval of about two months between the onset of symptoms and diagnosis of tuberculosis. Significantly, in diagnosing pulmonary tuberculosis, over three-quarters of all the patients in private clinics are not subjected to sputum examination at all, the reliance being always on an X-ray of the chest. Their treating doctors do not reveal the diagnosis of tuberculosis directly to a large proportion of patients, more so in rural areas. All the patients in private clinics receive drugs used in short course chemotherapy but they receive these in a variety of regimens, some of which are inadequate and inappropriate, including a single drug or two drugs. Having started on treatment in private clinics, about 60% of patients stick to the private sector. Patients who are regular in taking treatment during the first two months tend to be adherent throughout, unlike the ones who default treatment in the initial period. The treatment adherence rate of patients who remain with the private sector is around 55%, as compared to less than 40% in the public sector and, on average, patients with pulmonary tuberculosis spend Rs. 5,500 (US$160) on diagnosis and treatment.

There is a great discrepancy between what private practitioners state that they practice and what their patients actually experience. While over three-quarters of practitioners reported that they based their diagnosis of tuberculosis on a sputum test and X-ray, over three-quarters of patients had undergone only chest X-rays. When practitioners reported drug regimens containing excess drugs for longer durations, their patients were actually consuming fewer drugs than prescribed. Private practitioners take little action, if any, when a patient on treatment fails to attend (Uplekar et al., 1998).

Practices in other countries do not differ greatly. In spite of accommodating their views about treatment regimens, the private physicians in the Philippines have never organised themselves into a system to facilitate tuberculosis control. No central tuberculosis registry for private tuberculosis patients exists, so there is no notification of cases to the Department of Health. Individual practitioners are free to prescribe any treatment of their choice and, indeed, surveys have shown that private practitioners in the Philippines use a wide variety of mostly inappropriate regimens for the treatment of tuberculosis. Beyond patient education of questionable quality, no case-holding mechanisms are in place in private doctors' clinics. The responsibility of completing therapy is placed on the patients shoulders (Romulo, 1997).

Questionnaire surveys of 923 private general practitioners in 29 health centres in Korea showed that 47% had an unfavourable opinion of the National Tuberculosis Programme (NTP), over 50% did not consider sputum examination essential in diagnosis, and 75% did not consider it essential to monitor treatment response. For initial treatment of active tuberculosis, only 11% were prescribing the current Korean NTP's six-month regimen; 73% were giving currently non-recommended regimens, and 16% were giving unacceptably bad regimens (Hong *et al.*, 1995).

The situation in affluent, low-prevalence countries does not differ greatly. The Hong Kong Chest Service/British Medical Research Council (1984) noted that a great majority (86%) of their patients originally attended a private practitioner when symptoms occurred. Only 18% had had their sputum examined, although 76% had had a chest radiograph; 65% of the smear positive and 71% of the smear negative patients had been told that they had or might have tuberculosis. For 40%, there was an interval of more than one month between their first attendance at a private practitioner's clinic and at a government chest clinic. In all, 19% of the patients were definitely or probably prescribed an anti-tuberculosis regimen, although this was not always an adequate regimen. Byrd and colleagues (1977) reported very similar practice deficiencies in the USA that were still present 16 years later (Mahmoudi and Iseman, 1993). In both these studies, delays in diagnosis and errors in treatment and follow up resulted in an increased risk and likelihood of disease transmission, more advanced and complicated disease, and lengthened hospital stays with increased medical costs as well as the development of multidrug-resistant tuberculosis. Sumartojo and her colleagues (1993) questioned 3,600 US physicians and found that only 75% were aware of any tuberculosis treatment and control recommendations, only 50% used recommended treatment regimens, 71% incorrectly interpreted skin test results, and 16% used an incorrect regimen for preventive treatment.

Clearly, the positive aspects of the private practitioners' tuberculosis related practices — their proximity to the patients, the confidence patients have in them, the relatively better treatment adherence of patients under their care compared to those under the public health services, and the patients' acceptance of their services despite costs — are all countered in poor countries by poor practices such as excessive reliance on X-rays for diagnosis, a disregard of recommended drug regimens, a lack of effective action with regard to treatment default, and a failure to keep even minimum essential records (Uplekar, 1997; Uplekar *et al.*, 1998).

India's Revised National Tuberculosis Programme and the Private Medical Sector Involvement

With the help of a huge loan from the World Bank, India's National Tuberculosis Programme (NTP) is being revitalised and the revised NTP (RNTP), using the Directly Observed Therapy, Short Course (DOTS), strategy is being put in place in phases. It seems that the very strengths of the revised NTP of India are the main weaknesses of the management of tuberculosis in private practice. To be specific, a very strong emphasis on sputum examination for diagnosis, directly observed treatment with standardised short course regimens, and utmost stress on treatment completion rather than treatment initiation are the strengths of the revised NTP and at the same time the weaknesses in private doctors' present approach to managing tuberculosis.

Should the aim of involving the private sector in tuberculosis management be to shift a large number of patients from the private sector to the public sector? If interventions are directed with this objective, it could well result in alienation of the private practitioners from the RNTP, and would also swamp the public sector with large numbers of patients in a very short time, many of whom would be chronic cases and treatment failures who are not the first priority of a treatment programme in its early days. Rather, the aim should firstly be to inform private practitioners about the recommended diagnostic criteria and treatment regimens, to ensure proper detection of suspects, and to reduce both treatment failure and the risk of development of resistance, and then to create a conduit through which private practitioners can send those patients they wish, or whom they think should benefit from, the newly improved public sector services. If good-quality care available free of charge in the public sector is not matched by service of similar quality in the private sector, a natural pressure will build up for the movement of patients from the private to the public sector. What is required is a system to enable this flow to occur, assisting it where necessary.

Thus, a *sine qua non* of private sector involvement is a well functioning, high-quality local tuberculosis control programme. Nothing will be achieved without this first being established (Nunn, 1994). The degree to which private practitioners are prepared to refer their patients to the public sector will probably vary widely according to the practitioners' attitudes towards the public services, their previous experiences with referring patients, their expectations of remuneration from a given patient, and their concept of what constitutes proper tuberculosis care. Consideration will also need to be given to the possibility of offering some form of incentive to the private practitioners for refering patients. Such incentives need not to be financial: they could, for example, be educational — the offering of advanced courses on tuberculosis with some form of award on successful completion of the course which identifies that practitioner as being an expert in the management of the disease and therefore able to offer a wider and a better range of services than other practitioners not as well trained.

Engaging the Private Medical Sector in Tuberculosis Control: Practical Efforts

While much is being discussed about the private sector in tuberculosis control, documented literature on the *modus operandi* of institutionalising a meaningful public/private mix is extremely scanty and sketchy. The ensuing paragraphs provide a few examples, past and present, of private sector engagement in tuberculosis control in greatly different settings. One example dates way back to the pre-chemotherapy days and may sound irrelevant today. Yet, it offers useful insights into the approach to tuberculosis control within the private sector.

The Japanese Example

According to Shimao (personal communication), very few countries have succeeded in integrating the NTP into currently existing health care systems, including the private sector. Japan was able to achieve 80% success in this problem and the strategy employed was as follows: an NTP in Japan was launched in 1951 and, from the very beginning, it was integrated into the then-existing health care system including the private sector, essentially since it would have been impossible for the public sector, with just one centre for every 100,000 population, to cope with the huge number of tuberculosis cases on its own. Moreover, the general practitioners' network had already covered the whole country including the rural areas and, hence, the diagnostic and treatment services could be available through the private sector.

In the early 1950s, 28% of the national medical expenditure of Japan was devoted to tuberculosis and, taking into account the seriousness of the problem, the Japan Medical Association was very co-operative with the government tuberculosis control activities. One half of the expenses for treating tuberculosis was covered by the public subsidy offered by the

Tuberculosis Control Law, and most of the remaining expenses were covered by various health insurance schemes. Patients needing the subsidy had to approach the Tuberculosis Advisory Committee at the health centres, consisting of five members, including the director of the health centre, two tuberculosis experts and two representatives of the local medical associations. This committee checked the appropriateness of the treatment strategy employed, comparing it with the standard guidelines, and then sanctioned the public subsidy. The guidelines offered the best method of treatment available, and these were revised periodically taking into consideration the advances in chemotherapy. Thus, the best available treatment was given to the patients with minimum cost to the patients themselves.

The New York Story

The famous New York City (NYC) operation in 'turning the tide' of re-emergent tuberculosis in the city is now well known (Frieden *et al.*, 1995). Not much is known about the way the private sector was involved in tuberculosis control in NYC. Conscious steps were taken by the NYC's Department of Health to improve interaction which yielded positive results (Fujiwara, 1996; Frieden, personal communication). In doing so, the Department of Health offered standard treatment recommendations, medical conferences, updates on epidemiology and treatment issues, data from its registry, free tuberculosis-related services, and case management of every patient in NYC.

A review by the NYC Department of Health of tuberculosis program indicators of 5,737 patients with fully drug-susceptible pulmonary tuberculosis treated in the public and private sectors showed, from 1992 to 1995, significant improvements in most indicators including sputum culture conversion within three months, the percentage of patients completing treatment, the percentage of patients receiving Directly Observed Therapy (DOT) and the percentage started on the recommended four-drug regimen of isoniazid, rifampicin, pyrazinamide and ethambutol (HRZE). Table 1 shows the results achieved.

Table 1.   Improvement in the indicators of tuberculosis treatment in New York City between 1992 and 1995*.

Indicator	1992	1995
Patients started on HRZE (%)	69	90
Patients receiving DOT (%)	11	33
Proportion completing treatment (%)	54	65
Sputum culture conversion (%)	18	65

*Adapted from Frieden *et al.* (1995).

All yearly trends were also significant ($p = 0.01$) for the private sector. The review demonstrated that, in the NYC setting, tuberculosis care in the private sector can be standardised, the DOT strategy can be used and the local health department can be a partner in care.

The Mumbai Projects

It is not that the Indian private sector is absolutely unresponsive to the needs of their tuberculosis patients. In our study of voluntary organisations engaged in tuberculosis control, we came across two groups of private doctors who had organised themselves to provide tuberculosis care to needy patients (Rangan *et al.*, 1995).

One organisation is formed by a group of 350 private doctors registered with a local medical association of a municipal ward area of Mumbai (Bombay) City. Tuberculosis control is a part of a wide range of activities including holding camps to detect and treat, for example, hypertension and anaemia and to provide continuing medical education. The tuberculosis programme is being conducted in the space provided in the clinic of one of the enthusiastic member doctors. The beneficiaries of the programme are sputum positive pulmonary tuberculosis patients who are newly diagnosed by any of the member doctors and who cannot afford the cost of anti-tuberculosis treatment. The treatment strategies are standardised. The tuberculosis programme is recognised by the City Tuberculosis Programme and the organisation receives 10%

of its drug requirements and stationary from the programme. In return, they are expected to maintain and submit monthly records to the City Programme.

The second organisation is a panel of doctors who came together to help tuberculosis patients in the suburbs of Mumbai. It consists of a loose network of doctors including consultants and general practitioners who offer free or subsidised tuberculosis services to poor and needy patients from their clinics with the help of drugs provided by the organisation. This programme also receives about 10% of its annual drug requirement from the City Programme in return for submission of regular reports.

The two programmes are compared in Table 2. Undoubtedly, there is scope for considerable improvement in the functioning of both the organisations. The point to be made is that it is possible to organise doctors and enable them to contribute constructively to the control of tuberculosis. It may be easier to provide support to a group of doctors than offer laboratory and drug support to individual practitioners. The first organisation, which appears to be concerned more about the quality of the service than the number of beneficiaries, obviously achieved better results.

Another significant way that the private sector participates in tuberculosis control is through various private non-profit organisations, called non-governmental organisations, in India. A full discussion on non-governmental organisations is outside the scope of this chapter, but they could well be used as an interface between the for-profit practitioners and the tuberculosis programmes managed by the local public health services. Private doctors can either form an organisation for the purpose of tuberculosis control or make use of other non-governmental organisations to facilitate functions such as counselling of patients, retrieving defaulters, keeping records and monitoring the outcomes of treatment — tasks which a busy practising doctor has little inclination, training or time to accomplish. Undoubtedly, regardless of whether health interventions occur in the public or private sectors, it is the attention to the non-medical or para-medical aspects of tuberculosis control that decisively determines the quality of the outcome.

Table 2. Comparison of two private sector-based tuberculosis control programmes in Mumbai, India.

	Organisation 1	Organisation 2
Case-Finding	From among patients attending clinics of member GPs.	From among patients attending clinics of doctors on the panel of the organisation.
Diagnosis	Sputum examination and chest X-ray by member doctors, the cost of which is borne by the patients. Sputum-positive patients who cannot afford treatment are referred to a centre operated from a member doctor's clinic.	Chest X-ray and sputum examination at patient's expense. Poor and needy tuberculosis patients are registered in the organisation's tuberculosis programme being run from the clinics of panel doctors.
Treatment	Standardised short course regimens followed for all patients: 2SHR/6HE or 2HER/6HE. Patients need to attend the central clinic once a fortnight for drug collection. Streptomycin injections and treatment of associated minor ailments are given by the referring doctors free of charge.	The regimens recommended (but not mandatory) are 2SHRZ/4HR or 2EHRZ/4HR for all patients. Drugs being offered are free or at subsidised rates. Nutritional supplements (milk powder) are also given to all patients.
Case-Holding	Treatment cards are prepared and maintained at the central tuberculosis clinic by a part-time social worker of the organisation. When patients do not report on due dates, the referring doctors are duly informed for retrieval actions. Follow up sputum examinations and chest X-rays are done free of change. Referring doctors continue giving them vitamin and calcium supplements until six months after treatment. To improve treatment adherence, some patients are made to pay a refundable deposit.	No standardised treatment cards are made for the patients. Individual doctors maintained information. Treatment regimens not strictly adhered to. In case of default, reminder postcards are sent. Follow up investigations at subsidised rates are performed by radiologists and pathologists on the panel. The free distribution of nutritional supplements is believed to positively influence adherence to treatment.

Table 2. Continued

	Organisation 1	Organisation 2
Records/ Reports	Standardised treatment cards and drug registers are maintained at the central clinic. Monthly reports are prepared and submitted to the City Programme.	Records and registers are maintained by individual panel doctors. Every month the doctor is expected to file a return. Volunteers help in record keeping.
Treatment Completion/ Cure Rates	About 60% of 120 sputum-positive patients in the year 1993.	About 30% of 592 patients in 1992, both sputum positive and negative.

Conclusions

There can be no doubt that, considering the magnitude of the problem of tuberculosis in poor countries, the size of the private sector, the share of the caseload it deals with and its continued alienation can only hamper current efforts towards global tuberculosis control. The important question to be raised is how can those mismanaging tuberculosis be left out of tuberculosis control efforts and allowed to continue to (mis)manage tuberculosis patients the way they see fit, unhindered? Further, need we wait until the National Tuberculosis Programmes are revitalised and start functioning efficiently, and hope that they will automatically wean patients away from the private sector?

The issue of how to involve private doctors in local tuberculosis control programmes may be addressed through research and experimentation. Orienting private doctors may not be very simple, as there are two processes involved. They will have to be first de-oriented on what they have been doing and then re-oriented about what they ought to do. Efforts in this direction must begin and be followed vigorously.

That private practitioners need educational input is very clear. The tuberculosis management practices of private practitioners are at a great variance with even standard textbooks of medicine, not to mention specific national or international recommendations which rarely, if at all, get effectively communicated to them. Many practitioners in our studies justified their actions by pointing to the conformity between their practices and those of their seniors and consultants, including their teachers in medical colleges.

Several shortcomings brought out explicitly by the investigations referred to above can be addressed forthwith without waiting for results of future research. The glaring gaps in the knowledge and practices of private practitioners and their patients are now known. Producing relevant educational material for practitioners, identifying district-level or subdistrict-level teams of eloquent programme managers and experts to address groups of private practitioners to answer their queries directly, convincing them of the broader implications of their actions, and at the same time supplying them with educational material does not have to wait for any research results. Simple formats for record keeping in private clinics can also be devised, tested, modified and brought into practice. Identifying locally existing laboratories with high-quality sputum microscopy facilities, and making practitioners aware of these, could be a rewarding initial step. Such places may not exist at all, in which case strengthening sputum microscopy services at conveniently located public as well as private laboratories need not wait for the outcome of any research.

Diagnostic facilities should be an in-built component of the local programme. It may be too late to first wait for the local tuberculosis programmes to perfect their functions and then open their doors to the private practitioners. Brought down to the level of a rural village or town, or a manageable municipal ward in an urban setting, programme managers may achieve some success if they work from the beginning with a few enthusiastic private practitioners (always available everywhere) to set up local and mutually acceptable mechanisms facilitating key programme functions. Again, provision of precise norms and guidelines is necessary but not sufficient; a system for supervising and evaluating both the private and the public systems is essential (Chaulet, 1987).

Some policy issues also need to be addressed and quick decisions taken to facilitate private sector involvement in matters of public health importance. One such issue is the place of practitioners trained in systems other than modern Western medicine. Yet, efforts to involve different types of health providers with very clearly spelt out roles and responsibilities should proceed pending policy decisions which may take a long time to arrive at. Also, isolated disciplinary actions against private practitioners in order to oblige them to improve their tuberculosis management practices are unlikely to be beneficial if the issues of regulation of the private sector and continuing education linked to re-certification of private practitioners are not addressed simultaneously. Another issue could be that of incentives to non-specialist private practitioners as tuberculosis patients generally form only a small part of their clientele. Preferably, non-monetary incentives should be considered first for ease of implementation and these might work very well.

Finally, no programme is likely to bear fruits if its beneficiaries are kept ignorant about it. As is clearly brought out by our own and several other studies, it has been ingrained on peoples' minds that tuberculosis is diagnosed from a chest X-ray, and its treatment, as for most other illnesses, has to be tailored to individual patients. People still believe that disappearance of illness or symptoms is synonymous with disappearance of the disease. On the other hand, peoples' wrong notions about tuberculosis are often perpetuated by the actions of the providers. If simple truths about tuberculosis and its treatment, including what to expect and what not to expect from the health care providers, can be conveyed to the lay people effectively, it could empower them to make their own decisions — whether to continue to pay a private practitioner and extract appropriate services in return, or to demand service from the public health sector, or to make judicious use of both, as it suits their informed needs and purpose. So long as people get the services they require, at an affordable cost and in a manner acceptable to them on a sustainable basis, it is immaterial whether the public or private sector, or a mix of the two, make these available. Since it is well known that people use the private sector overwhelmingly, it is imperative that the tuberculosis care they receive in the private clinics meets the desired standards. And these standards must first be set and rigorously followed by the public health services.

References

Bennett, S. (1992) Promoting the private sector: A review of developing country trends. *Hlth. Pol. Plann.* **7**, 97–110.
Bennett, S., McPake, B. and Mills, A. (1997) The public/private mix debate in health care. In: Bennett, S., McPake, B., Mills, A., eds. *Private Health Providers in Developing Countries: Serving the Public Interest?* London and New Jersey: Zed Books Limited, pp. 1–18.
Byrd, R. B., Horn, B. R., Solomon, D. A., Griggs, G. A. and Wilder, N. J. (1977) Treatment of tuberculosis by the non-pulmonary physician. *Ann. Int. Med.* **86**, 799–802.
Chaulet, P. (1987) Compliance with anti-tuberculosis chemotherapy in developing countries. *Tubercle* **68**, 19–24.
Duggal, R., *et al.* (1995) Health expenditure across states — Part I. *Economic and Political Weekly* **30**, 834–844.
Frieden, T., Fujiwara, P. I., Washko, R. M. and Hamburg, M. A. (1995) Tuberculosis in New York City — Turning the tide. *New Engl. J. Med.* **333**, 229–233.
Fujiwara, P. I., Cook, S. V., Osahan, S. S. and Frieden, T. R. (1996) Working with the private medical sector: Improvements in tuberculosis control. *Tubercle Lung Dis.* **77** (Suppl. 2), 72.
Government of India, Central Bureau of Health Intelligence (CBHI), Ministry of Health and Family Welfare. 1993. *Health Information of India 1993*. Delhi: Government of India.
Hong Kong Chest Service/British Medical Research Council. 1984. Survey of the previous investigation and treatment by private practitioners of patients with pulmonary tuberculosis attending government chest clinics in Hong Kong. *Tubercle* **65**, 161–171.
Hong, Y. P., *et al.* Survey of knowledge, attitudes and practices for tuberculosis among general practitioners. *Tubercle Lung Dis.* **76**, 431–435.
India Today. (1997) Quacks in the box. *India Today* **XXII**(30), 74–77.
Kapil, I. (1988) Doctors dispensing medication: Contemporary India and 19th Century England. *Soc. Sci. Med.* **26**, 691–699.
Mahmoudi, A., Iseman, M. D. (1993) Pitfalls in the care of patients with tuberculosis. Common errors and their association with acquisition of drug resistance. *J. Am. Med. Assoc.* **270**, 65–68.

McPake, B. (1997) The role of the private health sector. In: Bennett, S., McPake, B., Mills, A., eds. *Private Health Providers in Developing Countries: Serving the Public Interest?* London and New Jersey: Zed Books Limited.

Nunn, P. (1994) *Background Paper for the World Health Organization-World Bank Protocol Development Workshop for Invovlement of Private Sector in Tuberculosis Control, Bombay.* Geneva: World Health Organization Global Tuberculosis Programme.

Prakash P. (1996) Editorial: Overburdened under-utilised. *Rad. J. Hlth.* **2**, 199–200.

Rangan, S. and Uplekar, M. (1993) Community health awareness among recent medical graduates. *Natl. Med. J. Ind.* **6**, 60–64.

Rangan, S., et al. (1995) *Non Governmental Organisations in Tuberculosis Control in Western India.* Mumbai: The Foundation for Research in Community Health.

Reichman, L. B. (1997) Tuberculosis elimination — What's to stop us? *Int. J. Tuberc. Lung Dis.* **1**, 3–11.

Romulo, R. L. C. (1997) Tuberculosis Control: Collaboration in the Philippines. *Proceedings of the Second Mid-Year Conference of IUATLD, North American Region.* Paris: International Union Against Tuberculosis and Lung Disease, pp. 60–65.

Roth, G. (1987) *The Private Provision of Public Services in Developing Countries* Oxford: Oxford University Press, pp. 122–157.

Sumartojo, E., et al. (1993) Physician practices in preventing and treating tuberculosis: Results of a national survey. *Am. Rev. Resp. Dis.* **147**, A702.

Thavar, I. H. and Harpham, T. (1997) Private practitioners in slums of Karachi. In: Bennett, S., McPake, B., Mills, A., eds. *Private Health Providers in Developing Countries: Serving the Public Interest?* London and New Jersey: Zed Books Limited.

Uplekar, M. (1997) Tuberculosis in India: Engaging the private sector. *Proceedings of the Second Mid-Year Conference of IUATLD, North American Region.* Paris: International Union Against Tuberculosis and Lung Disease, pp. 49–59.

Uplekar, M. and George, A. (1993) Access to health care in India: Present situation and innovative approaches. A state-of-art paper for the UNDP project: Strategies and financing for human development. New Delhi: United Nations Development Programme.

Uplekar, M. and Rangan, S. (1993) Private doctors and tuberculosis control in India. *Tuberc. Lung Dis.* **74**, 332–337.

Uplekar, M. and Rangan, S. (1996) *Tackling TB: The Search for Solutions.* Bombay: Foundation for Research in Community Health.

Uplekar, M. W. and Shephard, D. S. (1991) Treatment of tuberculosis by private general practitioners in India. *Tubercle* **72**, 284–290.

Uplekar, M., Juvekar, S., Morankar, S., Rangan, S. and Nunn, P. (1998) Tuberculosis patients and practitioners in private clinics in India. *Int. J. Tuberc. Lung Dis.* **2**, 324–329.

World Health Organization (1997) *Global Tuberculosis Control*. Geneva: World Health Organization.

World Health Organization (1994) *Report of the WHO-World Bank Protocol Development Workshop for Involvement of Private Sector in Tuberculosis Control, Bombay*. Geneva: World Health Organization.

World Health Organization (1979) *Alma-Ata 1978: Primary Health Care. Report of the International Conference on Primary Health Care. Alma-Ata, USSR*. Health for All Series No.1 Geneva: World Health Organization.

World Bank (1993) *Investing in Health: World Development Report 1993*. Washington DC: World Bank.

World Bank (1987) *Financing Health Services in Developing Countries: An Agenda for Reform*. Washington DC: World Bank.

CHAPTER 9

COMPLIANCE VERSUS ADHERENCE: JUST A MATTER OF LANGUAGE? THE POLITICS AND POETICS OF PUBLIC HEALTH

Jessica A. Ogden

"Scientific thought succumbed because it violated the first law of culture, which says that 'the more man controls anything, the more uncontrollable both become'" (Tyler, 1986: p. 123)

This chapter is an exploration, not of the effects of tuberculosis on people, but of the effects of history, language and culture on the ways in which people affect tuberculosis. It is an awkward project not least because it requires a shift in perspective: from seeing tuberculosis as something outside of ourselves — the image of the skull-faced grim reaper, looming over us and threatening apocalypse — to an acceptance of the disease as being present, and as being something of our own creation. It is also awkward because it exposes our power to ourselves, and in realising this power we are then charged with the onus to wield it responsibly: to make better choices, responsible choices, indeed moral choices, about how to cope with the existence of tuberculosis in our world.

Why Politics and Poetics?

The words politics and poetics have been used in the title of this chapter in order to situate it historically (that is to call attention to the fact that it is being written in a particular historical period) and philosophically (that it derives from the theoretical fashions of our current post-structure/post-modern period). These words have also been used because this seems an appropriate forum and an appropriate moment to begin to challenge and expose some of the language of public health — in particular to take a deeper look at some of its discourses of *control*. The author has borrowed the phrase[a] here to draw attention to, and provide the basis for a critical reappraisal of, the discourse of power and control insinuated in the language of public health and the effects of this discourse on the kinds of interventions developed. Specifically, this chapter addresses the discursive trail that has led 'us' to the re-invention of directly observed therapy not as *a* but as *the* gold standard approach to the 'eradication' of tuberculosis. This chapter, though more indirectly than others in this book, will question the foundations on which this 'gold standard' was built, as well as the appropriateness of *eradication* as a goal in public health.

Tuberculosis control and other dilemmas in public health

> '*Infectious disease which antedated the emergence of human kind will last as long as humanity itself, and will surely remain, as it has been hitherto, one of the fundamental parameters and determinants of human history*'.
> (McNeill, 1976, cited in Wall and Stanwell Smith, 1997, p. 137)

---

[a]The phrase has been borrowed, though reversing its order, from the title of a book which has been influential in shaping the recent critique within anthropology (Clifford and Marcus, 1986).

In 1854, John Snow effectively, dramatically and apparently single-handedly proved his theory of disease transmission. His removal of the Broad Street pump handle in London during the cholera epidemic of that year saved many lives and has subsequently become the defining gesture of modern epidemiology and public health. Over a century later, in 1977, as the result of a concerted global effort, the last case of smallpox was reported, and the disease was declared 'eradicated': smallpox had been effectively "expunged from the earth" (Ogden, undated, p. vii) — the first, and last, known epidemic disease ever to disappear completely from the human race. Two decades on from the disappearance of smallpox the goal of eradication remains the ultimate objective of many infectious disease programmes. The smallpox 'crusade' proved it could be done with sufficient commitment at all levels of society and in all corners of all communities.

Tuberculosis has proved a thorn in the side of the eradication enthusiasts. Effective chemotherapeutic treatment for the disease has existed since the early 1950s, and yet the disease continues to flourish, and is even enjoying something of a comeback in communities previously thought 'safe': according to the Advisory Council for the Elimination of Tuberculosis, morbidity from tuberculosis rose by 14% in the USA between 1985 and 1993 (Centers for Disease Control and Prevention, 1995). Yet the problem is thornier still. Biomedicine has not only failed to eradicate this disease, but has contributed to its increased virulence: multidrug resistance to tuberculosis therapy is likely to be one of the greatest challenges to disease control (see Garrett, 1995).

Changes in the historical, political and bacteriological/virological landscape have impacted changes in public health perspectives and in the locus of blame for public health 'failures'. In practice, this has created a shift in the locus of responsibility for effective public health programming (from the services to the patients) without an accompanying shift in agency, power or knowledge (see Weeks, 1985). Disturbingly, for example, growing evidence of a strong link between social inequalities and disease (e.g. Wilkinson, 1996; Davey Smith *et al.*, 1990, 1996) has not yet been translated into policies or programmes which effectively take this into account. This would necessarily entail a broadening of perspective — embracing the multiple agencies, multiple levels of responsibility for the public's health, and their interconnections. It would entail perceiving of 'state', 'community' and 'individual' as neither perpetrators nor victims, but as *participants*. It would entail a more equitable distribution of key resources (such as knowledge) and a more enlightened perspective on what knowledges are most legitimate, most meaningful, most useful in the production of health (see Golds *et al.*, 1997). Ultimately, it means letting go of 'control' — both as an end in itself, and as means to an end. And this may be the greatest challenge of all.

Compliance Research: Controlling Disease/Controlling Patients

Historians in the future may well look back on this period in our technological evolution as being exceptionally short-sighted. It may seem incomprehensible that in our quest for biomedical 'magic bullets' we continue to create 'superbugs' — bacteria and viruses capable of killing their human hosts and against which we have neither effective medicine nor natural defences. Yet how can we stop creating new drugs when we have the technological and intellectual capability to do so? If we do not develop new drugs, people will die of these diseases, and we cannot allow people to die if we have the capabilities to prevent those deaths. And yet, how can we NOT stop? For as long as we are creating these drugs we will also be creating the bugs, and where will it all end (cf. Garrett, 1995)?

Not surprisingly, perhaps, there does not seem to be a move toward the rational use of technology: so far, no one seems to be proposing that control be exerted over the pharmaceutical industries and research institutes developing, producing and marketing their new 'improved' drugs (see Kamat and Nichter, 1997). Nor does there seem to be an effective or concerted effort, yet, to control or regulate the freedoms and behaviours of many of those dispensing and/or prescribing these drugs, particularly within the burgeoning private health care sectors in developing countries (Bennett, 1997; Bennett *et al.*, 1997). Thus, we are left, apparently, with little choice but to control these diseases by controlling the people who have become infected with them and who suffer from them most — the patients. Herein lies the discourse and the performance of 'compliance'.

'Compliance': Definition and discourse

As a number of excellent reviews already exist, no attempt will be made to review the compliance literature here (see Homedes and Ugalde, 1993; see also Volmink and Garner, 1997, who focus on adherence to tuberculosis treatments). Perusal of these reviews indicates that over the past 20 years there has been an enormous outpouring of interest in 'compliance' with medical advice. At least two writers have investigated this trend in some detail (Trostle, 1988; Donovan and Blake, 1992). Today, a simple search on *Medline* reveals that between 1990 and 1997, over 16,000 articles concerned with compliance have been published, over two-thirds of which were published between 1992 and 1996. Between the months of January and September 1997, over 2,000 publications are cited.

What, then, is meant by compliance? Within medical texts, there seems to be an implicit assumption that "we all know what it means". Generally, these texts seem to prefer to define 'non-compliance', which is simply understood as "any departure from intended treatment" (Pocock, 1989, p. 179). Donovan and Blake (1992, p. 507) appeal to the dictionary definition: to "obey, submit, defer or accede to instructions". Haynes (1979, quoted in Lerner, 1997, p. 1427) defined compliance as 'the extent to which a person's behaviour (in terms of taking medications, following diets, or executing lifestyle changes) coincides with medical or health advice'. Behind these definitions is an assumption that all patients *should* comply with the instructions given to them by medical professionals and that "in an ideal world non-compliance would not occur" (Donovan and Blake, 1992, p. 507).

This assumption has been challenged in recent years, notably by social scientists concerned with uncovering and legitimising the agency of patients suffering from non-communicable diseases such as epilepsy (Conrad, 1985) and rheumatoid arthritis (Donovan and Blake, 1992). What has been implied in this literature is that the language of compliance has failed to recognise patients' active participation in their own health care; that whether doctors like it or not, patients are not passive or powerless but

> "are quite capable of making choices about treatments
> and lifestyles rationally within the context of their beliefs,
> responsibilities and preferences ... **Non-compliance may
> thus not be deviance, but reasoned decision-making**".
> (Donovan and Blake, 1992: p. 508, emphasis added)

It is interesting to note that 'compliance' is an important area of overlap between the social and biomedical sciences. Social science researchers have been asked to identify, for example, an explanation for the apparently wide variations in 'compliance behaviour'. Two themes have emerged from this work: one argues that the source of the 'problem of compliance' is the doctor-patient relationship (see, e.g. Zola, 1973) while the other identifies patient's health beliefs as the main 'cause' of non-compliance (e.g. DiMatteo and DiNicola, 1982; Barnhoorn and Adriaanse, 1992; Becker, 1979). Critics such as Conrad (1985) and Donovan and Blake (1992) might argue, however, that both perspectives fundamentally miss the point because both take for granted that non-compliance is in some way 'deviant', that it is something that can be measured and overcome. The notion of 'compliance' is problematic for these writers, not least because it is a notion developed to solve doctors' problems — mainly by placing the fault for treatment failures on patients (Conrad, 1985).

While some social scientists continue to pursue the 'health belief model' perspective in their analyses (e.g. Barnhoorn and Adriaanse, 1992; Rubel and Garro, 1992; Mull et al., 1989) others are highly critical of this approach. Farmer (1997), for example, argues that focusing on patient's health beliefs unduly privileges 'culture' and patient agency, while at the same time masking the central reason for treatment failure which has to do with social inequalities and 'structural violence'. Thus, while these social science perspectives endeavour to take patient perspectives and realities into account, they ultimately fail to overcome the assumptions about power, knowledge, legitimacy and agency which are embedded in the discourse itself.

'Compliance' as ideology and historical construction

> *'If true tragedy lies in the failure to achieve that which can be achieved, then true non-compliance is a tragic flaw in our efforts to reap the benefits of treatments that work when taken'.* (Haynes, 1987, quoted in Lerner, 1997: p. 1427)

A decade ago Trostle (1988) wrote provocatively about the language of compliance. His suggestion that medical compliance is an ideology, "a system of shared beliefs that legitimise particular behavioural norms and values at the same time that they claim and appear to be based on empirical truths" and that "ideologies help to transform power (potential influence) into authority (legitimate control)" (Trostle, 1988: p. 1300), remains relevant today. It is also a useful notion in relation to the current project, because Trostle manages to persuade us that though presented as a literature about improving medical services, the research literature about compliance is pre-eminently, although covertly, a literature about power and control (Trostle, 1988: p. 1299). More specifically, he asserts (p. 1300) that

> *"Compliance is an ideology that transforms physicians' theories about the proper behaviour of patients into a series of research strategies, research results, and potentially coercive interventions that appear appropriate, and that reinforce physicians' authority over health care".*

Trostle goes on to argue that the contemporary concern for compliance is in part a product of "the growing monopoly of the medical profession over the past century" as well as the "growth and sales strategies of the pharmaceutical and proprietary drug industries". Thus "a concern for market control combined with a concern for therapeutic power [has] evolved into a concern for patient compliance" (ibid, p. 1301).

It will be shown below how this appears to be playing itself out in relation to tuberculosis control. Trostle also makes the point that as much as this agenda may be fuelled by existing relations of power and control, so it may be driven by fear — by the very present fear confronting the medical profession since the appearance of HIV that their authority may be on the decline (ibid, p. 1303).

This perspective resonates with a more recent appraisal of the compliance literature in which Lerner (1997, p. 1429) notes that "by examining the historical construction of language we remind ourselves how a social agenda may be concealed within scientific terminology". He argues that "in demonstrating the social construction of the term 'non-compliance', the historical record suggests that we may be over-emphasising the current strategy of identifying certain patient behaviours as deviant and then attempting to correct them" (ibid, p. 1423).

In his analysis of the discourse on compliance with tuberculosis therapies over the last century Lerner found that after the appearance of antibiotics there was a shift in public health writing from a focus on the social status and ethnicity of patients as an explanation for non-compliance, to "the act of disobedience itself". Patients who did not comply with their physicians instructions were classified as 'recalcitrant', or "obstinately defiant of authority or restraint" (ibid, p. 1425). Lerner notes that:

> *"This emphasis on defiant behaviour is not surprising.*
> *The new antibiotic agents greatly enhanced the author-*
> *ity of physicians treating tuberculosis. Patients who*

> *disregarded therapeutic recommendations posed a direct
> challenge to this authority".*

According to Lerner the notion of 'compliance', and its foil, non-compliance, achieved popularity in the 1970s through the work of David Sackett and Brian Haynes (See Sackett and Haynes, 1976; Haynes *et al.*, 1979). Although these writers attempted to develop less judgmental ways of classifying patient behaviour, their basic assumptions (that patients *can* and *should* obey their doctor's orders) did not change, and so they did not ultimately achieve their stated aim.

As the work of Conrad (1988), Donovan and Blake (1992) and Lerner (1997) demonstrate, another shift in the discourse of compliance has occurred over the past ten years. In acknowledging the power of language, as well as the power of patients, a number of writers have attempted to once again steer the course of compliance discourse in a more meaningful and equitable direction. This effort is discussed briefly below.

'Adherence': Acknowledging Patient Agency?

In an influential overview of the causes of treatment failure for tuberculosis, Sumartojo (1993, p. 1311) argues that:

> *"The word compliant, typically used to refer to a patient who completes treatment, has the unfortunate connotation that the patient is docile and subservient to the provider.... A better word, which reflects the active role of the patient in self-management of treatment and the importance of co-operation between the patient and the provider, is adherence".*

Yet, a dictionary definition of 'to adhere' is "1. To stick to as if glued; 2. To maintain loyalty, as to a person; 3. To follow without deviation". Thus, on the surface, it does not appear that simply replacing the word compliance with the word adherence will create the desired change in meaning/emphasis/implication.

Adherence in relation to non-infectious disease

The critique of 'compliance' has two main threads; one has grown out of an awareness of the importance of patient-provider communication, and the other, not unrelated, line of argument has to do with patient agency. In their study of patients with arthritis, for example, Donovan and Blake (1992) found that patients listened to medical advice and integrated it into their own theories/understandings about their disorder and into the exigencies of their everyday lives. Most patients in this study expressed a desire for more information about their condition and its treatment, but did not feel able to direct their questions and concerns to their provider. Thus, these authors conclude that "the key to improving compliance (although effectively doing away with the concept), is the development of active, co-operative relationships between patients and doctors" with doctors endeavouring to acknowledge and take account of their patients' decision-making capabilities, and patients being more active in stating their needs, expectations and constraints (Donovan and Blake, 1992, p. 512). Central to this approach, therefore, is the sharing of information and knowledge, and this entails something of a shift in the nature of the therapeutic relationship and balance of power between doctor and patient.

Conrad (1985) found that for epilepsy patients the medications themselves had more meaning than the doctor-patient interaction. He argues that a better way of conceptualising the patient's approaches to the doctor's advice would be to think of it in terms of 'medication practice'. This perspective, he maintains, is patient-centred, and looks at the ways in which patients "create their own medication practice based on the doctor's prescription". This perspective, he argues, sees patients as active agents rather than *passive recipients* of doctor's orders. Indeed, his study showed that "regulating medication represents an attempt to assert some degree of control over a condition that appears at times to be completely beyond control" (Conrad, 1985, p. 36).

It is notable that these writers are dealing with non-communicable diseases. Neither epilepsy nor arthritis are conditions of 'public health importance': the implications for non-compliance stop at the patient-provider interface. While it might frustrate doctors to have their advice ignored, and while there may be repercussions in terms of expenditure for the patient, the state or for insurance companies, the choices these patients make about their treatment do not pose any direct health threat to their families, communities or nations.

Lerner's historical account of non-compliance to tuberculosis therapy is instructive in understanding the implications of this issue. While initially concerned with the demonstration that the compliance discourse essentially serves to protect the privileged power position of the health care professions *vis à vis* their patients, he then asks us to consider the possibility that the criticisms he has made are not actually valid. "After all", he writes:

> *"as physicians are highly trained professionals who have earned the cultural authority to treat illness, there is good reason why they might expect that patients would choose to follow their recommendations. Moreover, in the case of certain contagious diseases, a societal consensus exists that non-compliance cannot be tolerated"*. (Lerner 1997, p. 1427, emphasis added)

He notes that while the forcible detention of tuberculosis patients is "no longer a viable option in the US" (ibid: p. 1428),

> *"[n]evertheless, with the resurgence of tuberculosis and the emergence of multidrug-resistant strains, health officials have come to rely on another restrictive intervention, directly observed therapy"*.

This shift from legitimising patient agency in relation to compliance with therapies for epilepsy and arthritis, to discomfort with this agency in the face of infectious disease is telling. Within this discourse it is apparently permissible to acknowledge and support patient agency and capacity as long as there is no danger to the community should that agency lead to a lack of 'control'. On the other hand, the exercise of force, the existence and persistence of imbalances in power and knowledge — the lack of respect for, and recognition of, patient agency — is an acceptable price to pay for the 'control' of the disease and the 'protection' of the community. This is an awkward scenario, and it begs the question: if it can be accepted that the people's everyday lived realities will have an effect on the choices they make — and are able to make — about physicians' prescriptions, why should this be less so for tuberculosis than for epilepsy?

Somewhere in the shift from individual to public health there is a subtle but crucial shift in locus of responsibility and agency: people cannot be trusted to act for the good of the community and therefore it is legitimate to deny them control. Happily this is not a position universally accepted in the literature on adherence to tuberculosis therapy.

Adherence in relation to tuberculosis

There is little controversy that incomplete treatment for tuberculosis poses "serious risks, both for the individual patient as well as the community, and contributes to a failure in eradicating the disease globally" (Volmink and Garner, 1997, p. 1). It has become almost a truism that "patient non-compliance is the most important cause of treatment failure and relapse" (Snider, 1982). The recent literature looking at adherence, however, asks important and difficult questions about what this scenario means, and what it *should* mean to patients and communities affected by tuberculosis. The implicit assumption that once a person acquires an infectious disease he or she steps outside of humanity is being challenged on various fronts. In fact, as Sumartojo (1993) points out, adherence issues are not only multi-faceted and complex, but range from the characteristics of the individual patients to qualities of the social and economic environment; that "in most settings where TB is prevalent, the degree to which patients are able to comply is significantly limited by forces quite beyond their control" (Farmer, 1997, p. 350). In short, the trend among this school of social scientists is to bring our understanding of 'adherence' into articulation with our growing understanding of social inequalities and their impacts on health.

An effect of this approach is that it begins to expose *and confront* the political biases which are couched and hidden within the discourse of 'compliance' — whether it is being used by clinicians, or indeed by social scientists themselves. Farmer (1997) finds compliance to be a problematic concept, not only because it implies docility and subservience of patients relative to providers, as Sumartojo (1993) argues, but even more insidiously, that it assumes that all patients are equally able to comply — or refuse to comply — with anti-tuberculosis therapies. Farmer argues that in fact there are radical differences in the ability of different populations *and different individuals within populations* to comply with these demanding therapeutic regimens. Factors which increase people's vulnerability to infection, to developing disease and their access to care are structured by forces outside their control. The profound effects of poverty and/or economic inequity, racism, gender inequalities, drug use, homelessness, overt political violence and war, are all key factors in the ability of patients to obtain, maintain and complete therapy. Farmer refers to the effect of these forces as 'structural violence', and argues that they are everywhere more important in shaping 'patient compliance' than are illness beliefs or the patient-provider relationship. 'Structural violence', not patient beliefs and behaviours, for example, will influence the presence or absence of monotherapy, regular or erratic drug supplies, and better or worse access to adequate care facilities. Farmer drives home his point with the following key message, that

> *"Throughout the world, those least likely to comply are those least able to comply ... these settings are crying out for measures to improve the quality of care, not the quality of patients".* (ibid, p. 353)

The Global Emergency: Public Health or Public Fear?

Assumed all but conquered for many years after the introduction of effective chemotherapy, tuberculosis re-emerged dramatically onto the international health agenda in the 1990s. In 1993, the World Health Organization (WHO) declared tuberculosis a 'global emergency'. They estimated that nearly 90 million new cases of tuberculosis and 30 million deaths may occur between 1990 and 1999; that tuberculosis kills more adults each year than any other communicable disease; and that it may be the largest single cause of death in the developing world. In response to this situation, the WHO developed the DOTS strategy, where DOTS stands for directly observed treatment, short course. This strategy is discussed and described elsewhere in this volume (see Chapter 6). In this section, and by way of closure, it is argued that the introduction of DOTS and its aggressive marketing as the central feature of the WHO's strategy, may have the effect of improving 'compliance' in some patients, but it does so without respecting patient agency and it may actually reinforce — or at least does nothing to redress — the fundamental issues underlying the persistence of tuberculosis in populations: structural violence and social inequality.

Compliance and the re-emergence of directly observed therapy

In an editorial in the *International Journal of Tuberculosis and Lung Disease*, Grange (1997) discusses the international response to the WHO's recent 'breakthrough in TB control', DOTS. He notes that concern has been expressed among tuberculosis workers for two principal reasons: that this claim would discourage funding agencies from supporting basic research on diagnostics, vaccines and drugs, and that DOTS is merely the familiar and well-used strategy of direct observation in new clothes. Uplekar and Rangan (1995) suggest that while DOTS has been found effective in improving patient adherence to chemotherapy in some settings, it's usefulness and sustainability in resource-poor settings where tuberculosis is endemic (such as India) may be limited.

It is important not to confuse DOTS (the WHO's strategy containing the five main points outlined in Chapter 6) and DOT, which is an approach to treatment administration that has been around for many decades (Grange, 1997; see also Bayer and Wilkinson, 1995). Part of the controversy over DOTS, however, has been generated by the aggressive way in which the strategy has been promoted by the WHO, and the fact that they have foregrounded DOT as the primary 'selling point' of their new strategy. This has reawakened concern from some corners about the suitability of DOT itself as an element of the standardised, international response to tuberculosis.

In their systematic review of the literature on promoting adherence to tuberculosis treatment, Volmink and Garner (1997, p. 2) note that:

> *"from a theoretical standpoint, DOT can be criticised as it moves away from adherence models of communication and co-operation between patient and provider (Sumartojo, 1993) back to a traditional medical approach with the patient as the passive recipient of advice and treatment. (Ogden, 1996)"*

This concern is based at least in part on the fact that the WHO requires supervision to be undertaken only by a trained health professional. In many settings, the patient is not given possession of the drugs, but must appear at the clinic or DOT facility where they are handed the requisite pills by the provider who then literally watches as the patient swallows the medicine. It is an authoritarian approach which makes a certain kind of sense in, for example, prison settings in which patients lack autonomy anyway (the scenes of patients queuing up for their supervised therapy in Russian gulags are a graphic illustration of this), but have very different kinds of implications when applied to regular out-patients in, for example, urban settings of India. In both settings agency, authority and power over cure belong solely to the biomedical system and its workers and are removed entirely from the patient and community. The patient's autonomy and, therefore, his or her personhood (see Ogden, 1991) is essentially removed from the healing process.

Indeed, direct observation has been criticised on the grounds that it is unethical as an infectious disease control strategy. Porter and Ogden (1997, p. 118), for example, note that DOT is a public health intervention which embodies "the imbalance of power and capacity between the public health profession and the infected person, and lead(s) to a moral debate over public health and civil liberties". They also ask whether "DOT is an appropriate health intervention or merely a means for us to avoid tackling the major public health issues of poverty and inequality" (ibid, p. 125).

Ironically, despite criticisms that DOT represents a return to the 'medicalisation' of tuberculosis treatment (Ogden, 1996), DOTS has been lauded by enthusiasts as a move *away* from the medical model (e.g. Kochi, 1996). But is it? When DOT for tuberculosis was first introduced by Fox in Madras, it was part of an overall package aimed at reducing the need for long-term hospitalisation of tuberculosis patients (see Fox, 1962). According to Bayer and Wilkinson (1995, p. 1545), Fox found that

> *'Despite the fact that the patients involved came from a poverty-stricken community in a city with a poor transport system and that travel of up to 5 miles was necessary, it was possible to get patients to come to a clinic 6 days a week for treatment'.*

This is indeed a telling illustration of the power of biomedicine and people's desire to get well, but does it justify the method? Is it not appalling to think of those desperately poor, desperately ill people undertaking such an arduous and expensive journey six days a week — or even three days a week — in order to obtain their medicines? Is letting tuberculosis patients out of hospital only acceptable if there is not a concomitant loss of control, by doctors, over the daily administration of their treatment?

There is a notable lack of evidence by which the importance of the DOT component of the DOTS strategy, relative to the other components, in different settings can be assessed (Volmink and Garner, 1997). A number of studies conducted in India in the 1970s, for example, investigated the relationship between drug collection and drug consumption (Savic, 1967; Gothi *et al.*, 1971; Gehani *et al.*, 1984). These studies demonstrated that, as Gothi *et al.* (1971, p. 107) note:

> *"those who take the trouble of collecting drugs would also consume them. It therefore suggests that in the National Tuberculosis Programme, it is more important to prevent default in drug collection than to supervise drug consumption".*

Evidence from India also suggests that if other supports are in place (such as a regular supply of drugs and a motivated cadre of health workers), direct observation does not substantially improve adherence to therapy (e.g. Banerji, 1967).

So what is DOTS all about? At its roots it is about protecting communities from infection with tubercle bacilli and, more urgently, with multidrug-resistant tubercle bacilli. This is a laudable aim. But what *else* is DOTS about? The strategy itself is comprehensive. The commitment of governments and health care structures to supporting this aim figure centrally. Oddly, however, DOT has become its marketing focus. The reason for this would be an interesting avenue of research. Nevertheless, the effect of this choice has been to capitalise on the discourse of compliance — a discourse which comforts doctors because it reaffirms and legitimates their authority and their sense of being 'in control', as well as the general public in whom fear has been instilled that tuberculosis represents a 'global emergency': that this disease is spinning out of 'control' and is threatening communities and individuals previously thought safe.

Concealed within the discourse of DOT are biomedicine's existing relations of power (over microbes, patients and communities) and control (over microbes, patients and communities). The complex daily lives of real people, who also happen to have contracted tuberculosis, are not addressed. The complexity of the people themselves — their knowledge, their multiple and sometimes conflicting needs and priorities, the fragility and culturally constructed nature of their bodies — are subsumed and simplified down to the lowest common denominator: the presence of the tubercle bacilli in their lungs or other organs. The underlying assumption of direct observation — that tuberculosis patients cannot be trusted with responsibility for the social good — presupposes a fundamental lack of responsibility on the part of patients and that they lack respect for their bodies, their families and their communities.

To return to the argument that opened this chapter, the word and notion of 'compliance' has made policy makers behave in a particular way in relation to tuberculosis. Adopting a different vocabulary — replacing the word 'compliance' with the word 'adherence' — may be one step in the right direction. Such a shift addresses only part of the problem, however. More fundamentally, what is needed is a shift away from the reductionist tendencies of biomedicine. It is time for the scientific community to turn the mirror inward, to look more critically at our own 'beliefs and behaviours' in relation to infectious disease; our own structures of control; and our own assumptions about power: ours and that of the individuals and communities we are trying to support.

Tuberculosis is with us but it does not have to be a grim reaper. We do not have to wage a 'war' against it. The time has come for us to accept the limits of our control over this microbe and to ask difficult questions, moral questions, about how we may learn to live with it, and each other, in a more realistic, creative and healthy way.

References

Banerji, D. (1967) Behaviour of tuberculosis patients towards a treatment organisation offering limited supervision. *Ind. J. Tuberc.* **14**, 156.

Barnhoorn, F. and Adriaanse, H. (1992) In search of factors responsible for noncompliance among tuberculosis patients in Wardha District, India. *Soc. Sci. Med.* **34**, 291–306.

Bayer, R. and Wilkinson, D. (1995) Directly observed therapy for tuberculosis: History of an idea. *Lancet* **345**, 1545–1548.

Becker, M. H. (1979) Patient perceptions and compliance: Recent studies of the health belief model. In: Haynes, R. B., Taylor, D. W., Sackett, D. L., eds. *Compliance in Health Care.* Baltimore: Johns Hopkins University Press.

Bennett, S. (1997) Health-care markets: Defining characteristics. In: Bennett, S., McPake, B., Mills, A., eds. *Private Health Providers in Developing Countries: Serving the Public Interest?* London: Zed Books. pp. 85–101.

Bennett, S., McPake, B. and Mills, A. (1997) The public/private mix debate in health-care. In: Bennett, S., McPake, B., Mills, A., eds. *Private Health Providers in Developing Countries: Serving the Public Interest?* London: Zed Books. pp. 1–18.

Centers for Disease Control and Prevention (1995) Essential components of a tuberculosis prevention and control program; and screening for tuberculosis and tuberculosis infection in high risk populations: Recommendations of the Advisory Council for the elimination of tuberculosis. *Morb. Mort. Wkly. Rep.* **44**, (RR-11), September 8.

Clifford, J. and Marcus, G. E., eds. (1986) *Writing Culture: The Poetics and Politics of Ethnography.* Berkeley: University of California Press.

Conrad, P. (1985) The meaning of medications: Another look at compliance. *Soc. Sci. Med.* **20**, 29–37.

Davey-Smith, G., Shipley, M. J. and Rose, G. (1990) Magnitude and causes of socio-economic differentials in mortality: Further evidence from the Whitehall Study. *J. Epidemiol. Commun. Hlth.* **44**, 265–270.

Davey-Smith, G., Neaton, J. D. and Stamler, J. (1996) Socio-economic differentials in mortality risk among men screened for Multiple Risk Factor Intervention Trial. White men. *Am. J. Publ. Hlth.* **86**, 486–496.

DiMatteo, M. R. and DiNicola, D. D. (1982) *Achieving Patient Compliance.* New York: Pergamon Press.

Donovan, J. and Blake, D. R. (1992) Patient non-compliance: Deviance or reasoned decision-making? *Soc. Sci. Med.* **34**, 507–513.

Farmer, P. (1997) Social scientists and the new tuberculosis. *Soc. Sci. Med.* **44**, 347–358.

Fox, W. (1962) Self-administration of medicaments: A review of published work and a study of the problem. *Bull. Int. Union Tuberc.* **32**, 247–271.

Garrett, L. (1995) *The Coming Plague: Newly Emerging Diseases In a World Out of Balance.* London: Virago.

Gehani, S., Perumal, V. K. and Mathur, G. P. (1984) A study to determine the reliability of assessing the regularity of self-administration of drugs at home by patients at the clinic. *Ind. J. Tuberc.* **31**, 74.

Golds, M., King, R., Meiklejohn, B., Campion, S. and Wise, M. (1997) Healthy aboriginal communities. *Aust. NZ. J. Publ. Hlth.* **21**, 386–390.

Gothi, G. D., *et al.* (1971) Collection and consumption of self-administered antituberculosis drugs under programme conditions. *Ind. J. Tuberc.* **18**, 107.

Grange, J. M. (1997) DOTS and beyond: Towards a holistic approach to the conquest of tuberculosis. *Int. J. Tuberc. Lung Dis.* **1**, 293–296.

Haynes, R. B., Taylor, D. W. and Sackett, D. L. eds. (1979) *Compliance in Health Care.* Baltimore: Johns Hopkins University Press.

Haynes, R. B. (1987) Patient compliance then and now. *Patient Education and Counselling* **10**, 103–105.

Homedes, N. and Ugalde, A. (1993) Review Article: Patients compliance with medical treatments in the third world: What do we know? *Hlth. Pol. Plann.* **8**, 291–314.

Kamat, V. and Nichter, M. (1997) Monitoring product movement: An ethnographic study of pharmaceutical sales representatives in Bombay, India. In: Bennett, S., McPake, B., Mills, A. eds. *Private Health Providers in Developing Countries: Serving the Public Interest?* London: Zed Books, pp. 124–140.

Kochi, A. (1996) Editorial: TB control isn't what it used to be. *The TB Treatment Observer*, Tuesday, November 5th, No. 1, p. 2.

Lerner, B. H. (1997) From careless consumptives to recalcitrant patients: The historical construction of non-compliance. *Soc. Sci. Med.* **45**, 1423–1431.

McNeill, W. (1976) *Plagues and Peoples.* Garden City, NY: Anchor Press.

Mull, D. J., Shear, C., Wood C. S., Gans, L. P. and Mull, D. S. (1989) Culture and 'compliance' among leprosy patients in Pakistan. *Soc. Sci. Med.* **29**, 799–811.

Ogden, H. G. Undated, *CDC and the Smallpox Crusade.* Atlanta:US Department of Health and Human Services, Centers for Disease Control and Prevention.

Ogden, J. (1991) *Autonomy and Interdependence in Two Kenyan Societies: A Challenge to the Universal Domination of Women.* MA Thesis, University of Manchester.

Ogden, J. (1996) *Health Psychology: A Textbook.* Buckingham: Open University Press.

Pocock, S. J. (1989) *Clinical Trials: A Practical Approach.* Chichester: J. Wiley and Sons.

Porter, J. and Ogden, J. (1997) Ethics of Directly Observed Therapy for the control of infectious diseases. *Bull. Inst. Pasteur* **95**, 117–127.

Rubel, A. J. and Garro, L. C. (1992) Social and cultural factors in the successful control of tuberculosis. *Publ. Hlth. Rep.* **107**, 626–636.

Sackett, D. L. and Haynes, R. B., eds. (1976) *Compliance with Therapeutic Regimens.* Baltimore: Johns Hopkins University Press.

Savic, D. (1967) Relationship between drug collection and intake among tuberculosis patients in ambulatory chemotherapy. *Proceedings of TB Worker's Conference*, Hyderabad.

Snider, D. E. (1982) An overview of compliance in TB treatment programmes. *Bull. Int. Union Tuberc.* **57**, 247.

Sumartojo, E. (1993) When tuberculosis treatment fails: A social behavioural account of patient adherence. *Am. Rev. Resp. Dis.* **147**, 1311–1320.

Trostle, J. A. (1988) Medical compliance as an ideology. *Soc. Sci. Med.* **27**, 1299–1208.

Tyler, S. A. (1986) Post-modern ethnography: From document of the occult to occult document. In: Clifford, J. and Marcus, G. E., eds. *Writing Culture: The Poetics and Politics of Ethnography.* Berkeley: University of California Press, pp. 122–140.

Uplekar, M. and Rangan, S. (1995) Alternative approaches to improve treatment adherence in tuberculosis control programmes. *Ind. J. Tuberc.* **42**, 67–74.

Volmink, J. and Garner, P. (1997) Promoting adherence to tuberculosis treatment. In: Garner, P., Gelband, H., Olliaro, P., Salinas, R., Volmink, J., Wilkinson, D., eds. *Infectious Diseases.* Module of The Cochrane Database of Systematic Reviews [updated March 4th, 1997]. Available in The Cochrane Library [database on disk and CD ROM]. The Cochrane Collaboration; Issue 2. Oxford: Update Software. Updated quarterly.

Wall, P. and Stanwell Smith, R. (1997) Communicable disease challenges and control. In: Scally, G. ed. *Progress in Public Health.* London: FT Healthcare, pp. 137–155

Weeks, J. (1985) *Sexuality and its Discontents.* London: Routledge.

Wilkinson, R. (1996) *Unhealthy Societies: The Afflictions of Inequality.* London: Routledge.

Zola, I. K. (1973) Pathways to the doctor — From person to patient. *Soc. Sci. Med.* **7**, 677–689.

Travis, A. (1989) Medical complications in the elderly. 29 Dec. Med. 21, 1290-1298.

Tyler, S.A. (1986) Post-modern ethnography: from document of the occult to occult document. In: Clifford, J. and Marcus G. Ebers. Writing Culture. The Politics and Culture of Ethnography. Berkeley University of California Press, pp. 122-140.

Umberson, and Terling, S. (1864) Alternative approaches to injury treatment and the risks in inpatient drugs control programmes. Br. J. Psychol. 43, 67-74.

Valentine, J. and Clinch, P. (1994) Fracture reduction and reduction treatment. In: Vestium, K., Oxford, R., Olsten, T., Vestium, R., Vestium, J., Wilkinson, P. The Hypnosis Disease Module of The Cochrane Database of Systematic ... He Review (updated March 44th, 1994). Available in The Cochrane Library 2000 Issue on md and ... [CD-ROM]. The Cochrane Collaboration Issue 2 Oxford: Update Software, Up dated quarterly.

Wall, P. and Stanwell-Smith, R. (2001) Contamination and disease: hygiene and control. Br. J. of Program for Professional Abortion, CT Healthcare, pp. 131-147.

Webb, J. (1999) Sexuality and its Discontents. London: Routledge.

Whitman, R. (1990) Consuming Society. The Affection of Inability. London: Routledge.

Zola, I. K. (1973) Pathways to the doctor. Biomedicine to patient. Soc. Sci. Med. 7, 677-689.

PART III

TUBERCULOSIS TREATMENT FROM THE PATIENT'S PERSPECTIVE: SOCIAL AND ECONOMIC DIMENSIONS OF TREATMENT-SEEKING FOR TUBERCULOSIS

Chapter 10

The Economics of Tuberculosis Diagnosis and Treatment

Susan Foster

Introduction

After several decades of neglect, tuberculosis is now widely acknowledged to be one of the world's biggest and most pressing health problems: in 1990, it contributed approximately 3% to overall morbidity and mortality. Calculations made for the global burden of disease based on data from 1990 showed that, globally, approximately 46.5 million

Table 1. The global burden of tuberculosis in 1990 (in millions of DALYs).

Region	Men	Women	Total	% of Total
Established market economies	0.10	0.05	0.15	0.3
Former socialist countries of Europe	0.31	0.05	0.36	0.8
Middle East, North Africa, and South-West Asia	2.17	1.88	4.04	8.7
India	6.28	4.50	10.80	23.2
China	3.47	2.45	5.91	12.7
Other Asia Pacific countries	5.17	3.78	8.94	19.2
Latin America and the Caribbean	1.51	1.06	2.57	5.5
Sub-Saharan Africa	7.46	6.21	13.67	29.4
Total	**26.47**	**19.98**	**46.45**	**100**

Note: Totals may not agree due to rounding.
Source: Adapted from Murray (1994, p. 195).

237

disability adjusted life years (DALYs) were lost to tuberculosis (Murray, 1994). Table 1 shows the estimated regional and gender distribution of these DALYs.

Thus, although Africa has only about 10% of the world's population, it had 29% of all DALYs due to tuberculosis in 1990 — and these figures reflect data collected prior to the full-blown AIDS-related tuberculosis epidemic. India, China, the Asia Pacific, and the Middle East are other areas with high rates of tuberculosis — all of them predominantly low-income regions. Tuberculosis is therefore primarily a disease of lower income and low-resource base countries.

Since these data were collected, tuberculosis notifications in some countries have doubled, tripled, or even quadrupled. The economic implications of this unprecedented rise in the caseload have yet to be fully grasped. The resources for treatment and control of tuberculosis have, perhaps, increased slightly as a result of the increasing awareness of the threat posed by tuberculosis. But unless resources have kept pace with the increase in cases at country level — in other words, unless they have doubled or tripled — the result is that, in the majority of cases, any increase in resources has been absorbed by the increase in cases, and thus *there has been no increase in resources per case of tuberculosis.* Nor is there likely to be any increase in the near future, and the prospect for a *decrease* in real resources per patient is real. Furthermore, as Fryatt (1997) points out, it is likely that resources which have been saved by adoption of more cost-effective tuberculosis treatment practices, such as the increasing use of out-patient treatment and more effective drugs, have not been reallocated to tuberculosis treatment and control, but rather have been absorbed by the overstretched health services. This is the reality of tuberculosis treatment today, and the situation makes it all the more crucial to make the very best possible use of available resources. It is in that spirit, of questioning the rationale behind existing patterns of resource use at every step in the process, that this chapter is written.

The Advent of HIV and its Implications for the Economics of Tuberculosis Control

There are a number of important implications of the fact that tuberculosis has accompanied the AIDS epidemic, especially in Africa. It has brought a rise in new and unusual presentations of tuberculosis, as has been documented elsewhere in this book (see Chapters 1 and 12). But in terms of the health services and the care of people with tuberculosis it has meant that treatment of tuberculosis forms part of a huge wave of additional HIV-related illnesses which the health services must treat. In one district hospital in Zambia, tuberculosis accounted for nearly half of hospital expenditures on HIV-related illnesses (Foster *et al.*, 1992). Health staff, including medical practitioners, nurses, and laboratory technicians have not been spared from HIV infection — mortality among female nurses rose by a factor of 13 at two hospitals in Zambia between 1980 and 1991, most of it attributable to HIV (Buvé *et al.*, 1994). Although data are difficult to collect due to the small numbers, anecdotal reports are that laboratory technicians have also been heavily affected by HIV, and vacancies are becoming increasingly difficult to fill. Attrition in some countries greatly exceeds the training capacity for laboratory technicians. Moreover, bed occupancy in hospitals is well above 100% in most African hospitals, with patients often having to share beds.

Time to 'Think Beyond the Box' and Break Some Rules

Tried and trusted methods which have worked so well in the past are having to yield to the new realities. Two-month in-patient admissions are no longer possible, even if there are two persons in every bed. Laboratories are groaning under the weight of hundreds of sputa to be examined each week — in addition to the increase in blood testing for HIV and the other routine work, such as malaria smears. Under such conditions, the services responsible for the control of tuberculosis are completely overwhelmed. They lack the human and financial resources to treat the cases which present and are unable to 'get ahead' of the situation by taking measures to prevent transmission and thus the creation of future cases. Yet the picture may not be as bleak as this suggests. More effective ways of using existing resources can be found.

Consensus is emerging among some tuberculosis experts that new ways can and must be found to use existing resources more effectively — and to develop new tools. As one expert put it at a meeting on tuberculosis, "If you do what you always did, you'll get what you always got" (Dixie Snider quoted in McAdam, 1994). Young (1997) points out that "DOTS is the best we have at present" and warns of the risk that "promotion of DOTS as the only answer to tuberculosis control will become a self-fulfilling prophecy. If no case is made for development of new tools, no new tools will be made".

Available Evidence on the Costs of Diagnosis and Treatment of Tuberculosis

Treatment of tuberculosis is in a state of change in the developing world, as the figures in Table 2 show. In 1991, the issue was the relative costs and effectiveness of standard versus short course treatment, whereas by the mid 1990s the issues had shifted to the use of DOTS and the advantages of decentralised treatment in terms of lower patient costs. These figures are by no means a comprehensive review of the costs of tuberculosis treatment, but rather are given as an indication of the range of costs of different strategies in different settings. Some include the costs of diagnosis and capital costs, while others do not and thus they are not directly comparable, although they have all been updated to 1997 US$. Several key points, however, emerge. One is that the costs of drugs under all strategies and settings account for less than half of the overall health services costs, ranging from 6% to a high of 39% in the decentralised Ugandan model. Where substantial periods of hospitalisation are included, this accounts for a high percentage of the overall

Table 2.　Costs of treatment through different strategies in three settings (1997 US$).

Health services costs	Tanzania (a) 1986 Standard	Tanzania (a) 1986 Short course	South Africa (b) 1992 DOT	Uganda (c) 1992 Short course	Uganda (c) 1992 Decentralized
Diagnosis	8.69	8.69	–	9.74	14.48
Drugs	23.22	54.64	36.28	35.50	45.81
DOT costs	–	–	46.64	–	–
Administration	3.89	3.89	97.63	–	–
Hospitalisation	92.41 (d)	123.21 (d)	582.14	22.36	
Out-patient costs	(d)	(d)	–	19.49	33.69
Transportation	27.8	27.80	–	–	–
Training	3.24	3.24	–	–	–
Supervision	3.96	3.96	6.77	6.59	13.19
Capital costs	4.40	4.40	–	(e)	(e)
Other costs				3.05	7.64
Sub-total	167.61	229.83	769.45	96.73	114.81
Patient costs	–	–	109.70	234.03	85.70
Overall total	167.71	229.83	879.19	330.76	200.50

(a) Murray *et al.* (1994). 1986 costs adjusted to 1997 US$.

(b) Floyd *et al.* (1997). 'Post-1991' strategy costs adjusted to 1997 US$.

(c) Saunderson (1995). 1992 costs in UK£ adjusted to 1997 US$. In 'decentralised' model, ethambutol replaces streptomycin.

(d) In-patient and out-patient costs were not separated in the Tanzania estimates.

(e) Capital costs were included under other headings.

costs, both to health services and to patients. Another point to note is that where patient costs have been estimated, they are substantial — accounting for approximately 29–42% of total costs in Uganda and 12% in South Africa. Finally, one point which cannot fail to emerge from the table is that tuberculosis treatment, under whatever strategy, is expensive for both the health services and the patients. This makes it all the more important to improve diagnosis, thereby ensuring that those who are treated for tuberculosis actually do have tuberculosis.

Some of the issues which these data raise are examined below.

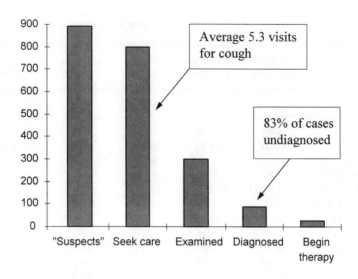

Fig. 1.   The 'Piot' model of the treatment process.

A Model of the Diagnosis and Treatment Process

First, it is useful to refer to the many steps involved in the chain of
events leading a patient with a cough through to a complete cure. A
model of the treatment-seeking process was originally developed in the
1970s by Maurice Piot of the World Health Organization (WHO). In
an adapted and simplified form it has proven useful in illustrating the
issues in the treatment process for several different diseases other than
tuberculosis, such as sexually transmitted infections (Adler *et al.*, 1998).
The model (Fig. 1) begins with the percentage of the whole population
which is infected with the disease, of whom a certain percentage are
symptomatic, and of whom yet a smaller percentage seek care for their
illness. Of those who seek care, some get appropriate diagnosis at the
first contact, while many do not. Not all of those who are diagnosed
actually begin treatment, and of those who begin treatment, a smaller
percentage actually complete it. The percentage finally cured depends
on the 'losses' at each step of the way, and is clearly a small fraction of
the number infected.

The model is useful in helping to locate problem points and areas for intervention. The problem areas may be briefly summarised as:

- Some people with symptoms of tuberculosis are not coming forward for treatment.
- Many people who *do* come forward are not properly and promptly diagnosed. As a result, many people who have sought care for tuberculosis are not on treatment, and remain infectious.
- Some people being treated for tuberculosis do not have, or no longer have, tuberculosis.
- In some cases, sub-optimal regimens and obsolete drugs continue to be used — many of which are less effective, more toxic, and more costly than available alternatives.
- Many people do not continue their treatment until they are cured.
- Relapses are common and increasingly difficult to treat.

Figure 1 illustrates these problems. At every step of the way, infected people exit the process and are lost to the health services, but continue to be infectious and transmit disease to their neighbours and colleagues. The model also has a major advantage in that it shows the impact of 'upstream' improvements — the difference between increasing the percentage of people seeking health care who get diagnosis, compared with increasing the percentage of patients who are cured through the use of more effective drugs.

The economic issues that the process raises will be examined in more detail.

Economic Barriers to Access to Treatment

The first problem is that many people with tuberculosis are not coming forward for treatment. What are the possible reasons for this? In some

cultures there is such a stigma associated with tuberculosis that people
wait until the last possible minute before coming forward for treatment.
The gender imbalance and, in some cultures, greater mortality among
female patients suggests that this is an even greater problem for women
(see Chapter 14). They may become unmarriageable, or divorced, following a diagnosis of tuberculosis. Indeed, tuberculosis is becoming
synonymous with HIV in some countries, adding to the stigma of coming forward with suspected tuberculosis.

In many cases, however, the reason for not coming forward may relate to real or imagined barriers to access — either financial in the
sense of user fees, hospital and drug charges, or more broadly economic
in terms of, for example, travel expenses and lost time and opportunity to earn money. In these cases there are economic remedies to be
applied — to reduce or eliminate the charges for diagnosis and treatment of tuberculosis. Saunderson (1995) in Uganda, and Needham and
Godfrey-Faussett (1996) in Zambia found that people spent a good deal
of their own money trying to get a diagnosis and in some cases had to
persist quite hard in order to finally get on treatment. Of course, many
infected patients must have given up before diagnosis. Similarly, Aluoch
et al. (1982) in Kenya found that patients had visited health services
complaining of cough more than five times before their tuberculosis was
finally diagnosed.

Charging patients for tuberculosis treatment can be a very costly policy in terms of incomplete treatments and possible emergence of drug
resistance — yet it continues in a number of countries. In China, when
economic liberalisation hit the health sector, a policy of requiring patients to pay for anti-tuberculosis drugs was introduced. Not only did
the number of people coming forward for treatment decline significantly,
leading to a rise in the number of new cases, but the prescribers took
advantage of the situation to prescribe unnecessarily expensive drug
regimens — a percentage of the cost being kept by them (World Bank,
1993). The role of exemptions and incentives in tuberculosis treatment
needs to be carefully monitored and remedial actions taken if the situation requires it.

In India, most patients begin their treatment-seeking in the private sector, and studies there have confirmed that over-diagnosis and over-prescription are common problems. Uplekar and Shepard (1991) found that 100 doctors prescribed 80 different regimens, most of which were inappropriate and unnecessarily expensive. Following on this and other studies, Pathania and colleagues (1997) found that patients in India pay out of pocket expenses estimated at between US$100–150, a substantial proportion of the annual income of a daily labourer of US$200.

In other cases people fear coming forward for treatment knowing that they may be more or less confined to hospital for two months (or more) — and they cannot afford that amount of time away from their work. Some may, as a result, lose their jobs and possibly their housing and other benefits.

There is an increasing awareness of the tremendous efforts made by patients in order to get diagnosis and treatment for tuberculosis. In India, the process of seeking care for tuberculosis may last for several years (Pathania *et al.*, 1997). Every effort to minimise the inconvenience experienced by patients, and the real costs they may face in coming forward for treatment, is essential if more people are to be successfully treated. In Uganda, Saunderson (1995) found that the patients' costs of seeking and receiving treatment for tuberculosis amounted to 70% of the total cost, when lost wages were taken into account.

Removing Barriers to Rapid and Accurate Diagnosis

The three main tools of tuberculosis diagnosis in the developing world are microscopy, culture, and radiography. Culture takes too long for results to be of use in deciding on treatment and radiography is often inconclusive, or not available. Microscopy remains the mainstay of diagnosis in most settings. Yet microscopy "is a grossly insensitive tool for detection of persons with active tuberculosis" (Iseman, 1997). As a result, many of the people who do seek treatment are not properly diagnosed. Much more effort, and money, should be spent on improving diagnosis. Looking at Fig. 1 again, it is clear that in many settings perhaps the biggest problem with tuberculosis is *not* that patients default from treatment, but rather that so many people who *do* come forward are lost before they even get on treatment because they are not properly, and promptly, diagnosed.

The problem of diagnosis has three main consequences. The first is that people who do have tuberculosis are missed and return untreated to the community to spread their infection. Many of those who have a first sputum examination do not return for the results, or to give a second or third sample. In Malawi, 499 'suspects' gave a first on-spot specimen, but only 185 (37%) of suspects completed the full submission of three specimens and returned for their results. Of the 185 who did return, 69 were found to be smear positive, and of these, 63 (91%) were identified by the first smear (Squire *et al.*, 1996). Assuming the same proportion of smear positives of 37% in the whole group (69/185) there would have been 185 smear-positive suspects in the original group of 499. If treatment had been offered to the estimated 91% (168) who were smear positive on the basis of the first smear, 168 could have been started on therapy, rather than the 69 who started after three sputum smears — a net gain of 99 cases.

Alternatively, patients are sick enough, or wealthy enough, to continue to seek care elsewhere. Many turn to the private sector. They continue to spend their own money on seeking care, and in the process continue to consume health care resources (such as antibiotics) which are not leading to an eventual cure. This is an especially tragic situation — they come into contact with the health services which send them away untreated to contribute to the growing burden of new infections.

The special problem of what to do about sputum-negative patients is part of this issue. Sputum negative simply means that the bacilli, if there are any, are not numerous enough to be detected — there are something less than 10,000 per ml — and quite a lot depends on the luck, skill and fatigue level of the microscopist. There could still be perhaps 5,000 or 8,000 bacilli per ml. All sputum-positive patients must have been sputum negative at some point. If that was the case on the day on which a patient happened to be near the hospital — for example to go to the market — he or she would be classified as 'sputum negative' and the diagnosis of tuberculosis might therefore be missed. Bacilli could be detectable on the next day, but it would be too late.

Samb *et al.* (1997) proposed a simple method for detecting tuberculosis in sputum-negative patients, based on four easily ascertained symptoms: (1) cough for >21 days; (2) chest pain >15 days; (3) expectoration of sputum, and (4) shortness of breath. In two hospitals in Africa, diagnosis based on two of the four symptoms gave a sensitivity of 88% and specificity of 67%; while three symptoms reduced sensitivity to 49% but raised specificity to 86%.

A second aspect of the problem of diagnosis is that some people who do not have tuberculosis are misdiagnosed as having this disease and are put on 'trial treatment'. In Zambia a few years ago, the tuberculosis control officer estimated that as much as 10–15% of tuberculosis drugs were not being used for notified patients but rather were being used for 'trial treatments' for people, many of whom probably did not have tuberculosis. Clinicians who have to rely on results from overworked and understaffed laboratories often lack confidence in the laboratory and do not believe a negative sputum microscopy result.

A third consequence of the diagnosis situation is that some patients are already cured of their tuberculosis, but treatment continues because there is currently no reliable way of determining whether they are cured, and because that is the protocol.

The above situation cries out for improvement. Patients have come forward for treatment and the system fails them. What can be done to improve diagnosis? Given the current state of tuberculosis diagnosis, and bearing in mind that each untreated 'false negative' case means additional cases for the future, while each 'false positive' case means that one less 'true positive' patient can be treated with available resources, we could quite usefully and economically spend a lot more time and effort on getting diagnosis right at this point. Health workers at peripheral facilities do not suspect tuberculosis often enough, and fail to refer patients for investigation, thus returning infectious patients to their families and communities. Possibilities include the development and dissemination of diagnostic algorithms to the lower level of the health services (where the majority of patients are seen). The 'four symptoms' approach outlined above (Samb et al., 1997) could form the basis for such an algorithm. At least more sensitive referral criteria could be developed, and an attempt made to raise the profile of tuberculosis in the minds of the health workers at the point of first contact. An unconventional approach would be the provision of an incentive, or other encouragement (either monetary or non-monetary), for the peripheral health workers for each suspected case of tuberculosis referred upwards to the appropriate diagnostic level and confirmed as having tuberculosis. This would certainly raise the profile of tuberculosis at local level, but the risk is that tuberculosis services would be swamped with 'tuberculosis suspects'.

Laboratory technicians in developing countries are an extremely scarce resource, in some countries more scarce than doctors and more difficult to replace. Thus, although they are paid very little, they should be thought of more as a scarce resource than as a cheap cadre of manpower. A laboratory technician at a district hospital in Zambia is responsible on average for the laboratory needs of about 50,000 of the population, compared with his or her counterpart in Britain, responsible for about 1,000. The laboratory technician in Britain may be called upon to do many more analyses, but can also rely on a highly-automated laboratory. It is estimated that a laboratory technician can examine up to 20 sputa per day — if he or she has no other duties (Murray et al., 1990). By comparison, the situation facing a district hospital laboratory technician is sobering — he or she is facing as many as 50 sputa for examination per day (Squire SB, personal communication) and has the same to look forward to every day of the week.

The increase in workload is not limited to the rise in sputum examinations. An example will show the impact of the rise in laboratory workload. At a district hospital laboratory in southern Zambia, the total number of analyses rose from 21,000 to 50,545 from 1991 to 1993. Along with a rise in tuberculosis cases from 439 in 1991 to 885 in 1993, the number of sputa for examination doubled in three years, from 1,700 in 1991 to 3,190 in 1993 (Monze Hospital, 1991–93). In the same three-year period, the number of laboratory staff fell from four to three due to illness. Thus, in a 220-working day year, in 1993 each laboratory assistant was responsible for 77 tests a day, compared with 24 in 1991.

Rather than blaming laboratory technicians for not doing their jobs thoroughly there should be a major effort undertaken to find ways to make more efficient use of the scarce resource they represent — and this is likely to include use of improved and advanced diagnostic methods.

In some countries, the microbiology services have deteriorated so much that it will be a long time before the clinicians actually trust, and are willing to act upon, the results from the laboratories. It is a vicious circle — the laboratory is overwhelmed, quality begins to suffer, clinicians stop trusting the results, the laboratory staff know the clinicians are not paying attention to the results, and the incentive to do good work declines. Laboratory technicians are crucial to the diagnosis of tuberculosis and yet they appear to be undervalued — and misused to some extent. Often it is said that there is no need for new diagnostic methods, but that it is simply a matter of using the existing methods 'properly.' Such an approach ignores the realities of many developing country laboratories today.

What is really needed is a better, simpler, easier and faster diagnostic method, and it would be a real advantage if it were cheap enough to be readily and widely adopted. We could actually afford to pay quite a lot for such a test if it were sensitive and specific enough to be trusted, and clinicians were willing to act upon it. But how much would be worth paying?

Phillips and Phillips-Howard (1996) have developed a formula for estimating the threshold of cost-effectiveness. It is based on the assumption that diagnosis is worth doing when the cost of diagnosis (Cd) plus the cost of selective treatment (Ct × P/100, where P is the proportion of diagnosed cases) is less than the cost of presumptive treatment (Ct). Applying this formula to tuberculosis, and assuming that tuberculosis treatment costs the health services US$200 on average, and that 80%

of suspects truly have tuberculosis but most of the other 20% would nonetheless be put on tuberculosis treatment, it would be worth paying up to US$40 per test (200 × (100-80)/100). These figures do not take into account the public health impact of further transmission from cases which have presented for diagnosis but have not been picked up by microscopy. Neither do they take into account the very significant costs incurred by the patients in seeking diagnosis of tuberculosis, as mentioned previously.

Removing Economic Barriers to Effective Treatment and Cure

In other cases, people who do not have, or no longer have, tuberculosis are continuing on treatment. By the fourth month of short course therapy, approximately 70–90% of patients are cured. If it was possible to determine *reliably* who was and who was not cured, the resources spent on the last two months of treatment could be used to treat other patients. Given the more expensive initiation phase and the need to hospitalise some critically ill tuberculosis patients, the profile of costs of treatment would taper off at the end, with the last two months of a six-month course of treatment representing about 10–20% of the total cost to the health services.

In Singapore, 11% of patients treated for four months on SHRZ/HRZ relapsed — but 89% were cured (Singapore Tuberculosis Service/MRC, 1981). What would be saved if it was possible to stop treatment for them at that point, and to continue treatment for the 11% who were not cured? Suppose that drugs for short course treatment costs on average US$40: US$12 per month in the initiation phase, and US$4 per month in the continuation phase. Suppose also that, of 100 patients under treatment, it were possible to stop treating the 89 who are already cured by four months. This would give a theoretical gross savings of US$712, i.e. 89 patients × 2 months remaining of treatment × US$4/month. Continuing to treat the 11 who are not cured would cost US$88 (11 × 2 months × US$4/month), so the net gain would be US$624 per 100 patients. Of course, it would be necessary to pay the costs of the testing — but how much would it be worth paying for increased certainty of diagnosis? A reliable test which could distinguish between those who still need treatment and those who are cured, would allow treatment to be stopped for the 89 who are cured, and save US$624 in treatment costs. This US$624 could be reallocated to improved diagnosis at the fourth month for the 100 patients, and the system could afford to spend up to about US$6 per patient in order to find out who still has tuberculosis and who does not, without adding to the overall programme costs.

Choice of Treatment Regimen

A chapter on the economics of tuberculosis written ten years ago would probably have focused primarily on the cost-effectiveness of short course regimens containing rifampicin as compared with longer regimens which were widely used at that time. Fortunately, that issue has now been conclusively dealt with. Fryatt (1997) concludes a review of the literature on the cost effectiveness of tuberculosis treatment programmes and summarises the current situation: "There is consistent evidence that effective, shorter, rifampicin-based regimens are more cost-effective from both a provider and household perspective, despite the higher cost of drugs. Ambulatory care is more cost-effective than hospitalised care from a users perspective. From a provider's perspective, however, it may depend on the costs of providing an effective community-based service" (Fryatt, 1997, p. 107).

The costs of individual drugs and drug regimens are shown, respectively, in Tables 3 and 4. Excluding the thiacetazone-containing regimen in Table 3, the drug costs of the five recommended regimens for the initiation phase amount to an average of US$9.75 per month, and those of the continuation phase to about US$3.18 per month. Health services and patients' own costs (but excluding hospitalisation) would easily add US$2 per month, bringing these totals to US$12 and US$4

Table 3.   Recent prices of commonly-used drugs for the treatment of tuberculosis (cost per 1,000 units).

Drug	Formulation	UNICEF price (US$)	Lowest price (US$)
Isoniazid	100 mg tablet	2.89	2.30
Rifampicin	150 mg tablet/capsule	39.00	33.00
	300 mg tablet/capsule	56.20	57.40
Pyrazinamide	500 mg tablet	35.07	31.50
Ethambutol	400 mg tablet	25.06	18.30
Streptomycin	Powder, 1 g base in vial	22.70	7.30
Water	5 ml vial	31.40	2.67
Disposable syringe and needle	unit	–	2.80
Thiacetazone + isoniazid	150 mg + 300 mg tablet	10.33	7.35
Ethambutol + isoniazid	400 mg + 150 mg tablet	–	22.00
Rifampicin + isoniazid	300 mg + 150 mg tablet	–	55.00
Rifampicin + isoniazid + pyrazinamide	120 mg + 50 mg + 30 mg tablet	–	40.00

Source: World Health Organization (1997).

per month respectively.   Drug costs for tuberculosis treatment would therefore total an average of US$40 for a six-month regimen. Drugs for 100 patients would cost approximately US$4,000.

Intermittent therapies and shorter course therapies have been the subject of study in several developing and middle-income countries. In Brazil, a twice-weekly continuation phase regimen (following 2RHP) of 900 mg isoniazid and 600 mg rifampicin was found to be as effective as daily therapy of 400 mg isoniazid and 600 mg rifampicin (Castelo et al., 1989). In Thailand, a comparison of three short course regimens showed that the most cost-effective treatment from both patients' and provider's perspectives was 2RHP followed by a twice weekly continuation phase of isoniazid and rifampicin (Kamolratanakul et al., 1993). The cost of direct observation of therapy per se was not examined in either of these studies, but clearly this cost for patients and providers would be significantly less if patients had only to be observed twice a week rather than seven times a week.

Table 4. Cost of World Health Organization-recommended treatment regimens (in US$)*.

Initial phase	Total Cost	Cost per month	Continuation phase	Total Cost	Cost per month
2 EHRZ	19.3	9.65	4 RH	15.4	3.85
2 SHRZ	32.6	16.3	4 R_3H_3	6.6	1.65
2 $E_3R_3H_3Z_3$	9.5	4.75	6 TH	2.0	0.33
2 $S_3H_3R_3Z_3$	14.2	7.10	6 EH	11.2	1.87
2 RHZ	14.5	7.25			
2 $R_3H_3Z_3$	7.0	3.50			
2 SERHZ/1 ERHZ	46.4	15.47	5 ERH	27.2	5.44
2 SERHZ/1 $E_3R_3H_3Z_3$	42.3	14.10	5 $E_3R_3H_3$	14.6	2.92
Average		9.75			3.18**

* Calculated on the basis of UNICEF prices in Table 3 above. Includes the cost of water and disposable syringes for injection.
** Excludes the thiacetazone-containing regimen (TH).
Source: World Health Organization, 1997.

The Costs of DOTS

It is important to be clear about what DOTS involves for patients. Depending on the regimen chosen, in South Africa it will involve five visits per week in the initiation phase and three or five per week in continuation phase, for a total of 40 in initiation phase and 48 or 80 visits in continuation phase — a total of 88 or 120. Many patients will spend their whole day getting to and from the treatment source, and thus be unable to resume their work even when they are well enough to do so. The key issue regarding DOTS as far as the health services are concerned is where the observation of therapy will be performed, and by whom. Floyd *et al.* (1997) investigated the cost of DOTS in South Africa at a district hospital in KwaZulu Natal province, at which patients are permitted a choice of 'observer' and the observer can be someone other than a health worker. They found that the overall cost of providing an observed dose at hospital level was US$6.43, compared with US$1.70 at lower levels of the health services or when done by the community 'observer' whom the patients had chosen. Average patients' costs per visit were estimated for hospital, health centre, and community-level observation as US$0.95, US$0.67, and US$0.36 respectively — a key consideration in a low-income setting, given that patients will have at least nearly 100 'observed' treatments. The average cost of transport to the hospital for patients was, however, US$10. This clearly shows the advantage of flexibility in choice of 'observer' and of having the therapy given close to the patient's home. Even the 'cheapest' alternative for the patient will involve costs of US$32. Provider costs at hospital level will amount to between US$566 and US$772 *per patient!* (Floyd *et al.*, 1997).

Adherence to Treatment — Feckless Patients or Faulty Services?

Tuberculosis specialists are becoming increasingly aware that the problem of patient compliance is more complex than simply patients not taking their drugs. Rouillon, cited by Reichman (1997), wrote in 1972 that "default by the patient is in fact rarely an isolated phenomenon; in reality it follows or flows from other failures, insufficiencies, or imperfections in the people or the system to whom or to which the patient has entrusted his fate.... His behaviour is... in large measure the result of the long chain of influences which he has undergone consciously or unconsciously within his system. It is the system that is mainly at fault when there is a large default of patients". Somehow Rouillon's central message — that often it is the system which is at fault — got lost over the years and blame began to be shifted directly on to the patient, and away from inefficient and thoughtless health services. An example will serve to demonstrate this.

One defaulting patient in Africa, interviewed nine months after discharge, was asked whether he had continued his tuberculosis treatment until the end. He explained that he had made the journey to the hospital three times to collect his drugs. Three times he had been told that the drugs were out of stock and he was to come back 'next week'. Each time he had sold one of his chickens to pay the taxi fare to get to the hospital and back, and each time he had come back empty handed. When he was interviewed he was destitute, having sold all his chickens, was no longer on treatment, and was thin and quite unwell. The hospital tuberculosis officer had been cavalier about his treatment — knowing that at the time rifampicin was out of stock and would be for some time, it would have been appropriate to try to switch the patient to another regimen — but not to tell him to come back when it was certain that the drugs would still be unavailable. Meanwhile, as far as the tuberculosis control programme was concerned, this patient had 'defaulted' and was 'non-compliant'. This figure was then fed into the national tuberculosis statistics and he became one of those feckless tuberculosis defaulters. The 'default' problem may be somewhat overstated in other respects as well. Many patients who 'fail to comply' or adhere are in fact cured. Perhaps they know that when they start to feel better, they are probably out of danger and can turn their attentions back to the business of life. In fact, such non-adherence saves considerable time and resources for the tuberculosis treatment services — they are not consuming any more drugs, diagnostics, or health personnel time. If 40% of patients are not complying with treatment and not picking up their drugs, then the health services are in fact making significant savings. In conditions when the services are stretched to their limit, is it possible that there is a subtle incentive for health staff to let defaulters default, especially the 'troublesome' ones?

If approaches to behaviour change can be categorised as either 'carrot' or 'stick' then DOTS represents the ultimate in the 'stick' model of behaviour change. Yet much more attention could be paid to the possibilities offered by the more gentle 'carrot' approach. A wide range of incentives for patients and providers could be envisioned. In some countries (notably the USA), patients are provided help with transport costs, or given a bonus at the successful completion of treatment. In Sierra Leone, patients paid a deposit at the beginning of treatment which was returned to them at the end of the in-patient phase (Foster and Salomao, 1994), and a similar system has been used in Bangladesh (see Chapter 16). Such an incentive need not be a huge percentage of the overall cost of treatment, yet might have a significant impact on the outcome. If treatment costs US$150 and 60% complete treatment, the cost per completed treatment is US$250. If adding a US$5 incentive to complete treatment raises compliance by 10%, to 70%, the overall cost per completed treatment actually *falls* to US$221. Even a US$10 incentive which achieves a 70% completion rate still means a lower cost per treatment completed of US$228. Patients would be motivated to complete treatment without the costly and burdensome need to make as many as 100 visits to the 'observer'.

Preventive Therapy

In the era of HIV, given the high probability of a dually infected person developing tuberculosis, preventive therapy for tuberculosis in people with HIV infection has great appeal. It has been established that not only does having HIV increase the risk of developing tuberculosis, but having tuberculosis increases the rate of progression of HIV disease as well. The synergy of the two is bad for the patient and also bad for the community. Work on the economics of tuberculosis preventive therapy shows that under certain circumstances — for example, an HIV-positive person with, should they develop tuberculosis, a high likelihood of infecting a number of other people either because of the nature of their work or their living circumstances — the benefits of provision of isoniazid preventive therapy exceed the costs by a factor of as much as four, especially in cases where HIV testing has been done for another purpose. This takes account of a relatively low uptake of preventive therapy and poor compliance, and of the need to test many in order to find a few eligible persons (Foster *et al.*, 1997). In South Africa, it was estimated for a mixed population of high (50%) and low (5–10%) tuberculosis infection prevalence that nearly two-thirds of expected cases could be prevented, and the benefits of isoniazid preventive therapy would exceed the costs by a factor of nearly two (Masobe *et al.*, 1995). People who either live or work in close contact with many others, such as teachers and students, health care workers, bus conductors, prisoners, soldiers, policemen, and miners, could therefore be considered for preventive therapy. The key issue is how to identify eligible persons early enough in their HIV disease to get the intervention to them in time for it to be useful.

Programme Issues

The economic and social environment of the late 1990s is not favourable to tuberculosis control. The exploding tuberculosis epidemic, the rise of HIV, the resulting shortages of health staff, not to mention structural adjustment and health sector reform and the consequent disruption of health services — all these give reason to believe that it will not be possible to use the old methods and tools of tuberculosis control as well as they were used in the past. It is essential to find ways to enhance productivity of laboratory and medical and nursing staff — and it is essential to realise the fact that even though such staff are paid little it does not mean their value to society is low. Quite the contrary, they are 'cheap but not plentiful' and therefore a scarce resource that must be used appropriately. It seems foolish to deny them new techniques and equipment which could enhance productivity. One aspect which is rarely discussed is that many laboratory technicians in developing countries are exposed to high quantities of infectious material including tuberculosis — infectious material which would be kept under a hood in a category-3 laboratory in an industrially developed nation is lined up on the bench, awaiting their attention. In fact, they are the unsung heroes of the piece.

On the issue of drug supply, there is considerable good news. Prices are falling (Chaulet, 1995), and as an example, the price of rifampicin has fallen by about 25% since 1990. Availability of essential drugs has improved significantly in many countries, due in part to the assistance of

multilateral and bilateral donors and the WHO. Other countries have
been driven to acceptance of essential drugs — generic drugs — by
economic necessity. There is still a need to procure drugs carefully — the
use of large-scale quality generic procurement agencies such as IDA in
the Netherlands or Echo in the UK can save literally thousands of dollars
on drug procurement. Prices of existing commonly-used tuberculosis
drugs are dropping and the trend may continue for a few more years. In
any case, the cost of tuberculosis drugs rarely exceeds 3% of a developing
country's drug budgets (Chaulet, 1992).

The resource implications of tuberculosis control are significant but
perhaps are not as overwhelming as is often thought. Murray (1994)
estimated the optimal budget allocation for cost-effective control of tuberculosis for four regions of the world, as shown in Table 5 below.

Table 5.   Optimal budget allocation for tuberculosis control.

Region	% of GDP spent by public sector on health	% of public sector health budget that should be spent on tuberculosis	Optimal tuberculosis expenditure per capita (US$)
Sub-Saharan Africa	3.0	8.4	0.86
Latin America/Caribbean	5.0	1.7	1.65
India	2.4	4.5	0.60
Other parts of Asia (including islands)	4.0	2.4	0.94

Source: Murray (1994, p. 204).

According to Murray (1994), therefore, a sub-Saharan African country should be spending about US$0.86 per capita on tuberculosis con-
trol, on the assumption that it spends US$10 per capita for all health
services. Clearly, this is far less than is currently being spent, but could
it be afforded? Other priorities would have to be cut back — a painful
process. Many African countries spend only US$5 per person on annual
drug expenditures. There is a tendency to view such a figure as a ceiling

— but it is an average. Most people will consume little or no drugs at all in a year, the majority will be consumed by seriously ill persons, and they will typically consume US$25–50 worth of drugs each. So the US$5 figure should not be taken as an upper limit.

Tuberculosis at present is a costly disease and new approaches — drugs, vaccines, and so on — which are more effective than current practice could, paradoxically, be fairly expensive *and cost-saving*. Eventually, it is not inconceivable that there could be a treatment which lasts six days rather than six months (Young, 1997). Such a treatment could be 30 times more expensive per day than current treatment and still be cost-neutral, and almost certainly cost-saving, when all the health service, and patient and household costs associated with tuberculosis treatment are taken into account. In other words, if tuberculosis treatment today costs US$200 approximately, a six-day treatment could cost nearly US$35 per day and still be advantageous.

However, the implementation of improvements, including cost-effective strategies is not automatic, as Fryatt (1997) points out. He notes in a review of cost-effectiveness studies that "conclusions on the cost-effectiveness of some programmes assumed an ability to transfer resources from one aspect of a programme (such as hospital or staff costs) to another (such as drugs or community supervision). In reality, any savings in hospital costs may go to investment in other, non-tuberculosis related, hospital services .... In practice... it may prove difficult for health services... to become technically more efficient for the same level of resources, even after theoretically cost-effective changes have been introduced".

Potential Gains from 'Breaking the Rules'

How much could be gained from 'breaking the rules' of current practice in tuberculosis diagnosis and treatment? Table 6 summarises some of the estimates of the potential gains to be made by 'breaking the rules', or changing established procedure in various ways. Each situation is

Table 6.   Estimates of potential gains to be made by changes to tuberculosis diagnosis and treatment procedures.

Measure	Estimated potential gain	Evidence/ source
Diagnosis		
Treatment on the basis of first on-spot positive sputum smear vs. three smears	Up to 50% of laboratory costs of examining sputum; possibly some gains in accuracy due to reduced laboratory workload? Doubling, or more, of cases detected and treated at health services	Author's estimates (see text)
Presumptive diagnosis and treatment on clinical grounds/using algorithm	Up to 70% of laboratory costs of examining sputum (where 90% of patients can be diagnosed clinically, plus increased coverage)	Author's estimates (see text)
New reliable diagnostic techniques	Improved accuracy, ?10% of tuberculosis treatment costs; reduced transmission and fewer new cases (little or no laboratory cost savings expected)	Author's estimates (see text)
Incentive for health worker to refer tuberculosis suspect cases appropriately (e.g. US$1 per confirmed tuberculosis case)	Improved case-finding and reduction in delay in getting appropriate care — longer term reduction in transmission?	Author's estimates (see text)
Treatment		
Intermittent short course therapy vs. regular short course	Up to 50% of drug costs; significant savings for patients and providers under DOT situation	Author's estimates

Table 6. (*Continued*).

Measure	Estimated potential gain	Evidence/ source
Stopping therapy at four months for those who are cured	10–15% of net drug costs; investment required in improved diagnostics	Author's estimates (see text)
Local DOT supervisor vs. Health services-based DOT vs. no DOT	26.1% of health services costs, 52.8% of patients costs 81% of hospital costs (assumes previously 120 days in hospital)	Floyd *et al.* (1997)
Hospital vs. ambulatory/ community treatment	Cost/cure reduced by 57%; cure rate improved from 50% to 70%	Saunderson (1995)

unique, and each local health service will have to consider what would be the most appropriate way of dealing with the tuberculosis situation they face. These may suggest some new avenues for operational research into better ways to diagnose and treat tuberculosis, given today's realities.

Conclusion

The existing situation of tuberculosis control in most countries is not an orderly, careful process but rather characterised by low levels of resources and vastly increasing numbers of patients requiring treatment. As a result, poor performance is widespread. The danger of multidrug resistance in the developing world is great — Carpels *et al.* (1995) have estimated that sub-Saharan Africa could be facing between 15,000 and 223,000 cases of multidrug-resistant tuberculosis by the year 2000. In such a situation, insistence on optimal procedures may be a case of 'the best being the enemy of the good'. In many countries, additional resources will be absorbed by the growing number of cases — resources per patient will remain stagnant or continue to decline. Referring back to the Piot model, the weakest points appear to be in the diagnosis of tuberculosis in those who come forward, and in keeping those diagnosed on treatment long enough to be cured. Scrutiny of every decision and procedure will reveal that resources — financial, but also human resources — can be used better, and indeed they must be used to best effect if any improvement in the present situation is to be seen. Getting the epidemic of tuberculosis under control will require imaginative and daring new approaches to the diagnosis and treatment of the disease.

References

Adler, M., Foster, S., Grosskurth, H., Richens, J. and Slavin, H. (1998) *Sexually Transmitted Infections: Guidelines for Prevention and Treatment*. Revised edition. London: Department for International Development.

Aluoch, J. A., Edwards, E. A., Stott, H., Fox, W. and Sutherland, I. (1982) A fourth study of case-finding methods for pulmonary tuberculosis in Kenya. *Trans. R. Soc. Trop. Med. Hyg.* **76**, 679–691.

Buvé, A., *et al.* (1994) Mortality among female nurses in the face of the AIDS epidemic: A pilot study in Zambia (short communication). *AIDS* **8**, 396.

Carpels, G., *et al.* (1995) Drug resistant tuberculosis in sub-Saharan Africa: An estimation of incidence and cost for the year 2000. *Tubercle Lung Dis.* **76**, 480–486.

Castelo, A., *et al.* (1989) Comparison of daily and twice-weekly regimens to treat pulmonary tuberculosis. *Lancet* **2**, 1173–1176.

Chaulet, P. (1992) The supply of antituberculosis drugs and national drugs policies. *Tubercle* **73**, 295–304.

Chaulet, P. (1995) The supply of antituberculosis drugs: Price evolution. *Tubercle* **76**, 261–263.

Floyd, K., Wilkinson, D. and Gilks, C. (1997) *Community-Based Directly Observed Therapy for Tuberculosis: An Economic Analysis*. Tygerberg, South Africa: Medical Research Council.

Foster, S. D., Buvé, A., Kleinschmidt, I. and O'Connell, A. (1992) *Costs of Treatment for HIV Disease at a District Hospital in Zambia*. VIIIth Conference on AIDS, Amsterdam, July 19–24.

Foster, S. D. and Salomao, A. (1994) Workshop Report. Control strategies and resource allocation. In: Porter, J. D. H., McAdam, K. P. W. J., eds. *Tuberculosis: Back to the Future*. Chichester: John Wiley, pp. 250–251.

Foster, S. D., Godfrey-Faussett, P. and Porter, J. D. (1997) Modelling the economic benefits of tuberculosis preventive therapy for people with HIV in Zambia. *AIDS* **11**, 919–925.

Fryatt, R. J. (1997) Review of published cost-effectiveness studies on tuberculosis treatment programmes. *Int. J. Tuberc. Lung Dis.* **1**, 101–109.

Iseman, M. (1997) Better means for the diagnosis of tuberculosis: 'In the mean-time...' *Int. J. Tuberc. Lung Dis.* 1, 2.

Kamolratanakul, P., *et al.* (1993) Cost-effectiveness analysis of three short-course anti-tuberculosis programmes compared with a standard regimen in Thailand. *J. Clin. Epidemiol.* 46, 631–636.

Masobe, P., Lee, T. and Price, M. (1995) Isoniazid prophylactic therapy for tuberculosis in HIV-seropositive patients — A least-cost analysis. *S. Afr. Med. J.* 85, 75–81.

McAdam, K. P. W. J. (1994) Back to the Future: 'The Ten Commitments.' In: Porter, J. D. H., McAdam, K. P. W. J., eds. *Tuberculosis: Back to the Future.* Chichester: John Wiley, pp. 267–276.

Monze Hospital. *Annual Report 1991, 1992, and 1993.* Monze, Zambia: Monze District Hospital.

Murray, C. J. L., Styblo, K. and Rouillon, A. (1990) Tuberculosis in developing countries: Burden, intervention, and cost. *Bull. Int. Union Tuberc. Lung Dis.* 65, 2–20.

Murray, C. J. L. (1994) Resource allocation priorities: Value for money in tuberculosis control. In: Porter, J. D. H., McAdam, K. P. W. J., eds. *Tuberculosis: Back to the Future.* Chichester: John Wiley, pp. 193–211.

Needham, D. and Godfrey-Faussett, P. (1996) Economic barriers for tuberculosis patients in Zambia. *Lancet* 348, 134–135.

Pathania, V., Almeida, J. and Kochi, A. (1997) *Tuberculosis Patients and Private for-Profit Health Care Providers in India.* Geneva: World Health Organization.

Phillips, M. and Phillips-Howard, P. (1996) Economic implications of resistance to antimalarial drugs. *Pharmacoeconomics* 10, 225–238.

Reichman, L. B. (1997) Tuberculosis elimination — What's to stop us? *Int. J. Tuberc. Lung Dis.* 1, 3–11.

Samb, B., *et al.* (1997) Methods for diagnosing tuberculosis among in-patients in Eastern Africa whose sputum smears are negative. *Int. J. Tuberc. Lung Dis.* 1, 25–30.

Saunderson, P. R. (1995) An economic evaluation of alternative programme designs for tuberculosis control in rural Uganda. *Soc. Sci. Med.* 40, 1203–1212.

Singapore Tuberculosis Service/MRC. (1981) Clinical trial of six-month and four-month regimens of chemotherapy in the treatment of pulmonary tuberculosis: The results up to 30 months. *Tubercle* 62, 95–102.

Squire, S. B., Nyasulu, I. K., Amali, R., Kanyerere, H. and Salniponi, F. M. L. (1996) Is smear microscopy functioning as a case-finding strategy for tuberculosis in Africa? *Tubercle Lung Dis.* 77(Supplement 2), 77.

Uplekar, M. W. and Shepard, D. S. (1991) Treatment of tuberculosis by private general practitioners in India. *Tubercle* 72, 284–290.

World Bank (1993) *World Development Report: Investing in Health.* Washington DC: World Bank.

World Health Organization (1997) *Treatment of Tuberculosis: Guidelines for National Programmes*, Second edition. Geneva: World Health Organization.
Young, D. (1997). New tools for tuberculosis control: Do we really need them? *Int. J. Tuberc. Lung Dis.* **1**, 193–195.

CHAPTER 11

SOCIO-CULTURAL DIMENSIONS IN TUBERCULOSIS CONTROL

Sheela Rangan and Mukund Uplekar

Sharda, a mother of four, living in a small village in Western India, never really recovered after her last pregnancy and child bearing. When her child was five months old, she started feeling weak and tired. A nagging cough was further worrying her. After a couple of weeks, she visited the local private doctor, who treated her with some cough mixtures, tonics and antibiotics for a month and a half, but later told her to get herself investigated in the nearby town or go to the local Primary Health Centre (PHC). Never finding the time to go to town to get the investigations, Sharda continued to take some home-made remedies suggested by her mother-in-law.

Over the next couple of months, her physical condition deteriorated and she was no longer able to carry on her day-to-day work. Her mother-in-law then decided to send her to her mother's house for treatment and rest. Her neighbour, a health worker attached to the local PHC, told her mother that she should get her sputum examined. This worried the family as only tuberculosis patients usually had their sputum examined. And if they did make her give her sputum to the health worker, the entire neighbourhood would come to know and talk about it. So her brother took her to a reputed private doctor in the city. The doctor advised some investigations and revealed that Sharda had tuberculosis and would need to take medicines for 6–8 months. The family could not believe it. How could Sharda have got tuberculosis? Since they could not accept the diagnosis, they consulted two more doctors, wasting time

265

and precious resources, before resigning themselves to the truth. They
reasoned that perhaps she had inherited it from her paternal grandfather.
Anyway, this fact had to be kept secret from her husband and in-laws.
If they knew the diagnosis, she would never be accepted back. Somehow
they needed to get her cured.

The medicines prescribed by the doctor were very expensive — her
brother wondered how long he could afford to buy them for her when he
had six mouths to feed on his meagre earnings. He was told by his friend
to check with the local PHC to see if they had these medicines, but they
had no stocks of drugs. So Sharda had the medicines as and when her
brother got them for her from the local chemist. Consequently, Sharda's
physical condition did not show any improvement. In the meantime, a
maternal uncle who came down to visit them heard about Sharda and assured them that he knew of a local traditional healer who could definitely
cure her. He took her to this healer who advised a series of indigenous
remedies consisting of goat's milk, goat's meat and pig liver, which gave
Sharda no relief though she followed them religiously. Three months
later, when her brother went to the PHC for some other problem, he
was informed that they had received a fresh supply of anti-tuberculosis
drugs. Sharda was registered with the PHC and started taking the drugs.
She had to go to the out-patient department once a month to collect her
medicines and face the barbed remarks of her neighbours as well as the
unsympathetic attitude of the PHC staff every time she had to go to the
PHC. Added to this were the adverse effects of the medicines she was
taking which she countered by eating some "cold" foods. It was only her
will to get well soon and return home to her husband and children that
kept her going. Soon she started getting better. Her parents felt that she
should stop taking the medicines, but her brother who had been informed
about the need for completion of the course of treatment, insisted on her
continuing it. Eight months later, Sharda was declared as cured from
tuberculosis.

A letter was immediately sent to Sharda's husband informing him
about this improvement. During the school holidays her husband came
with their elder children and his mother to visit Sharda. Seeing that

she was looking and feeling better, he wanted to take her back home. His mother, however, was keen to know the exact nature of Sharda's illness. Though Sharda's parents wanted to conceal her illness from her mother-in-law, her brother felt that they should not lie since it would be worse for Sharda if her in-laws found out from some other source about her illness; he also felt safe about revealing the diagnosis now that Sharda was totally cured. Sharda's mother-in-law, unfortunately, could not be convinced. She was angry with Sharda's parents for even trying to send her back. She did not want to return home with a daughter-in-law who was a tuberculosis patient and would endanger the health and reputation of her family. Sharda's brother pleaded with the husband reassuring him about her health. Her husband, however, kept remembering instances of various tuberculosis patients in his community who had either died of tuberculosis or who were living as social recluses. He did not want his family to be ostracised because of Sharda. They finally left for their home without Sharda.

A month later, Sharda was informed that her husband had decided to get remarried! The news shocked Sharda, who lost all interest in life. Her health was also subsequently affected — two months later a weak and malnourished Sharda once again developed cough and fever. When the doctor diagnosed her to be suffering from tuberculosis once again, she refused to take medicines. Her family watch helplessly as she gets weaker as each day passes.

Sharda's story illustrates many of the socio-cultural dimensions in tuberculosis control in India. Over the decades, the poor utilisation of the National Tuberculosis Programme by the people and the consequent inability of the programme to effectively control the problem of tuberculosis in various communities and in several developing countries, have led to some of the current dilemmas in global tuberculosis control. Why have programmes that were, apparently, so well conceived and aimed at relieving people from their suffering failed? An easy and logical answer to this question is that *people* had failed to accept and adhere to the guidelines of the programme because they were ignorant and were guided by their socio-cultural perceptions and practices. Formulating policies to address the problem then became easy — these had to be aimed at the illiterate and non-compliant people. The ensuing paragraphs look at people's understanding regarding tuberculosis, their treatment-seeking practices and the extent of the influence of their socio-cultural beliefs and practices on tuberculosis control.

Causation and Transmission Beliefs

A look at peoples' perceptions regarding the pre-disposing factors and causes of tuberculosis reveal the extent to which modern scientific facts are reflected by their causation beliefs. People generally attribute multiple causes to the disease. Germs, poor nutrition (including its association with alcoholism, poverty and food scarcity), physical exertion and weakness (including that due to excessive loss of semen induced by excessive sexual activity and 'worry'), and heredity are the most commonly quoted causes of tuberculosis (Liefooghe et al., 1995; Menegoni, 1996; Westaway, 1989; Uplekar and Rangan, 1996; Nichter, 1994; Rubel and Garro, 1992; Mata, 1985; Metcalf et al., 1990; Geetakrishnan et al., 1988). Belief in supernatural causes such as witchcraft and the wrath of gods and goddesses have also been reported by certain communities (Ndeti, 1972; Farmer et al., 1991; Pool, 1992).

The stigmatising nature of tuberculosis also leads people to believe that this disease is associated with socially and morally unacceptable behaviour including alcoholism, sex with prostitutes or with menstruating or elderly women, and eating certain prohibited food items (Uplekar and Rangan, 1996; Nichter, 1994). These beliefs could prevent people from accepting the diagnosis and could encourage them, as in the case of Sharda, to shop around for an alternate diagnosis. These beliefs could also result in self-stigmatisation by patients who believe they are 'impure' and could contaminate others. A study from Nepal describes respondents who say that tuberculosis is a disease that 'comes from within a person' as a result of hot/cold imbalances, witchcraft, the nature of cosmological configurations at birth and a condition known as 'soul loss' (Pool, 1992). African Americans believe that it is a 'dirty' disease that attacks 'bad' people (Rubel and Garro, 1992). Even among people who accept that the disease is infectious and is curable with appropriate treatment, the associations of the disease are with dirt, poverty and poor nutrition which are unacceptable to the family and the community (Westaway and Wolmarans, 1994).

These causation beliefs held by the people are also reflected in their perceptions regarding cure — it is believed that tuberculosis is curable so long as certain dietary, social and cultural norms are followed or some additional folk remedies are used (Liefooghe *et al.*, 1995; Uplekar and Rangan, 1996; Nichter, 1994). Though, in general, people maintain that tuberculosis is curable, this view is not reflected in their attitudes (Uplekar and Rangan, 1996; Geetakrishnan *et al.*, 1988). This is seen in Sharda's case — though she had improved physically, her husband and mother-in-law refused to believe that she was completely cured and hence did not take her back home.

It is such beliefs that people have regarding tuberculosis, along with their perceptions that tuberculosis is transmitted through contamination (by actual contact with articles and clothing used by tuberculosis patients) that lead to physical isolation and social stigmatisation of patients (Westaway, 1989; Uplekar and Rangan, 1996; Nichter, 1994; Mata, 1985; Metcalf *et al.*, 1990; Kim *et al.*, 1985). The medical fraternity may even contribute to this belief by its insensitive advice which stems from its cultural distance from the community (Uplekar and Rangan, 1996; Hong *et al.*, 1995; Volinn, 1983). Doctors recommend, for example, that the family members of tuberculosis patients should 'avoid close contact with patients, including sexual relations' to avoid 'catching' the disease, and that young mothers should stop breast feeding their infants. Such recommendations strengthen the belief that people have about the contaminating nature of the disease and, consequently, stigma (Uplekar and Rangan, 1996).

Yet another complicating aspect is the image that people still carry about tuberculosis patients — an image of people suffering from cough, bringing out blood in their sputum, taking medicines for years on end and wasting away. This is despite an advertised programme in place. And only until such time that people actually see tuberculosis patients (a large majority of them) improving and getting on with their lives, will health education messages alone reassure them about the curable nature of the disease. Sharda developed tuberculosis a second time and that too within months after she had completed the entire course of recommended treatment. It is this end result that would register in people's mind and not the fact that this relapse or re-infection that Sharda suffered was only because of the emotional trauma she had to face because of social rejection which led to the subsequent physical deterioration of her general health.

Symptom Awareness and Help Seeking for Tuberculosis

Banerji and Andersen (1963) showed that the level of worry because of symptoms suggestive of tuberculosis which prompted them to seek help from health providers was very high especially among the sputum-positive infectious cases of tuberculosis — the epidemiological target of any tuberculosis control measures. People do associate the cardinal symptoms and symptom complexes of tuberculosis with the disease (Uplekar and Rangan, 1996; Rangan, 1995; Narayan and Srikantaramu, 1987; Narayan *et al.*, 1976, 1979; Krishnaswamy *et al.*, 1977). While cough, fever, chest pain and weakness are the usual symptoms associated with the disease, haemoptysis has very often been viewed by people as a serious symptom which triggers action and is used as a prognostic indicator (Nichter, 1994; Ndeti, 1972; Pool, 1992). A common belief is that haemoptysis indicates that the disease has reached a 'serious stage' and requires admission to a large tuberculosis hospital (Uplekar and Rangan, 1996). The mental picture that people usually associate with tuberculosis is of a very weak, thin person having persistent cough

(Uplekar and Rangan, 1996). Could this be the reason why the early symptoms of tuberculosis still fail to raise the suspicion of the disease in people's minds?

Early chest symptoms, however, have been evoking prompt help-seeking actions by people (Rangan, 1995; Krishnaswamy *et al.*, 1977; Nagpaul *et al.*, 1970; Saxena *et al.*, 1987; Uplekar *et al.*, 1996). In fact, over the years, the speed of help-seeking has also improved. This could be due to better access to health care providers which is also echoed in the fact that action is taken much more speedily in urban than rural areas (Rangan and Ogden, 1997). In the case study given above, though her early symptoms did not lead her or her family to suspect tuberculosis, Sharda did visit a doctor within a couple of weeks. Unfortunately, in this and numerous other cases, the doctor himself has a very low suspicion index, thereby leading to a provider-induced delay in diagnosis and subsequent treatment.

Though tuberculosis itself is viewed as a major illness by people and hence is associated with hospitalisation or treatment under 'specialist doctors in big hospitals', its early symptoms such as persistent cough or fever lead people to seek help from their usual sources of health care providers — local doctors, health centres and chemists (Uplekar and Rangan, 1996; Banerji and Andersen, 1963; Narayan *et al.*, 1976, 1979; Narayan and Srikantaramu, 1981). Some communities also use self medication with home/folk remedies or over-the-counter drugs since they believe the early symptoms to be benign (Nichter, 1994; Rubel and Garro, 1992; Mata, 1985; Jaramillo, 1995).

Tribal people are known to have their own set of traditional beliefs and customs which very often differ from those of the population at large. But in case of tuberculosis, this does not appear to be true (Basu, 1995; Jagga *et al.*, 1996). Basu (1995) found that tribal populations studied in several Indian states did not have any extensive traditional knowledge of tuberculosis — they too believed in the concept of contagion and in the curability of the disease and preferred to take treatment from modern medical practitioners.

Stigma and Tuberculosis

The social stigma associated with the disease plays a major role in almost all its stages — from presenting for diagnosis to being labelled as cured. A closer look at the complex of problems leading to the social stigma associated with tuberculosis points out the various socioeconomic and structural factors which play a major role in the perpetuation of this stigma.

In many cases, patients and their families are shocked when the diagnosis of tuberculosis is disclosed to them and are unable to accept it easily (Liefooghe et al., 1995; Uplekar and Rangan, 1996; Dick et al., 1996). It is this that leads patients to shop around in the hope of getting a different diagnostic label. Accordingly, some doctors avoid labelling the patient as tuberculosis, for fear of driving the patient away from them. Even while the label of tuberculosis is not acceptable to patients, some of them continue to take the prescribed anti-tuberculosis treatment after being convinced by their health providers that the medicines are for prevention rather than cure (Uplekar and Rangan, 1996).

In Sharda's case, when she was first advised by her village physician to get herself investigated, it was the work and family pressures she faced as a woman in the family combined with the fact that her access to these investigations was poor, which led to her neglecting the doctor's advice. Later, however, when the health worker advised her to get her sputum examined, the fear of rejection by neighbours and the community because of the association between sputum examination and tuberculosis made the family choose to go to doctors in the city. This practice of choosing to take treatment from doctors not practising in their own community and avoiding use of the free services made available by the public health care system so as to conceal their disease from their communities has been shown in the case of other stigmatising diseases, including leprosy (Pearson, 1988).

Stigma differentially affects the weak in the community (Liefooghe et al., 1995; Uplekar and Rangan, 1996; Rubel and Garro, 1992; Barnhoorn and Adriaanse, 1992; Saunderson, 1995; Teklu, 1984). Women who have a low status within the household, those who are not economically productive, and those awaiting marriage are particularly vulnerable to stigmatisation, as are people from the lower social or economic groups and those not contributing to the family's economy (Uplekar and Rangan, 1996; Rangan and Ogden, 1997; Nair *et al.*, 1997; Hudelson, 1996; see also Chapter 14). This is true even in the case of tribal women (Basu, 1995). Married women either delay or do not come forward for diagnosis and treatment fearing disclosure of their illness and desertion by their husbands (Rubel and Garro, 1992; Connolly and Nunn, 1996). The gender issues related to tuberculosis are very complex. Smith concludes that access to modern medical care for women in Nepal is limited by a combination of factors — inferior social status, poor education, conflicting health beliefs and illness behaviour, dependency, discrimination, distance to health services, poverty, stigma, lack of decision making power, and gender of health workers (Smith, 1994).

In Sharda's case, even the fact that she was cured failed to convince her husband to take her back home since he was worried about his family being socially ostracised. Nichter (1994) reports that while people in Nepal think of tuberculosis as a bad mark against the family, within the family the stigma is less powerful. Stigma also results in patients losing their jobs or remaining unemployed (Jaramillo, 1995; Dick *et al.*, 1996; Johansson *et al.*, 1996). This stigma, consequently, affects their chances of access to tuberculosis diagnosis, treatment and cure.

Relationship Between Beliefs and Treatment Adherence

Several case studies and anecdotes show very clearly that people's beliefs regarding the disease and its treatment have a limited influence on their help-seeking practices for the initial symptoms of the disease and their subsequent behaviour during treatment. Analyses of the interaction of lay beliefs with adherence to treatment have shown a number of differing trends according to the settings. While a study in India showed that health beliefs such as perception of stigma and witchcraft were significantly related to nonadherence, such beliefs were not predictors of noncompliance in Haiti (Farmer *et al.*, 1991; Barnhoorn and Adriaanse, 1992). Another reason for patients not reporting to clinics for drug collections is because of their participation in social and cultural events such as marriages, births, deaths, religious festivals and fasts.

Among the factors which have been associated with poor adherence to treatment are the lack of resources, low per capita family income, poor housing, and reduced economic activity as a result of prolonged tuberculosis treatment (Liefooghe *et al.*, 1995; Barnhoorn and Adriaanse, 1992; Dick *et al.*, 1996; Saunderson, 1995; Johansson, 1996; van der Werf *et al.*, 1990). Many of the tuberculosis patients who report to clinics belong to the poorest of the poor, who have travelled long distances, spending their meagre resources to reach the clinic. Often, it is when such patients are unable to access appropriate tuberculosis care because of closed clinics, absent doctors or shortage of drugs, that they take recourse to their traditional beliefs and practices. Hence, the question to be asked is what dominates and dictates patient behaviour — the trouble and expense involved in reaching a treatment centre to collect drugs, the lack of social support and ostracism leading to a lack of will to live and get better, the overriding pressures of family and work, or their cultural beliefs? It is extremely essential for programmes to be less rigid so that local programme managers and health functionaries can be sensitive to these practical realities and to the 'problems of day-to-day living' that patients face and make appropriate modifications to help the patients to complete their treatment.

Cultural Dimensions of Provider Behaviour

An important aspect which has a direct bearing on patient behaviour, but has not yet received the attention it deserves, is the behaviour of providers — both in the private and public sectors. As seen in the discussions on patient practices, there are several pointers to the insensitive behaviour of providers which directly influence patients' help-seeking and behaviour during treatment. Providers may not understand the social and financial problems of patients which form the basis for their failure to follow advice on prevention and treatment, a problem often compounded by their inability to explain or advise in a language which patients can comprehend. This, in turn, leads providers to adopt rude and insulting behaviour and, at times, harsh and extreme actions which are harmful to patients, such as denying treatment or striking their names from treatment registers and labelling them as defaulters when patients report late or miss a few doses of medicines, and refusing to register such patients in the treatment programme since they would negatively influence the success rates of the programme. Are these actions of providers also culturally induced?

Doctors tend to believe that their training allows them to make decisions on behalf of the 'ignorant' masses as to the right actions to be taken to keep them disease-free. This belief is nurtured by the current system of medical education and training. It is further strengthened by the lack of accountability of health providers to the people. Since public health services are free, providers believe in their God-like role in doling out 'cure' to patients. Hence, when patients fail to 'comply', they believe it is their right to castigate them. Since health is a mystified topic, people have also failed to question this behaviour of providers; in fact, they often tend to justify their behaviour by saying "we are dirty and polluted, how therefore can we expect the doctor to behave nicely to us?"

Providers very commonly think of treatment failures as being synonymous with patient failures. Among the many reasons reported by them as to why patients fail to 'comply' to treatment are homelessness, illiteracy, alcohol or substance abuse, forgetfulness, emotional disturbances and behavioural problems, unemployment, low income, migrant or minority status (Sumartojo, 1993). These provider views clearly reflect their inability to appreciate the environmental, structural and operational factors which are beyond the control of the patients. This is one of the reasons why providers, in their enthusiasm to enhance their cure rates, deny care to tuberculosis patients having these attributes, and hence such patients may become 'high-risk patients' who, on the one hand, are denied access to the National Tuberculosis Programme and, on the other hand, are unable to afford the cost of obtaining anti-tuberculosis treatment from private providers.

Doctors, in their role as trainers, transmit these values to other health care workers. This is why even lower level workers, who are culturally closer to people and ought therefore to empathise with them, fail to behave in a sympathetic manner. A study of the tuberculosis control programme in a district in Western India shows very clearly the differences in the perceptions between medical officers of primary health centres and health workers as to why patients default — while doctors blamed the patients for being ignorant and careless, health workers pointed out practical problems that patients face in reporting to health centres for their monthly drug collections. Health workers were, however, as guilty as doctors in not spending time with patients explaining to them about the disease or motivating them to take uninterrupted treatment (Uplekar and Rangan, 1996). And even when advice is given, it reflects the beliefs of the health workers, which is very similar to the beliefs of people at large — beliefs which have remained unchanged by their formal training and which go on to strengthen people's belief that leading a morally and physically 'pure' life can help cure them and by avoiding physical contact they can avoid 'contaminating' others. Factors which explain the behaviour of public health workers, to some extent, are the 'work environment' and the 'work culture' of the public health system. Poor infrastructural facilities, limited career growth opportunities, unattractive remuneration scales and constant resource crunches lead to poor motivation to work and a lack of faith in the quality of their own services. Postings in remote villages with no scope for intellectual stimulation and peer group interaction further erode their knowledge and competence. These, in conjunction with the lack of accountability to the people and the indemnity they enjoy against job loss, contribute, to a large extent, to their insensitive and indifferent attitude to patients and their problems.

Doctors who enter into private practice are forced to change their behaviour since patients have a choice of accepting or rejecting them. A totally different set of economic factors guides their behaviour which is characterised by the excessive use of investigations and drugs and a failure to communicate to patients the diagnosis of tuberculosis and/or the length of treatment needed, since this may drive patients away from them to other providers in search of an alternative diagnosis and treatment. Thus, they often fail to realise the public health importance of the need for regular follow up and case holding in managing tuberculosis (Uplekar and Rangan, 1996).

A question that needs to be addressed is the extent to which provider-related factors influence patient perceptions and their behaviour. Successful tuberculosis programmes with high cure rates have been reported from both urban and rural situations where improved access to tuberculosis care — regular drug supplies and interactions with sympathetic providers — have shown cure rates to match those obtained using the rigorous new global strategy to control tuberculosis — the DOTS (Directly Observed Treatment, Short Course) strategy (Uplekar and Rangan, 1995). Hence, according to Chaulet (1994), "what has to be changed is the way treatment is organised and the way health personnel work". On the other hand, there are instances even within these 'successful' programmes, where despite all efforts to provide services in a 'patient-friendly' manner, there may be patients whose behaviour is harmful to themselves and to their communities. Such patients pose a constant challenge to programme implementers.

Lessons for Health and Tuberculosis Care Interventions

How does this understanding of the socio-cultural dimensions of tuberculosis translate into acceptable and effective interventions for global tuberculosis control? How important is an understanding of cultural beliefs and practices of people for the design, implementation and success of health care interventions? How far does culture influence people's help-seeking practices for illnesses and their adherence to prevention and treatment advice and care?

Though there are similarities in the manner in which communities across the world perceive tuberculosis and seek to rid themselves of the suffering caused by the disease, there is not much evidence to show that, at the macro level, these have a negative influence on tuberculosis control. People do have some misconceptions regarding the disease but these, though culturally determined, are modelled and strengthened by social, economic and structural forces. The literature clearly shows that socio-economic factors and access to tuberculosis care have a stronger influence on tuberculosis control than culturally determined behaviour of patients. Hence, attempts to correct these without combined efforts to deal with the structural forces which act as a barrier to effective tuberculosis control will be futile.

As often as we see similarities between communities, we also come across cultural variations between communities. A simple reminder letter to report to the tuberculosis clinic could strengthen stigma in some communities, while in others where literacy levels are very low, it could be seen to elevate the patients' status. While having health workers visiting a patient to administer the drugs could be viewed as an additional stigmatising factor in communities where the disease is already heavily stigmatised, it could be acceptable to others. Before instituting policies to make patients report every alternate day to the clinic to receive their drugs under direct observation or to send health workers to patients' homes, sensitivity to cultural (stigma) and socio-economic factors (cost of clinic visit — time, money, loss of wages), which could be barriers to adherence to treatment, is needed.

Disease control agencies must therefore be careful not to implement global intervention policies without making the necessary local changes. What could work and is necessary is global direction on how to procure drugs and to ensure that they reach the health centres but local policy is needed on the most effective means to get the drugs to the patients based on the socio-cultural milieu of the community. Such a policy can be determined by local authorities who are 'culturally close' to the people.

References

Banerji, D. and Andersen, S. (1963) A sociological study of awareness of symptoms among persons with pulmonary tuberculosis. *Bull. Wld. Hlth. Org.* **29**, 665–683.

Barnhoorn, F. and Adriaanse, H. (1992) In search of factors responsible for noncompliance among tuberculosis patients in Wardha district. *Soc. Sci. Med.* **34**, 291–306.

Basu, S. K. (1995) *Social Assessment Study: Perception, Attitude, Experience of Tribal Communities vis-à-vis the Role of Health Providers for the Acceptability and Demand for Tuberculosis Treatment in Tribal Areas.* Draft report submitted to the World Bank.

Chaulet, P. (1994) Tuberculosis control in developing countries: It is time for change. *World Health Forum* **5**, 103–119.

Connolly, M. and Nunn, P. (1996) Women and tuberculosis. *Wld. Hlth. Statist. Quart.* **49**, 115–119.

Dick, J., Van der Walt, H., Hoogendoorn, L., Tobias, B. (1996) Development of a health education booklet to enhance adherence to tuberculosis treatment. *Tubercle Lung Dis.* **77**, 173–177.

Farmer, P., Robin, S., Romilus, S. L. and Kim, J. Y. (1991) Tuberculosis, poverty and 'compliance': Lessons from rural Haiti. *Semin. Resp. Infect.* **6**, 254–260.

Geetakrishnan, K, *et al.* (1988). A study on knowledge and attitude towards tuberculosis in a rural area of West Bengal. *Ind. J. Tuberc.* **35**, 83–89.

Hong, Y. P., *et al.* (1995) Survey of knowledge, attitudes and practices for tuberculosis among general practitioners. *Tubercle Lung Dis.* **76**, 431–435.

Hudelson, P. (1996) Gender differentials in tuberculosis: The role of socio-economic and cultural factors. *Tubercle Lung Dis.* **77**, 391–400.

Jagga, R. K. *et al.* (1996) Health seeking behaviour, acceptability of available health facilities and knowledge about tuberculosis in a tribal area. *Ind. J. Tuberc.* **43**, 195–199.

Jaramillo, E. (1995) Knowledge, attitudes and practices of lay people about tuberculosis in Cali, Colombia. *Tubercle Lung Dis.* **76** (supp. 2), 106.

Johansson, E., Diwan, V. K., Huong, N. D. and Ahlberg, B. M. (1996) Staff and patient attitudes to tuberculosis and compliance with treatment: An exploratory study in Vietnam. *Tubercle Lung Dis.* **77**, 178–183.

Kim, S., *et al.* (1985) Study on the knowledge of tuberculosis and attitudes towards the disease. *Bull. Int. Union Tuberc. Lung Dis.* **60**, 131–132.

Krishnaswamy, K. V., *et al.* (1977) A sociological study of awareness of symptoms of pulmonary tuberculosis and action taken by the patients to seek relief. *Ind. J. Tuberc.* **24**, 15–20.

Liefooghe, R., Michiels, N., Habib, S., Moran, M. B. and De Muynck, A. (1995) Perceptions and social consequences of tuberculosis: A focus group study of tuberculosis patients in Sialkot, Pakistan. *Soc. Sci. Med.* **41**, 1685–1692.

Mata, J. (1985) Integrating the client's perspective in planning a tuberculosis education and treatment programme in Honduras. *Med. Anthropol.* **9**, 57–64.

Menegoni, L. (1996) Conceptions of tuberculosis and therapeutic choices in Highland Chiapas, Mexico. *Med. Anthropol. Quart* **10**, 381–401.

Metcalf, C. A., Bradshaw, D. and Stindt, W. W. (1990) Knowledge and beliefs about tuberculosis among non-working women in Ravensmead, Cape Town. *S. Afr. Med. J.* **77**, 408–411.

Nagpaul, D. R., Vishwanath, M. K. and Dwarakanath, G. (1970) A socio-epidemiological study of out-patients attending a city tuberculosis clinic in India to judge the place of specialised centres in a Tuberculosis Control Programme. *Bull. Wld. Hlth. Org.* **43**, 17–29.

Nair, D., *et al.* (1997) Tuberculosis in Bombay: New insights from poor urban patients. *Hlth. Pol. Plann.* **12**, 77–85.

Narayan, R., *et al.* (1976) Prevalence of chest symptoms and action taken by symptomatics in a rural community. *Ind. J. Tuberc.* **23**, 160–168.

Narayan, R., *et al.* (1979) A sociological study of awareness and action taking of persons with pulmonary tuberculosis (a re-survey). *Ind. J. Tuberc.* **26**, 136–146.

Narayan, R. and Srikantaramu, N. (1981) Symptom awareness and action taking of persons with pulmonary tuberculosis in rural communities surveyed repeatedly to determine the epidemiology of the disease. *Ind. J. Tuberc.* **28**, 126–130.

Narayan, R. and Srikantaramu, N. (1987) Significance of some social factors in the treatment behaviour of tuberculosis patients. *National Tuberculosis Institute Newsletter* **23**, 76–90.

Ndeti, K. (1972) Sociocultural aspects of tuberculosis defaultation: A case study. *Soc. Sci. Med.* **6**, 397–412.

Nichter, M. (1994) Illness semantics and international health: The weak lungs/ tuberculosis complex in the Phillipines. *Soc. Sci. Med.* **38**, 649–663.

Pearson, M. (1988) What does distance matter? Leprosy control in West Nepal. *Soc. Sci. Med.* **26**, 25–36.

Pool, H. M. (1992) *Illness Behaviour and Utilisation of the INF Tuberculosis Clinic in Surkhet, Nepal.* MSc Health Education and Health Promotion Dissertation, Leeds Polytechnic.

Rangan, S. (1995) User perspectives in urban tuberculosis control. In: Chakraborty, A. K., Rangan, S., Uplekar, M., eds. *Urban Tuberculosis Control: Problems and Prospects.* Bombay: The Foundation for Research in Community Health, pp. 97–106.

Rangan, S. and Ogden, J., eds. (1997) *Tuberculosis Control: A State-of-the-Art Review.* Bombay: The Foundation for Research in Community Health, and the London School of Hygiene and Tropical Medicine.

Rubel, A. and Garro, L. (1992) Social and cultural factors in the successful control of tuberculosis. *Pub. Hlth. Rep.* **107**, 626–635.

Saunderson, P. R. (1995) An economic evaluation of alternative programme design for tuberculosis control in rural Uganda. *Soc. Sci. Med.* **40**, 1203–1212.

Saxena, P., *et al.* (1987) Treatment taken before reporting at a tuberculosis clinic. *Ind. J. Tuberc.* **34**, 104–109.

Smith, I. (1994) *Women and Tuberculosis: Gender Issues and Tuberculosis Control in Nepal.* MA dissertation, Nuffield Institute for Health, University of Leeds.

Sumartojo, E. (1993) When tuberculosis treatment fails. A social behavioral account of patient adherence. *Am. Rev. Resp. Dis.* **147**, 1311–1320.

Teklu, B. (1984) Reason for failure of treatment of pulmonary tuberculosis in Ethiopians. *Tubercle* **65**, 17–21.

Uplekar, M. W. and Rangan, S. (1995) Alternative approaches to improve treatment adherence in tuberculosis control programme. *Ind. J. Tuberc.* **42**, 67–74.

Uplekar, M. W., Juvekar, S. and Morankar, S. (1996) *Tuberculosis Patients and Practitioners in Private Clinics.* Bombay: The Foundation for Research in Community Health.

Uplekar, M. W. and Rangan, S. (1996) *Tackling Tuberculosis: The Search for Solutions.* Bombay: The Foundation for Research in Community Health.

van der Werf, T. S., Dade, G. K. and Van der mark, T. W. (1990) Patient compliance with tuberculosis treatment in Ghana: Factors influencing adherence to therapy in a rural service programme. *Tubercle* **71**, 247–252.

Volinn, I. J. (1983) Health professionals as stigmatisers and destigmatisers of disease: Alcoholism and leprosy as examples. *Soc. Sci. Med.* **17**, 385–393.

Westaway, M. S. (1989) Knowledge, beliefs and feelings about tuberculosis. *Hlth. Educ. Res.* **4**, 205–211.

Westaway, M. S. and Wolmarans, L. (1994) Cognitive and affective reactions of black urban South Africans towards tuberculosis. *Tubercle Lung Dis.* **75**, 447–453.

CHAPTER 12

TUBERCULOSIS AND HIV — PERSPECTIVES FROM SUB-SAHARAN AFRICA

Andrew Ustianowski, Peter Mwaba and Alimuddin Zumla

Introduction

Tuberculosis has for centuries been a major health problem in developing countries but with the advent of the Human Immunodeficiency Virus (HIV) pandemic, it has become widespread in sub-Saharan Africa (World Health Organization, 1994). This region bears the brunt of both these diseases and this chapter considers co-infection from the view-points of the peoples, practising clinician/medical officer, health services and governments of sub-Saharan Africa, predominately using data derived from the region.

The Impact of the HIV/AIDS Pandemic on Tuberculosis

Several factors increase the risk of an infected person developing tuberculosis but over the last decade infection by the Human Immunodeficiency Virus (HIV) has emerged, by far, as the most important of these factors for two reasons (World Health Organization, 1994). First, it greatly increases the chance of a person already infected by the tubercle bacillus developing the disease. Non-immunocompromised people who have overcome the primary infection have about a 5% chance of developing post-primary tuberculosis sometime during the remainder of their lives. In a HIV-positive person, this chance is as high as 50%. As those infected with HIV have a shortened life expectancy, the annual risk of developing tuberculosis is around 8%, over 20 times higher than in HIV-negative persons (Dolin *et al.*, 1994).

Secondly, the chance of an HIV-infected person developing tuberculosis following exposure to an infectious source case, resulting in primary infection or in re-infection, is very high. Not only is the chance of infection very high, the subsequent progression from infection to overt disease occurs over a few months rather than years or even decades. The combination of the high ratio of infection to disease and the 'telescoping' of the progression of disease explains the explosive mini-epidemics reported among HIV-infected persons that originally drew attention to the serious nature of the interaction between the 'Cursed Duet' of HIV and the tubercle bacillus (Chretien, 1990).

The impact that the HIV pandemic is having on tuberculosis in sub-Saharan Africa reflects upon the number of persons infected with both this virus and *M. tuberculosis* — so-called dual infection. In 1996, the estimated number of dually infected persons had risen to six million and, as around 8% of these develop overt tuberculosis each year, it may be calculated that HIV was responsible for an additional 480,000 cases of tuberculosis in that year, of which at least 300,000 occurred in Africa (World Health Organization, 1996).

At the present time, it is estimated that about 10% of all cases of tuberculosis worldwide, and between 30 and 70% of those in Africa, are HIV related. By the year 2000, nearly 15% of all cases of tuberculosis could be HIV related, with about 1.4 million cases worldwide and 600,000 in Africa (Dolin *et al.*, 1994). This will have a very serious effect on health care provision, and already several African countries with reliable reporting systems (Burundi, Malawi, Tanzania and Zambia) have observed considerable increases in the incidence of tuberculosis over the last decade (World Health Organization, 1996). Beyond the year 2000, trends in HIV-related tuberculosis are not easily predicted as they depend on changes in the annual tuberculosis infection rate, the rate and prevalence of infection by *M. tuberculosis* in the at-risk age group, and the prevalence of HIV infection. Different scenarios applicable to Africa have been calculated (Schulzer *et al.*, 1992) and, in the worst-case scenario, one in 50 of the total population, and one in 25 of the at-risk population, could develop tuberculosis each year.

Changing Clinical Disease Pattern in HIV-Infected Adults

Co-infection with HIV influences the clinical course of tuberculosis and the past decade has witnessed a changing clinical pattern of tuberculosis presentation (Chaisson *et al.*, 1987; Chintu and Zumla, 1997; Huebner and Castro, 1995; Whalen *et al.*, 1995). The changing clinical presentation and the difficulties it presents to clinical practice have been highlighted in several reviews of clinical data and cross-sectional studies in which the differences in presentation of tuberculosis in HIV-infected and HIV-non-infected individuals in developed and developing countries have been compared (Elliot *et al.*, 1990; Lucas and Nelson, 1994). HIV-infected individuals have an increased susceptibility to reactivation of latent tuberculous infection. A rapid progression of clinical disease may occur following primary infection, reactivation or re-infection. A higher proportion of cases of extrapulmonary tuberculosis and lesions at more than one site occurs. Miliary tuberculosis, tuberculous lymphadenitis and bone and skin tuberculosis are more frequently seen. A lower rate of tuberculin skin test positivity, increased frequency of atypical chest radiographs and a lower frequency of sputum smear positivity have been documented. Adverse reactions to anti-tuberculosis drugs and mortality and relapse rates are increased in HIV-positive individuals with tuberculosis. The clinical differences in the disease between HIV-positive and HIV-negative children are not as striking as in adults.

Clinical Features of Tuberculosis in Children

One of the bugbears of paediatric clinical practice in Africa is the difficulties that arise in making an accurate diagnosis. The diagnosis of tuberculosis in children is conventionally based on a combination of clinical and laboratory criteria (Stegen et al., 1969). Sputum often cannot be obtained from children for examination by microscopy for acid-fast bacilli, and even when it can the diagnostic yield of is low. Examination of gastric aspirates is likewise often unrewarding. Even in countries where advanced diagnostic facilities are available, diagnosis can only be confirmed by culture in about 50% of cases (Starke and Taylor-Watts, 1989). Several of the signs and symptoms used in the clinical criteria for the diagnosis of childhood tuberculosis (such as prolonged cough, weight loss, failure to gain weight) are common features of other pulmonary illnesses which are consequences of HIV-induced immunosuppression. Radiographic changes may be misleading and often the distinction between *Pneumocystis carinii* pneumonia (PCP) and tuberculosis becomes difficult (Tshibwabwa-Tumba et al., 1997) especially in developing countries where advanced facilities for the diagnosis of PCP are not available. Tuberculin tests may be falsely negative and sometimes uninterpretable in HIV-positive cases. Against this background it is apparent that some children who do not have tuberculosis will satisfy the clinical criteria for the diagnosis of this disease and will receive a full course of anti-tuberculosis therapy. Others who have tuberculosis and present with atypical signs and symptoms may be missed by the current clinical criteria for tuberculosis, and will receive inappropriate treatment. Therefore, the clinical and laboratory criteria for the diagnosis of paediatric tuberculosis require re-evaluation. The potential use of more recently introduced molecular methods such as the polymerase chain reaction (Shaw and Taylor, 1998) and serodiagnostic test repeated (Wilkins, 1998) for the early and accurate diagnosis of paediatric tuberculosis also require further evaluation, although their applicability to the African situation may be limited by meagre health budgets.

Changing Pattern of Tuberculosis in HIV-Infected Children

Several diagnostic, therapeutic and epidemiological dilemmas are created by the inadequacy of the current clinical criteria for the specific diagnosis of respiratory infections in children. The changing clinical patterns of respiratory illnesses in children consequential upon the HIV epidemic have made the accurate diagnosis of tuberculosis even more difficult. Recent reviews on childhood tuberculosis (Starke, 1993; Coovadia, 1994; Donald, 1991; Chintu and Zumla, 1995) have brought to light the problems associated with assessing the magnitude of the tuberculosis problem in children. Studies from Zambia and those from West Africa (Bhat *et al.*, 1992; Chintu *et al.*, 1993a, 1993b, 1995; Luo *et al.*, 1994; Sassan-Morokro *et al.*, 1994; Lucas *et al.*, 1996; Vetter *et al.*, 1996; Lawrence *et al.*, 1996) show that pulmonary diseases are responsible for a large proportion of paediatric clinic attendances and hospital admissions.

It is generally recognised that, due to the overlap in symptoms and signs of several common respiratory illnesses, misdiagnosis is common, especially in HIV-infected children in whom opportunistic infections such as PCP may mimic tuberculosis (Tshibwabwa-Tumba *et al.*, 1997). Studies from Zambia show that the HIV seroprevalence rates among hospitalised children with tuberculosis have risen from 18% to 67% within the past eight years compared to a steady HIV seroprevalence rate of about 10% in children being treated for surgical conditions (Chintu and Zumla, 1995).

The only necropsy study on West African children (Lucas *et al.*, 1996) showed a low rate of tuberculosis in HIV-positive children, an observation which supports clinical data from the studies by Vetter and colleagues (1996) but conflicts with other clinical observations on childhood tuberculosis and HIV made in West and Central Africa (Cathebras *et al.*, 1988; Muganga *et al.*, 1991; Bhat *et al.*, 1993; Chintu *et al.*, 1993a, 1993b, 1995; Luo *et al.*, 1994, Sassan-Morokro *et al.*, 1994). Data from Bulawayo, Zimbabwe, where post-mortems were performed on children brought in dead, shows that tuberculosis was the post-mortem diagnosis in six out of 122 HIV-positive cases (5%) thus supporting the Côte d'Ivoire experience (Ikeogu *et al.*, 1997). Further post-mortem studies may provide information which will assist in developing diagnostic algorithms for the management of serious pulmonary illnesses in children.

Tuberculosis in Women of Reproductive Age

In sub-Saharan Africa, there have been rationalised and improved maternity services since the early 1980s. Increased antenatal care uptake and strengthened maternity services have led to a steady decline in the traditionally known 'direct obstetric' causes of maternal mortality. For example, in Lusaka, Zambia, in the years 1974, 1982 and 1989 the percentage of deaths from eclampsia declined from 37% to 20% to 12%. Despite improved antenatal services, maternal mortality rates have increased alarmingly from 118 in 1982 to 450 in 1993 per 100,000 live births. The rate is probably an underestimate as postnatal deaths may not be registered as maternity deaths. Clinical impressions were that this increase appeared to be mainly due to 'indirect non-obstetric' causes and were linked with the general increase in mortality of young Zambian adults seen over the past ten years as a result of the HIV epidemic. The tragedy of the situation is that the majority of the indirect causes of maternal deaths are due to two treatable and preventable diseases — tuberculosis and malaria. Urgent studies are required to delineate the problem further to develop stringent management guidelines for these two diseases in pregnancy.

Defining the Tuberculosis/HIV Relationship in Pregnancy

Up to 70% of deaths due to tuberculosis occur during the childbearing age group of 15 to 40 years (Connolly and Nunn, 1996). The specific problem of tuberculosis in pregnancy in sub-Saharan Africa has been sidelined and data on tuberculosis in pregnancy and the effects of dual infection with HIV on the mother and the neonate are not available. HIV infection is both widespread and increasing; with an estimated 30 million persons infected worldwide in December 1997. It has been estimated that 1% of people in the age range 15 to 45 are infected with HIV, though in some countries, notably those in parts of sub-Saharan Africa, the percentage infected is very much higher. In Zambia, for example, at least one in four pregnant women are HIV positive (Fylkesenes *et al.*, 1997). Despite this, there are no data on the number of these women co-infected with HIV and *M. tuberculosis*, nor on the number with overt tuberculosis. Given that around 50% of people in the child-bearing age range living in sub-Saharan Africa are infected by *M. tuberculosis* and that 25% are infected with HIV; then one in eight pregnant women would be co-infected. As a co-infected person has an 8% or more chance of developing overt tuberculosis each year, it is possible that around one in 100 pregnancies would be complicated by HIV-related tuberculosis. The actual percentage needs to be determined by epidemiological studies.

For many women in sub-Saharan Africa, pregnancy leads to an otherwise rare encounter with health services, often the first, thereby providing a unique opportunity to screen for tuberculosis and other infections. However, the diagnosis of tuberculosis may not be straight-forward. There is a similarity between certain symptoms and the physiological changes in pregnancy, i.e. fatigue and increased respiratory rate.

There is controversy as to whether pregnancy affects the presentation of tuberculosis. In one study (Margono, 1994), pregnancy did not appear to affect the presentation whilst a study in Cameroon indicated that it predisposed to lower lung field tuberculosis (Kuaban *et al.*, 1996). Lower lung lesions, as well as smear-negative, asymptomatic and non-cavitary disease, were also reported in Rhode Island, USA (Carter and Mates, 1994), although some of these patients could have been HIV positive. Certainly, the protean presentations of tuberculosis associated with HIV infection are likely to cause diagnostic difficulties. Guidelines for screening for tuberculosis in pregnancy are required but little research on the effectiveness and cost-effectiveness of various procedures has been conducted. Most of the literature is outdated (Bush, 1986) and applicable to developed countries such as the USA (Miller and Miller, 1996) rather than developing countries.

Unanswered Questions Regarding Tuberculosis in Pregnancy

The occurrence of tuberculosis in pregnant women raises several questions. Do pregnancy and/or childbirth have adverse effects on the clinical course of co-infection with HIV and tuberculosis? What are the particular risks and complications posed by HIV-related tuberculosis to the mother and the neonate? As a large percentage of antenatal women are HIV positive, and tuberculosis often indicates HIV infection in some countries, should all pregnant women be offered HIV testing, and what subsequent action should be taken to improve mortality rates due to tuberculosis? Are there opportunities for the early diagnosis of tuberculosis in the pregnant woman? Does anti-tuberculosis chemotherapy adversely affect the HIV-infected pregnant woman, foetus and, after delivery, the child? What is the role of preventive tuberculosis therapy in HIV-positive pregnant women? For centuries, pregnancy was thought to have a beneficial effect on pregnancy but around 1835, reports of an adverse effect of pregnancy on tuberculosis led to a considerable change in medical opinion. Indeed, many advocated therapeutic abortions. The advice was "for the virgin no marriage, for the married no pregnancy, for the pregnant no confinement, and for the mother no suckling". Perhaps we should add "for the HIV-infected, no pregnancy"?

Patient's Perspective

The patient's health-seeking behaviour depends on his or her perception of symptoms, the interpretation of their meanings and aetiologies, and the availability and type of healers and health care workers. There are also significant economic perspectives to the diagnoses of tuberculosis and HIV infection.

Misinterpretation of symptoms

Because many of the symptoms of tuberculosis are relatively non-specific, their import may not be recognised by the patient. They can develop insidiously and may not be noticed until they are relatively severe, by which time the disease may have progressed significantly. Even when noticed, symptoms such as weight loss and fatigue may be wrongly attributed to over-working, lack of sleep, excessive alcohol intake or poor diet, and symptoms such as cough and shortness of breath to benign conditions such as influenza or bronchitis (Rubel and Garro, 1992). This self-interpretation depends on the patient's own knowledge, experience and an assessment of liability or risk for the disease. As such, an individual may respond differently from expected by analysis of the community's perceptions of symptoms. For instance, a study in Kenya (Liefooghe *et al.*, 1997) established that the community viewed prolonged cough as the most characteristic and suggestive feature of tuberculosis, whilst tuberculous patients themselves ignored this symptom and most presented only after developing more severe symptoms such as chest pain or the coughing up of blood. In the presence of HIV co-infection these presenting symptoms may be even less specific. Also, in areas of particularly high HIV prevalence, some symptoms are more commonly recognised as consistent with AIDS than tuberculosis (especially weight loss, fever and sweats) and the consequent fear and anxiety contribute to denial and late presentations.

Perceptions of aetiology

Once the severity of symptoms has been appreciated, the person's concepts of disease aetiology have major roles in his or her consequent actions. The biomedical model of illness and disease is well known and recognised in Western culture and medicine, but is often not the prevailing view in other societies. Many have developed complex causation theories involving supernatural and divine forces. Examples include the Tswana peoples of central Africa who relate most illness to witchcraft, an ancestor's anger and pollution through the breaking of taboos (Ingstadt, 1990), and the powerful influences of ancestral spirits for the Yoruba peoples of western Africa (Caldwell et al., 1992). Tuberculosis is viewed as an ancient illness by many African cultures. It is frequently thought to be the result of either previous wrong-doings, unhygienic habits and lifestyles, witchcraft or poisoning. In one South African community 80% blamed tuberculosis on excessive beverages and smoking, 65% thought witchcraft had a role, 60% poor diet, 60% poisoning by enemies, and 5% adultery and infidelity. Alarmingly, 40% thought it was a direct result of having too many hospitals, doctors and nurses (Moloantoa, 1982). AIDS is often considered a modern and 'Western' disease. Aetiological theories vary from racist conspiracies of developed countries to the breaking of moral or cultural taboos and supernatural forces (Goldin, 1994). The Yoruba, mentioned above, relate AIDS, particularly in view of the prominent wasting often seen, to the eating of the life-soul by witches. The Swazi of southern Africa see it as the result of special medicines used by men-folk to ensure the fidelity of their wives and lovers and causing disease and illness in those that have sexual intercourse with them (Green, 1992).

Stigma

Stigma is largely related to the community's perceptions of the aetiology of the underlying disease. As causation theories are varied so there are variations in the causes and degrees of the resultant stigma. Tuberculosis may be associated with stigma secondary to the theories of unhygienic habits, excessive alcohol, lower class status, poverty, past wrong-doings and the breaking of taboos, and social isolation may result from the theories of supernatural forces, witchcraft or divine interventions as these powers are feared and best totally avoided. Exacerbating these is the perception that tuberculosis is highly infectious and transmissible by, for example, sharing eating utensils and close proximity, therefore contact is avoided and the patients are frequently shunned (Liefooghe *et al.*, 1997; Westaway and Wolmarans, 1994).

The community perception may also be that tuberculosis is not fully curable, so that any stigma continues indefinitely despite 'medical' cure (Liefooghe *et al.*, 1997). It is not surprising therefore that studies, such as one from East Africa (Ndeti, 1972), have shown that the association of tuberculosis with witchcraft, for example, has resulted in marked delays in health-seeking by patients and high rates of default. In most communities, the stigma related to HIV infection and AIDS is even greater than that of tuberculosis, predominately involving what are seen as deserved punishments for wrong-doings or powerful supernatural forces, and when dual infection is present the stigmas are often additive. Even those who are HIV seronegative, because of the frequent association of tuberculosis and AIDS in many areas, are often deemed by the community to suffer from both diseases when diagnosed with tuberculosis, and therefore suffer from the combined stigma.

Traditional healers and other source of medical advice and treatment

Health-seeking behaviour is largely related to the patient's perceptions of the aetiology of the underlying disease. Once the presence of symptoms has been appreciated he or she will usually decide to seek advice and treatment and there are several choices available. Most will initially seek advice from relatives and friends and self-medicate or attend pharmacies and acquire over-the-counter remedies. If there has been no resolution, traditional healers rather than orthodox health workers may be viewed as the best route to regain health depending on the predominant aetiological theories.

Tuberculosis is frequently seen as an ancient and 'African' illness and as such most amenable to traditional healing methods. This is supported by the fact that, in a group of South African tuberculosis patients, 55% admitted to seeking the opinion of traditional healers and self-medicating before seeking orthodox medical help (Moloantoa, 1982). Meanwhile, AIDS is mostly viewed as an outside and imported infection and successful treatment most likely with 'Western' biomedical therapies.

Other factors which help to determine the source of advice and care sought are the availability of the differing practitioners and the advantage that payment to many local healers is only required once cure is obtained (Liefooghe *et al.*, 1997).

Compliance

Compliance is the result of a subjective cost-benefit analysis which can be viewed from the position of the Health Belief Model (Becker and Maiman, 1975; Barnhoorn and Adriaanse, 1992). In order for a patient to be compliant with a treatment they must possess some minimal health knowledge and motivation towards health, the illness must be perceived as serious, the person must view themselves as vulnerable to it, and the treatment must be viewed as efficacious and affordable in both monetary and social terms. Acting upon these factors are enabling influences (such as geographical and economic accessibility of therapy), external influences (such as empathy of staff) and internal influences (such as health status and severity of symptoms). These perceptions are not static and vary with time and with the influence of competing events. In the presence of HIV co-infection these factors may be altered. A patient may view the prognosis of his HIV infection as dismal and treatment for his tuberculosis as not ultimately prolonging or improving his quality of life. This decreased health motivation and decreased perception of the efficacy of treatments will have adverse effects on compliance. Multiple pathologies and consequent increase in symptoms will alter the patients perception of his own health status and may result in decreased internal motivational factors. A study from the Ivory Coast showed that HIV-seropositive patients were significantly less likely than seronegative patients to complete treatment (Ackah *et al.*, 1995).

Economics

Information on the economic effects of dual infection with HIV and
M. tuberculosis on individual patients is scarce. In general, costs may
be divided into three categories — direct costs payable to the healthcare
worker and for drugs, associated costs involved in attending for medical care (transport, food etc.), and the indirect costs of, for example,
lost days of work and loss of employment. In Malawi, where a high
proportion of the population would be expected to be co-infected with
HIV, 44% of patients with tuberculosis had time off work previous to
admission and treatment (averaging four weeks). In 80% of those with
jobs the patient was the main wage-earner of the family and, even in
those with no job, financial difficulties were experienced by over half the
families (Pocock *et al.*, 1996). A study from Uganda demonstrated that
patients bore an estimated 70% of the total costs incurred up to the
time of cure (Saunderson, 1995) and in Zambia, in 1996, tuberculosis
patients made an average of seven tuberculosis-related trips to health
care providers with non-medical costs totalling US$14 (split between
food and transport), direct costs of US$24 and an average of 12.5 days
off work (20 days if self-employed). Median lost incomes were US$56
(US$89 in those not receiving benefits) in an area where the average
monthly income was US$60 (Needham and Godfrey-Faussett, 1996).

Doctor's Perspective

The predominant problems with tuberculosis and HIV co-infection from
the doctor's perspective are related to the diagnosis, the determination
of the best treatment for the patient, and whether programmes such as
preventive therapy should be instituted.

Diagnosis and treatment

As mentioned above, one of the major problems is the increased difficulty in diagnosing tuberculosis when there is HIV co-infection. Due

to the protean and varied manifestations of tuberculosis, the most important element of clinical practice in sub-Saharan Africa today is heightened clinical awareness. Once tuberculosis is diagnosed in the HIV-positive patient, several management issues need to be dealt with. The assessment of the suitability of a particular anti-tuberculosis regimen will depend on the availability of drugs, estimated efficacy, side effect profiles, pharmacokinetics and acceptability to the patient.

Side effect profiles. It was soon noticed in some regions that adverse events, sometimes fatal, were occurring with increasing frequency in HIV-infected patients on therapy for tuberculosis. Most common were skin rashes. The use of thiacetazone in particular appeared to be associated with adverse events. In Zaire, a 2.7-fold increase in skin rashes in HIV-positive patients compared to those who were HIV-negative was observed (Perriens *et al.*, 1991), and in Kenya 20% of the HIV-positive patients, as compared to only 1% of those who were HIV-negative, suffered cutaneous hypersensitivity reactions with several deaths occurring from toxic epidermal necrolysis (Nunn *et al.*, 1991). Further studies confirmed these findings (Pozniak *et al.*, 1992; Chintu *et al.*, 1993b). This increased adverse event rate, and hence diminished compliance, with thiacetazone was implicated as the main cause of the 34-fold increased relapse rate in HIV-seropositive patients observed in one study (Hawken *et al.*, 1993).

It is probable that adverse events, again mainly cutaneous, are more common with some of the other anti-tuberculosis agents in the HIV-infected patient (Small *et al.*, 1991) though to a much lesser degree and this does not appear to have a significant impact on management.

Pharmacokinetics and interactions. Research is presently on-going to assess if there are alterations in anti-tuberculosis drug absorption, distribution, metabolism or elimination in the HIV-infected patient. It is also important for the prescribing doctor to appreciate the many possible drug interactions that may occur. Most commonly these are related to the induction of the cytochrome P450 enzyme system by rifampicin, having possible implications for the uses of antibiotics, anti-fungal agents, anti-retroviral drugs and many other therapies (reviewed by Grange *et al.*, 1994).

Drug regimens and duration of therapy. Highly-effective anti-tuberculosis chemotherapy has been available for many years. Tuberculosis is among the most cost-effective of all diseases to treat (Floyd *et al.*, 1997; Murray *et al.*, 1990); a six-month course of anti-tuberculosis drugs costs only UK£18 (about US$30). Also, by curing one infectious patient, transmission of disease to several others is prevented. Currently recommended anti-tuberculosis drug regimens were developed from an extensive series of well controlled trials in large numbers of sputum-positive subjects with pulmonary tuberculosis well before the HIV epidemic. The standard recommended regimen for pulmonary and uncomplicated tuberculosis is a six-month course of rifampicin and isoniazid with an initial two months of pyrazinamide, together with ethambutol (or streptomycin) if initial resistance to one agent is suspected. For such six-month treatment regimens there appeared to be similar cure rates (in patients who complete treatment) regardless of HIV status (Kassim *et al.*, 1995) or CD4 lymphocyte count (Ackah, 1995). Studies from Zaire investigating the extension of treatment from six to 12 months have shown decreased rates of relapse (perhaps due to less re-infection from longer therapy) but no difference in survival rates (Perriens *et al.*, 1995). Thiacetazone should be avoided in HIV-infected patients due to increased adverse events (see above), and in areas without an adequate supply of sterile needles streptomycin would not be suitable. This optimum therapy may, however, not be logistically feasible due to problems of general availability, reliability of supply, and cost. Therefore, in developing countries, a number of different treatment regimens are used. In Zambia and Malawi, for example, the initial two month phase with quadruple therapy is followed by isoniazid and ethambutol for an additional six months. Research into the development of ultra-short course therapy is urgently required. Furthermore, advocacy for more tuberculosis programme support for African countries may yield the monies required to allow delivery of six-month

DOTS (Directly Observed Therapy, Short Course) to every section of the African population. As patients with HIV infection are more likely to relapse or acquire a new infection, preventive anti-tuberculosis therapy may be desirable after a full course of treatment.

Relapse on or soon after treatment. A major problem from the doctor's perspective is how to treat a patient that has a relapse of disease whilst either on treatment, soon after therapy, or when multidrug resistance is suspected. In most areas of sub-Saharan Africa there are no facilities available for culturing *M. tuberculosis* or for performing drug sensitivity tests. Clinical diagnosis of initial or developed resistance must therefore be made and the physician must assess possible treatments without the aid of investigations routinely available in the West. There are two options available to the doctor. Either routine therapy is re-instituted for a complete course or other second-line drugs must be used. The choice may be influenced by the suspected compliance of the patient and the availability and acceptability of the other drugs. If resistance is suspected, or known, then the new regimen must include at least two new drugs and compliance must be ensured by closely monitoring the patient.

Compliance

The vital role of the doctor in encouraging compliance in the patient is often overlooked. An awareness of local theories of aetiology, local healing customs, routes of health-seeking behaviour, expectations of patients, and the prevailing stigma are all required for the health practitioner to encourage adherence to a therapeutic regimen. Health education is vital and should aim to dispel some of the myths surrounding both HIV and tuberculosis as well as diminish predisposing factors and increase general awareness. Unfortunately, all too often treatment for tuberculosis is perceived as long, cumbersome and agonising by the community (Liefooghe *et al.*, 1997).

Portraying a biomedical causation and producing a conflict with local healers and local beliefs may not be acceptable. Stigma may be perpetuated and increased by the health care workers. The wearing of masks or the refusal to shake hands with patients only increases public concern and encourages social stigma. A Kenyan community perceived that, in hospitals, tuberculosis patients were often placed in isolation, had restricted visiting and that special precautions, such as the wearing of gloves and the impregnation of doormats with chemicals, were taken (Liefooghe *et al.*, 1997). The perceived interactions between the health services, health workers and patients are therefore important in establishing the attitude of a community to an illness and hence the potential stigma of a disease.

Preventive therapy

The case for prophylactic anti-tuberculosis chemotherapy in these patients has been the subject of intense debate (Angell, 1997; Msamanga and Fawzi, 1997). Given that HIV-infected patients are at increased risk of developing tuberculosis, the prevention of this disease in these individuals is a logical public health aim. Before the HIV epidemic, isoniazid preventive therapy was being recommended for contacts of patients with active disease. There was, however, concern about the increased side effects of anti-tuberculosis drugs in HIV-positive individuals and a number of clinical trials have now been performed in order to examine the safety and efficacy of chemoprophylaxis in HIV-infected individuals. Studies of varying design from Haiti (Pape *et al.*, 1993), Zambia (Wadhawan *et al.*, 1992; Foster *et al.*, 1997), Uganda (Whalen *et al.*, 1997) and elsewhere (Guelar *et al.*, 1993; O'Brien and Perriens, 1995; De Cock *et al.*, 1995) have shown that chemoprophylaxis in HIV-infected adults significantly reduced the incidence of tuberculosis. The cost-effectiveness of this intervention was shown in Zambia (Foster *et al.*, 1997) and in a computer model based on South African communities (Masobe *et al.*, 1995). A further potentially important aspect is that prevention of tuberculosis in the HIV-positive individual will prevent the adverse effect that this disease appears to have on the progression of HIV-infection itself. Some evidence for this comes from a study which showed that isoniazid preventive therapy not only decreased active tuberculosis but also delayed other opportunistic infections and death in these patients (Pape *et al.*, 1993).

There are, however, several points of caution. The optimum length of the preventive regimens are not known and there is a recognised incidence of severe or fatal hepatotoxicity with prophylactic isoniazid, particularly in older patients and those that drink significant amounts of alcohol (Kopanoff *et al.*, 1978). Nevertheless, severe reactions are infrequent and in 520 HIV-positive Ugandan patients there were no episodes of hepatotoxicity that required the discontinuation of treatment (Aisu *et al.*, 1995). There is also the ominous possibility of inducing resistant organisms (Twumasi, 1995). It is vital that active tuberculosis, which was found to be present in 6% of such persons in one study (Aisu *et al.*, 1995), be ruled out before commencing isoniazid monotherapy. Also, compliance must be maintained to allow any benefit and prevent the development of resistance. This may be difficult in practice (Godfrey-Faussett *et al.*, 1995) and, in Uganda, only 62% of patients took at least 80% of their medication (Aisu *et al.*, 1995). These problems may potentially be lessened by the use of alternative and shorter preventive regimens, often based on rifampicin (Halsey, 1998; Hong Kong Chest Service, 1992). Though most evidence supports its use, prophylactic therapy is rarely employed. This appears, as in many other situations, to be predominately due to a combination of lack of staff, adequate infrastructure support, accessible funds to improve these and, in some circumstances, a lack of political will (Walley and Porter, 1995).

Implications for the radiologist

Several studies published from Africa have documented the impact of HIV on tuberculosis and some of these illustrate associated changes in the clinical presentation of tuberculosis (Williame, 1988; Saks and Posner, 1992; Colebunders *et al.*, 1989; Rieder, 1994). These studies have drawn attention to the fact that HIV-related tuberculosis presents with atypical radiological changes which are more dramatic in some cases and not in others. A recent chest X-ray study of HIV-infected adult Zairian and Zambian patients shows a significantly increased incidence of lymphadenopathy, pleural effusions, parenchymal changes, consolidation and miliary disease, but significantly less cavitary disease and atelectasis (Tshibwabwa-Tumba *et al.*, 1997).

Similar trends were observed in a comparative radiological study of 61 HIV-positive South African tuberculosis patients with 50 HIV-negative tuberculosis patients (Saks and Posner, 1992). Lymphadenopathy on chest X-ray in previous studies has been reported at between 25–50% in HIV-infected adults with tuberculosis (Saks and Posner, 1992; Sumartojo, 1993; Grange and Festenstein, 1992). The available data to date suggests that the atypical changes seen on the chest X-rays of many HIV-infected patients with tuberculosis appears uniform across countries in sub-Saharan Africa. A wide range of chest X-ray features are, however, seen in both HIV-infected and HIV-non-infected individuals. Approximately one third of our HIV-infected patients showed classical chest X-ray findings of tuberculosis. The reasons why some HIV-infected individuals develop atypical features of tuberculosis while others continue to show classic chest X-ray features of tuberculosis are not clear. These may have implications for the radiologist (Scott and Darbyshire, 1997), especially in developing countries where accurate diagnosis of pulmonary infectious disease is often not possible. The atypical chest X-ray appearances of tuberculosis in a large proportion of HIV-infected adults makes it imperative to keep tuberculosis a prime diagnostic consideration in HIV-infected individuals with pulmonary disease.

Relative's Perspective

The influence of a diagnosis of either tuberculosis or HIV infection on the patient's relatives is frequently not considered. There is often a fear of infection and stigma, and there are economic implications.

Fear of infection

An understandable response of relatives to a diagnosis of either tuberculosis or HIV infection is the fear that they may also become infected. For tuberculosis, perceptions of possible methods of transmission include sharing of, for example, eating utensils, beds, bedding and rooms. All those in the home may therefore feel threatened. There is also the concept in many cultures that tuberculosis is at least partly genetically transmitted (Liefooghe *et al.*, 1997). For HIV, sexual partners are obviously at risk but many also feel that those in close acquaintance may be tainted by the same witchcraft and sorcery that caused the illness. Some relatives will be offered assessment at local health clinics and, if indicated, voluntary HIV testing but many will not be actively sought by the heath services and thus must seek medical attention themselves. Frequently, there is a significant degree of denial and often no active health-seeking occurs.

Stigma

The stigma acquired by the relatives of patients can be similar to that acquired by the patients themselves. Again, in view of the perceived mechanisms of transmission, many 'outsiders' and many within the family unit itself will regard those sharing abodes with patients as likely to be infected and those related by blood as being susceptible.

Economics

Often a significant degree of the financial burden of tuberculosis, whether the patient is HIV seropositive or negative, is borne by the family. Help with direct costs for consultation and treatment may be required and costs may be incurred in accompanying the patient to clinics. In one study from Zambia in 1996, these costs for the patient's guardians amounted to US$3.20 per patient (Needham and Godfrey-Faussett, 1996). The greatest effect, however, occurs when it is the main wage-earner that becomes ill or when it is one of the family that is involved in tending the farm, running the business or other commercial activity. The loss in income can then be substantial and particularly so at certain times of the year, such as harvest time.

Health Service Administrators' Perspective

Economic considerations

The main implications for administrators are associated with cost. HIV infection makes a patient infected with *M. tuberculosis* more susceptible to developing tuberculosis and also makes the development of disease and progression more rapid. Therefore, more cases of tuberculosis occur. Also, tuberculosis can be harder to diagnose in the context of HIV infection and this can result in an increased number of hospital attendances and a greater number of diagnostic tests. In other words, on average, more resources are required to diagnose a case. Then dually infected patients will not be optimally treated on the cheaper anti-tuberculosis regimens, particularly those including thiacetazone, and costs of treatment of each case may therefore be greater. The patients may be more severely unwell, particularly with the multiple pathologies associated with HIV infection, and therefore require increased hospital stays and consequent increase in bed requirements, staffing levels and other provisions. Several factors therefore increase the utilisation of health services and costs in dually infected patients (Nunn *et al.*, 1993). In South Africa, in 1996, estimated overall cost for treating each tuberculosis patient with conventional treatment was US$2047.70, though this figure was 2.8 times less if DOTS was implemented, as this was estimated to require only between a quarter and a third of the beds needed for conventional therapy (Floyd *et al.*, 1997).

Staffing and implementation of DOTS, contact tracing and tuberculin testing

Unfortunately, both tuberculosis and HIV are also exerting tolls upon health care workers. Therefore, a further problem for the hospital administrator may be the maintenance of adequate levels of staffing with adequately trained individuals.

The decision as to whether to implement DOTS is often left to local, regional or national administrators. It has been shown time and again to be a cost-effective strategy (Floyd et al., 1997) and is achievable in practice (Westaway et al., 1991; Iseman et al., 1993; Wilkinson, 1994) but its adoption has been very slow. This is partly due to the lack of political will, partly because of insufficient funds and also because an adequate health infrastructure, including laboratories, has to be established (Grange and Zumla, 1997). It is not as simple as just having every dose of medication observed.

It is often the decision of the local and regional health administrators whether to implement screening of contacts of tuberculosis cases and tuberculin skin testing of HIV-positive patients. If funds are available then both these procedures, the first to detect people infected by the index case and the second to help predict who may benefit from preventive therapy, are important for the public health. Both have, in a variety of studies, been shown to be cost effective in many circumstances. Unfortunately, there are formidable operational problems in setting up and running such programmes (Aisu et al., 1995), the accessible funds to implement them are seldom available, and these procedures are often low amongst the local health priorities.

Governments' Perspective

The main problems of HIV and M. tuberculosis co-infection at the national level are directly or indirectly economic. The majority of those infected with HIV, and hence prone to dual infection, are in the sexually-active age groups and hence the most economically active. The implications of this for the national economy are difficult to assess. Another burden on the state is the increase in orphans that results from the significant mortality due to both HIV and tuberculosis. In most societies, the care of orphans is often taken over by the extended family

(Rutayuga, 1992; Kamali *et al.*, 1996). Where HIV has affected large proportions of the populace this is no longer viable and it depends on the state to house, support and educate these children. The financial implications of this are also hard to assess.

Conclusions

HIV has had a profound influence on the epidemiology of tuberculosis and on control programmes throughout the developing world. It has also had an impact on clinical practice and has had a devastating socio-economic effect on the populations affected and their respective countries. Patients, doctors, relatives, medical administrators and governments have all been affected by this 'cursed duet'. Consideration of the factors discussed above are important if the morbidity associated with tuberculosis is to be decreased, compliance and control are to be improved, and the disease ultimately controlled in areas such as sub-Saharan Africa, where dual infection with *M. tuberculosis* and HIV is far too common. Tuberculosis should be placed high on the agendas of developing country health programmes and on donor country aid packages for developing countries.

References

Ackah, A. N., *et al.* (1995) Response to treatment, mortality and CD4 lymphocyte counts in HIV-infected persons with tuberculosis in Abidjan, Cote d'Ivoire. *Lancet* **345**, 607–610.

Aisu, T., *et al.* (1995) Preventive chemotherapy for HIV-associated tuberculosis in Uganda: An operational assessment at a voluntary counselling and testing centre. *AIDS* **9**, 267–273.

Angell, M. (1997) The ethics of clinical research in the third world. *N. Engl. J. Med.* **337**, 847–849.

Barnhoorn, F. and Adriaanse, H. (1992) In search of factors responsible for non compliance among tuberculosis patients in Wardha District, India. *Soc. Sci. Med.* **34**, 291–306.

Becker, M. H. and Maiman, L. A. (1975) Sociobehaviour determinants of compliance with health and medical care recommendations. *Med. Care* **8**, 11.

Bhat, G. J., Diwan, V. K., Chintu, C., Kabika, M. and Masona, J. (1993) HIV, BCG and TB in children: A case control study in Lusaka, Zambia. *J. Trop. Pediatr.* **39**, 219–223.

Bush, J. J. (1986) Protocol for tuberculosis screening in pregnancy. *J. Obstet. Gynecol. Neonatal. Nurs.* **15**, 225–230.

Caldwell, J. C., Orubuloye, I. O. and Caldwell, P. (1992) Under-reaction to AIDS in sub-Saharan Africa. *Soc. Sci. Med.* **34**, 1169–1182.

Carter, E. J. and Mates, S. (1994) Tuberculosis during pregnancy. The Rhode Island experience, 1987–1991. *Chest* **105**, 1466–1470.

Cathebras, P., *et al.* (1988) Tuberculosis et infection par le virus de l'immunodeficience humaine en Republique Centrafricaine. *Med. Trop.* **48**, 401–407.

Chaisson, R. E., *et al.* (1987) Tuberculosis in patients with acquired immunodeficiency syndrome. *Am. Rev. Resp. Dis.* **136**, 570–574.

Chintu, C., *et al.* (1993a) Seroprevalence of HIV-1 in Zambian children with tuberculosis. *Pediatr. Infect. Dis. J.* **12**, 499–504.

Chintu, C., *et al.* (1993b) Cutaneous hypersensitivity reactions to thioacetazone in the treatment of tuberculosis in Zambian children infected with HIV. *Arch. Dis. Child.* **68**, 665–668.

Chintu, C. and Zumla, A. (1995) Childhood tuberculosis and infection with the Human Immunodeficiency Virus. *J. R. Coll. Phys. Lond.* **29**, 92–94.

Chintu, C., *et al.* (1995) Impact of HIV on common paediatric illnesses in Zambia. *J. Trop. Pediatr.* **41**, 348–353.

Chintu, C. and Zumla, A. (1997) Paediatric TB and AIDS in Africa. In: Zumla, A., Johnson, M., Miller, R. F. eds. *AIDS and Respiratory Medicine*. London: Chapman and Hall ITP, pp. 153–163.

Chretien, J. (1990) Tuberculosis and HIV. The cursed duet. *Bull. Int. Union Tuberc. Lung Dis.* **65**(1), 25–28.

Colebunders, R., *et al.* (1989) HIV infections with patients with tuberculosis in Kinshasa, Zaire. *Am. Rev. Resp. Dis.* **139**, 1082–1085.

Connolly, M. and Nunn, P. (1996) Women and tuberculosis. *Wld. Hlth. Statist Quart.* **49**, 115–119.

Coovadia, H. M. (1991) Tuberculosis in Children. In: Coovadia, H. M., Banatar, S. R., eds. *A Century of Tuberculosis — A South African Perspective*. Cape Town: Oxford University Press. Chapter 5, pp. 91–105.

De Cock, K. M., Grant, A. and Porter, J. D. H. (1995) Preventive therapy for tuberculosis in HIV-infected persons: International recomendations, research, and practice. *Lancet* **345**, 833–836.

Dolin, P. J., Raviglione, M. C. and Kochi, A. (1994) Global tuberculosis incidence and mortality during 1990–2000. *Bull. Wld. Hlth. Org.* **72**, 213–220.

Donald, P. R. (1991) Diagnostic considerations in management and epidemiology. In: Coovadia, H. M., Banatar, S. R., eds. *A Century of Tuberculosis — A South African Perspective*. Cape Town: Oxford University Press. Chapter 15, pp. 243–257.

Elliot, A., Luo, N. and Tembo, G. (1990) Impact of HIV in tuberculosis in Zambia: A cross study. *Br. Med. J.* **301**, 412–415.

Floyd, K., Wilkinson, D. and Gilks, C. F. (1997a) Health system costs. In: Floyd, K., Wilkinson, D., Gilks, C. F. eds. *Community-Based Directly Observed Therapy for Tuberculosis: An Economic Analysis.* Tygerberg, South Africa: Medical Research Council, pp. 50–63.

Floyd, K., Wilkinson, D. and Gilks, C. F. (1997b) Comparison of cost effectiveness of directly observed treatment (DOT) and conventionally delivered treatment for tuberculosis: Experience from rural South Africa. *Br. Med. J.* **315**, 1407–1411.

Foster, S. D., Godfrey-Faussett, P. and Porter, J. (1997) Modelling the economic benefits of tuberculosis preventive therapy for people with HIV: The example of Zambia. *AIDS*, 919–925.

Fylkesnes, K., *et al.* (1997) The HIV epidemic in Zambia: Socio-demographic prevalence patterns and indications of trends among childbearing women. *AIDS* **11**, 339–345.

Godfrey-Faussett, P., *et al.* (1995) Recruitment to a trial of tuberculosis preventive therapy from a voluntary HIV testing centre in Lusaka: Relevance to implementation. *Trans. R. Soc. Trop. Med. Hyg.* **89**, 354–358.

Goldin, C. S. (1994) Stigmatization and AIDS: Critical issues in public health. *Soc. Sci. Med.* **39**, 1359–1366.

Grange, J. M. and Festenstein, F. (1993) The human dimension of tuberculosis control. *Tubercle Lung Dis.* **74**, 219–222.

Grange, J. M., Winstanley, P. A. and Davies, P. D. O. (1994) Clinically significant drug interactions with antituberculosis agents. *Drug Safety* **11**, 242–251.

Grange, J. M. and Zumla, A. (1997) Making DOTS succeed. *Lancet* **350**, 157.

Green, E. C. (1992) Sexually transmitted disease, ethno-medicine and health policy in Africa. *Soc. Sci. Med.* **35**, 121–130.

Guelar, A., *et al.* (1993) A prospective study of the risk of tuberculosis among HIV infected patients. *AIDS* **7**, 1345–1349.

Halsey, N., *et al.* (1998) Randomised trial of isoniazid versus rifampicin and pyrazinamide for prevention of tuberculosis in HIV-1 infection. *Lancet* **351**, 786–792.

Hawken, M. P., *et al.* (1997) Isoniazid preventive therapy for tuberculosis in HIV-1 infected adults: Results of a randomised controlled trial. *AIDS* **11**, 875–882.

Hawken, M. P., *et al.* (1993) Increased recurrence of tuberculosis in HIV-1 infected patients in Kenya. *Lancet* **342**, 332–337.

Hong Kong Chest Service/Tuberculosis Research Centre, Madras/BritishMedical Research Council. 1992. A double-blind, placebo-controlled clinical trial of 3 antituberculosis chemoprophylaxis regimens in patients with silicosis in Hong Kong. *Am. Rev. Resp. Dis.* **145**, 36–41.

Huebner, R. E. and Castro, K. G. (1995) The changing face of tuberculosis. *Ann. Rev. Med.* **46**, 47–55.

Ikeogu, M. O., Wolf, B. and Mathe, S. (1997) Pulmonary manifestations in HIV seropositivity and malnutrition in Zimbabwe. *Arch. Dis. Child.* **76**, 124–128.

308 A. Ustianowski, P. Mwaba and A. Zumla

Ingstadt, B. (1990) The cultural construction of AIDS and its consequences for prevention in Botswana. *Med. Anthropol. Quart.* **4**, 28.

Iseman, M. D., Cohn, D. L. and Sbarbaro, J. A. (1993) Directly observed treatment of tuberculosis: We can't afford not to try it. *N. Eng. J. Med.* **328**, 576–578.

Kamali, A., *et al.* (1996) The orphan problem: Experience of a sub-Saharan African rural population in the AIDS epidemic. *AIDS Care* **8**, 509–515.

Kassim, S., *et al.* (1995) Two year follow-up of persons with HIV-1 and HIV-2 associated pulmonary tuberculosis treated with short-course chemotherapy in West Africa. *AIDS* **9**, 1185–1191.

Kopanoff, D. E., Snider, D. E. and Caras, G. J. (1978) Isoniazid-related hepatitis. A US Public Health Service cooperative surveillance study. *Am. Rev. Resp. Dis.* **117**, 991–1001.

Kuaban, C., Gonsu Fotsin, J., Koulla-Shiro, S., Ekono, M. R. G. and Hagbe, P. (1996) Lower lung field tuberculosis in Yaounde, Cameroon. *Central Afr. J. Med.* **42**, 62–65.

Lawrence, H., *et al.* (1996) Three year mortality in a cohort of HIV-1 infected and uninfected Ugandan children. Abstract We.B.312. *Digestive Diseases Week.* Vancouver AIDS Conference.

Liefooghe, R., Baliddawa, J. B., Kipruto, E. M., Vermeire, C. and De Munynck, A. O. (1997) From their own perspective. A Kenyan community's perception of tuberculosis. *Trop. Med. Int. Hlth.* **2**, 809–821.

Lucas, S. and Nelson, A. M. (1994) Pathogenesis of tuberculosis in human immunodeficiency virus-infected people. In: Bloom, B. R., ed. *Tuberculosis: Pathogenesis, Protection and Control.* ASM Press, Washington. Chapter 29, pp. 503–513.

Lucas, S. B., *et al.* (1996) Disease in children infected with HIV in Abidjan, Cote-d'Ivoire. *Br. Med. J.* **312**, 335–338.

Luo, C., *et al.* (1994) Human immunodeficiency virus type-1 infection in Zambian children with tuberculosis: Changing seroprevalence and evaluation of a thiacetazone-free regimen. *Tubercle Lung Dis.* **75**, 111–115.

Margono, F., *et al.* (1994) Resurgence of active tuberculosis among pregnant women. *Obset. Gynecol.* **83**, 911–914.

Masobe, P., Lee, T. and Price, M. (1995) Isoniazid prophylactic therapy for tuberculosis in HIV-seropositive patients — A least cost analysis. *South Afr. Med. J.* **85**, 75–81.

Miller, K. S. and Miller, J. M. (1996) Tuberculosis in pregnancy: Interactions, diagnosis and management. *Clin. Obstet. Gynecol.* **39**, 120–142.

Moloantoa, K. E. (1982) Traditional attitudes towards tuberculosis. *South Afr. Med. J.* November 17, 29–31.

Msamanga, G. I. and Fawzi, W. W. (1997) The double burden of HIV infection and tuberculosis in sub-Saharan Africa. *N. Engl. J. Med.* **337**, 849–851.

Muganga, N., Nkuadiolandu, A. and Mashako, L. M. (1991) Clinical manifestations of AIDS in children in Kinshasha. *Paediatrie.* **46**, 825–829.

Murray, C. J., Styblo, K. and Rouillon, A. (1990) Tuberculosis in developing countries: Burden, intervention and cost. *Bull. Int. Union Tuberc. Lung Dis.* **65**, 6–24.

Ndeti, K. (1972) Sociocultural aspects of tuberculosis defaultation: A case study. *Soc. Sci. Med.* **6**, 397–412.

Needham, D. M. and Godfrey-Faussett, P. (1996) Economic barriers for tuberculosis patients in Zambia. *Lancet* **348**, 134–135.

Nunn, P., *et al.* (1991) Cutaneous hypersensitivity reactions due to thiacetazone in HIV-1 seropositive patients treated for tuberculosis. *Lancet* **337**, 627–630.

Nunn, P., *et al.* (1993) The impact of HIV on resource utilization by patients with tuberculosis in a tertiary referral hospital, Nairobi, Kenya. *Tubercle Lung Dis.* **74**, 273–279.

O'Brien, R. J. and Perriens, J. H. (1995) Preventive therapy for tuberculosis in HIV infection: The promise and the reality. *AIDS* **9**, 665–673.

Pape, J. W., Jean, S. S., Ho, J. L., Hafner, A. and Johnson, Jr. W. D. (1993) Effect of isoniazid prophylaxis on incidence of active tuberculosis and progression of HIV infection. *Lancet* **42**, 268–272.

Perriens, J. H., *et al.* (1991) Increased mortality and tuberculosis treatment failure rate among human immunodeficiency virus (HIV) seropositive compared with HIV seronegative patients with pulmonary tuberculosis treated with 'standard' chemotherapy in Kinshasa, Zaire. *Am. Rev. Resp. Dis.* **144**, 750–755.

Perriens, J. H., *et al.* (1995) Pulmonary tuberculosis in HIV-infected patients in Zaire: A controlled trial of treatment for either 6 or 12 months. *N. Eng. J. Med.* **32**, 779–784.

Pocock, D., Khare, A. and Harries, A. D. (1996) Case holding for tuberculosis in Africa: The patients' perspective. *Lancet* **347**, 1258.

Pozniak, A. L., MacLeod, G. A., Mahari, M., Legg, W. and Weinberg, J. (1992) The influence of HIV status on single and multiple drug reactions to antituberculous therapy in Africa. *AIDS* **6**, 809–814.

Rieder, H. L. (1994) Drug-resistant tuberculosis: Issues in epidemiology and challenges for public health. *Tubercle Lung Dis.* **75**, 321–323.

Rubel, A. J. and Garro, L. A. (1992) Social and cultural factors in the successful control of tuberculosis. *Publ. Hlth. Rep.* **107**, 626–636.

Rutayuga, J. B. (1992) Assistance to AIDS orphans within the family/kinship system and local institutions: A program for East Africa. *AIDS Edu. Prev.* Fall; Suppl: 57–68.

Saks, A. M. and Posner, R. (1992) Tuberculosis in HIV positive patients in South Africa: A comparative radiological study with HIV negative patients. *Clin. Radiol.* **46**, 387–390.

Sassan-Morokro, M., *et al.* (1994) Tuberculosis and HIV infection in hildren in Abidjan, Cote d'Ivoire. *Trans. R. Soc. Trop. Med. Hyg.* **88**, 178–181.

Saunderson, P. R. (1995) An economic evaluation of alternative programme designs for tuberculosis control in rural Uganda. *Soc. Sci. Med.* **40**, 1203–1212.

Schulzer, M., Fitzgerald, J. M., Enarson, D. A. and Grzybowski, S. (1992) An estimate of the future size of the tuberculosis problem in sub-Saharan Africa resulting from HIV infection. *Tubercle Lung Dis.* **73**, 52–58.

Scott, G. M. and Darbyshire, J. H. (1997) Management of mycobacterial infections. In: Zumla, A., Johnson, M., Miller, R. F. eds. *AIDS and Respiratory Medicine.* London: Chapman and Hall ITP. Chapter 12, pp. 177–197.

Shaw, R. J. and Taylor, G. M. Polymerase chain reaction: Applications for diagnosis, drug sensitivity and strain identification of *M. tuberculosis* complex. In: Davies, P. D. O., ed. *Clinical Tuberculosis,* 2nd. edition. London: Chapman and Hall. Chapter 7, pp. 97–110.

Small, P. M., *et al.* (1991) Treatment of tuberculosis in patients with advanced human immunodeficiency virus infection. *N. Eng. J. Med.* **324**, 289–294.

Starke, J. R. and Taylor-Watts, R. T. (1989) Tuberculosis in the paediatric population in Houston, Texas. *Pediatr.* **84**, 28–35.

Starke, J. R. (1993) Childhood tuberculosis. A diagnostic dilemma. *Chest* **104**, 393–404.

Stegen, G., Jones, K. and Kaplan, P. (1969) Criteria for guidance in the diagnosis of tuberculosis. *Pediatr.* **43**, 260–263.

Sumartojo, E. (1993) When tuberculosis treatment fails. A social behavioural account of patient adherence. *Am. Rev. Resp. Dis.* **147**, 1311–1320.

Tshibwabwa-Tumba, E., Mwinga, A., Pobee, J. O. M. and Zumla, A. (1997) Radiological features of pulmonary tuberculosis in 963 HIV-infected adults at three central African hospitals. *Clin. Radiol.* **52**, 837–841.

Twumasi, P. (1995) Preventive therapy for tuberculosis (letter). *Lancet* **345**, 1439.

Vetter, K. M., *et al.* (1996) Clinical spectrum of human immunodeficiency virus disease in children in a West African city. *Pediatr. Infect. Dis. J.* **15**, 438–452.

Wadhawan, D., Hira, S., Mwnasa, N. and Perine, P. (1992) Preventive tuberculosis chemotherapy with isoniazid among persons infected with HIV-1. Abstract. *8th International Congress on AIDS/STD Congress.* Amsterdam, July 19–24.

Walley, J. and Porter, J. (1995) Chemoprphylaxis in tuberculosis and HIV infection: Is it feasible in developing countries? *Br. Med. J.* **310**, 1621–1622.

Westaway, M. S., Conradie, P. W. and Remmers, L. (1991) Supervised outpatient treatment for tuberculosis: Evaluation of a South African rural programme. *Tubercle* **72**, 140–144.

Westaway, M. S. and Wolmarans, L. (1994) Cognitive and affective reactions of black urban South Africans towards tuberculosis. *Tubercle Lung Dis.* **75**, 447–453.

Whalen, C. C., *et al.* (1995) Accelerated course of human immunodeficiency virus infection after tuberculosis. *Am. J. Resp. Crit. Care Med.* **151**, 129–134.

Whalen, C. C., *et al.* (1997) A trial of three regimens to prevent tuberculosis in Ugandan adults infected with the human immunodeficiency virus. *N. Engl. J. Med.* **337**, 801–808.

Wilkins, E. G. L. (1998) Antibody detection in tuberculosis. In: Davies, P. D. O., ed. *Clinical Tuberculosis*, 2nd. edition, London: Chapman and Hall. Chapter 6, pp. 81–96.

Wilkinson, D. (1994) High-compliance tuberculosis treatment programme in a rural community. *Lancet* **343**, 647–648.

Willame, J. (1988) Tuberculosis and anti-HIV seropositivity in Kinshasa, Zaire. *Ann. Soc. Belg. Med. Trop.* **68**, 165–167.

World Health Organization (1994) *TB — A Global Emergency.* Geneva: World Health Organization (WHO/TB/94.177).

World Health Organization (1996) *Tuberculosis in the Era of HIV. A Deadly Partnership.* Geneva: World Health Organization (WHO/TB/96.204).

CHAPTER 13

TUBERCULOSIS IN ETHNIC MINORITY POPULATIONS IN INDUSTRIALISED COUNTRIES

Freda Festenstein and John M. Grange

Ethnic Minority Populations Worldwide

Ethnic minority populations, which are found in virtually all countries throughout the world, are divisible into three main groups. First, there are the original indigenous peoples, such as the Inuit and Amerindian populations of the North American subcontinent, who were displaced and marginalised by subsequent colonising populations which became numerically, politically and economically dominant. Secondly, there are more recent immigrants who have become permanent residents of their adopted country, yet in many cases remain more or less culturally and socially distinct from the majority population. Thirdly, there are those who reside in a country for relatively short periods as refugees or for purposes of study or employment, such as the *Gastarbeiter* (Guest worker) in Germany.

Indigenous, aboriginal or 'First Nation' communities are found in many countries and in 1997 comprised a total of 350 million persons worldwide (Report, 1997). A characteristic of many such communities is the possession of a very similar vision of the cosmos. There is a strong belief in the essential spiritual nature of all things, the sanctity of created nature and the dependence of human existence and well-being on the

313

integrity of the environment. This vision brings indigenous peoples into conflict with the industrialised world in which the environment is being sacrificed, perhaps irredeemably, on the altar of high technology, monetary growth and luxurious lifestyles. The health systems of indigenous peoples, largely based on herbalism and the attempted manipulation of spiritual forces, proved largely ineffective against the major epidemics of influenza, smallpox and tuberculosis which were introduced by those who colonised their lands. To this day, indigenous peoples are wary of the authoritarian and reductionist approach of Western medicine, not least on account of the ruthless suppression of their own systems of healing and spirituality by colonial authorities and missionaries. Thus, "The arrival of the Gospel was not always 'Good News' for indigenous populations" (Report, 1997). These and other factors reduce the access to, and utilisation of, healthcare services by these peoples. According to the 1996 United Nations Working Group on Indigenous Populations, life expectancy is lower while infant mortality and disability are much higher in these than in non-indigenous communities (see Report, 1997). The incidence of infectious disease, notably tuberculosis, is also much more common in the former group, with incidences of tuberculosis being ten times higher in some communities.

Somewhat different, but not unrelated, health considerations apply to migrant peoples. About one in 50 people move across national frontiers on a fairly permanent basis and others may become displaced within their own country. In 1996, about 85 million people were residing outside their country of birth. Their distribution is shown in Table 1.

While some migrant people choose to move as a result of socioeconomic factors, many are forced into migration by violence, persecution, famine or war. This is a problem that has haunted mankind for centuries. The sufferings of the Jews since the Diaspora are well described by Paul Johnson (1987) in his *History of the Jews*. Amongst the earliest migrants who became permanent residents of their adopted country were the French Huguenots who fled religious persecution in the years immediately after 1685 and mostly settled in Holland and England.

Table 1. Estimated number of people currently residing outside their country of origin. (The estimates include undocumented migrants; i.e. those who enter countries clandestinely or remain after expiration of their visas.)

Region	Number of migrants
Africa	20,000,000
North America	17,000,000
Central and South America	12,000,000
Asia	16,000,000
Europe	20,000,000
Total	85,000,000

It was hoped that, after the Second World War with its appalling Holocaust, all racial, religious and political oppression would cease, but this was not to be and we have continued to witness such horrors in Africa, the Indian subcontinent, the Far-East and the former Yugoslavia. As a consequence, victims from these and other countries where there is war, famine, and religious and political persecution are forced to seek security in the industrialised democratic countries of Northern Europe and North America.

In recent years, voluntary migration to the traditional industrialised receiving countries has become more restricted and an increasing proportion of migrants are now refugees or asylum seekers. Whether enforced and sudden or voluntary and planned, the psychological stresses of migration are enormous and, as a result, stress-related illnesses are common. Separation from family and friends is painful; disruption of a former network of social support increases vulnerability, and adaptation to a new set of cultural norms, roles and responsibilities is both demanding and difficult (Bollini and Siem, 1995). Another cause of considerable stress is the negative stereotyping of some migrant groups in host countries and the racism and discrimination which this generates, sometimes even within the health services.

Migrant women from developing countries are especially vulnerable to stress. They tend to have little schooling at the time of their move and this will restrict them to low-status jobs and will limit their possibility of interacting with the host community. In particular, they may experience unnecessary distress within the gender-insensitive Western medical services (see Chapter 14).

For these reasons, the health of immigrant peoples, even those preselected on grounds of initial good health and ability to find gainful employment, is often worse than that of the native population (Bollini and Siem, 1995). This problem is compounded by their reduced ability to establish 'entitlement' to good health care. In this technical sense, 'entitlement' refers to the ability of a person within a given social environment to establish ownership or right of use of given commodities, such as health services, or decent living and working conditions. Even when access to health facilities is unrestricted by geographical or economic factors, there are often racial, cultural and linguistic barriers to effective use of these facilities and adherence to treatment regimens (Sumartojo, 1993).

Some groups may also have reduced entitlements to services because of their legal status in the receiving country. The most extreme situation is that of 'irregular' migrants (those who enter the country clandestinely or remain after expiration of their visas) for whom access to health care, especially for a disease such as tuberculosis that requires repeated consultations, is extremely difficult (Rieder *et al.*, 1994).

An additional population requiring consideration consists of internally displaced persons within a society. These, who may or may not belong to ethnic minorities, reject the materialistic values and lifestyles of the industrialised nations and become 'travellers'. Some earn a living by simple craftsmanship while others rely on begging or on the state welfare system. Some 'travellers' adopt so-called 'New Age' beliefs which, paradoxically, closely resemble the ancient environment-conscious belief systems held by many indigenous peoples (see above). Their itinerant lifestyle coupled to their belief systems and their intrinsic hostility towards 'authority' compromise their access to long-term medical care and, in common with the groups discussed above, their general level of health is lower than in the more settled population (Bunce, 1996).

The Nature of Tuberculosis in Ethnic Minority Populations

Experience in many countries has shown that tuberculosis in ethnic minority groups differs from that in the indigenous population in both prevalence and presentation. In the UK, a relatively high prevalence of tuberculosis has, at various times, been observed among immigrants from Ireland, China, Africa the Caribbean, and the Indian subcontinent. In 1993, over half the notified cases of tuberculosis in England and Wales occurred in ethnic minority groups although these comprised only 6% of the population (Kumar *et al.*, 1997). Similar peaks in the prevalence of tuberculosis, related to ethnic minority groups, have been observed in several other developed countries. For further details see Advisory Committee for Elimination of Tuberculosis (1990), Davies (1998), Broekmans (1993), Enarson *et al.* (1979, 1987, 1990) Gaudette and Ellis (1993), Rieder (1989), Tala (1989), Wang *et al.* (1991), and Zuber *et al.* (1996).

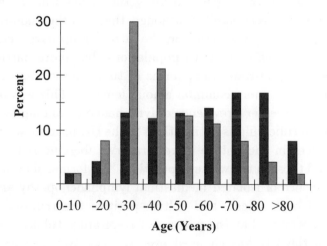

Fig. 1. The age distribution of patients of European ■ and Indian subcontinent ethnic origin ▨ in South-East England.

Tuberculosis patients in ethnic minority groups in the industrialised countries are usually in a younger age range than those in the majority population. An example is given in Fig. 1 which shows the age distribution of patients of European and Indian subcontinent ethnic origin in South-East England. Similar variations in age distribution between ethnic minority population and non-Hispanic whites have been reported in the USA (Centers for Disease Control, 1989).

Another characteristic of tuberculosis in ethnic minority groups that has been observed in many countries is the relatively high incidence of non-pulmonary forms of the disease, notably lymphadenitis. In a study of cases of bacteriologically-confirmed tuberculosis in South-East England between 1984 and 1991, 1,593 of 3,451 (46%) of patients of Indian subcontinent (ISC) ethnic origin and 772 of 4,805 (19%) of indigenous white patients had non-pulmonary manifestations of the disease (Table 2; Grange *et al.*, 1995). Lymphadenitis and tuberculosis involving bones and joints were particularly common in the ISC patients whereas genito-urinary tuberculosis was relatively uncommon. When stratified by age, the incidence of genito-urinary tuberculosis in the white and ISC patients was very similar although that of other non-pulmonary forms of the disease was higher in the latter group irrespective of age (Grange *et al.*, 1995). In both populations, but more particularly in the ISC group, non-respiratory forms of tuberculosis were, relative to respiratory forms, more common among females. This was principally due to a much greater prevalence of lymphadenitis among females.

Surveys of tuberculosis notifications in the UK have shown that there are differences in the nature of respiratory tuberculosis between ISC patients and those in the white population. The former show a relatively higher incidence of isolated mediastinal lymphadenopathy and a lower incidence of both smear- and culture-positive tuberculosis. There is evidence, however, that the pattern of respiratory tuberculosis in ISC patients in the UK has changed over the last two decades, with an increasingly higher proportion being smear positive and therefore more likely to be infectious (Ormerod *et al.*, 1997).

Table 2.   Anatomical site of bacteriologically-confirmed tuberculosis in patients of European (white) and Indian subcontinent ethnic origin in South-East England, 1984–1991. (Adapted from Grange *et al.*, 1995.)

Site of disease	European			Indian subcontinent		
	Female	Male	Total	Female	Male	Total
Lymph node	171	104	275	488	406	894
Bone and joint	76	68	144	141	155	296
Genito-urinary	61	136	197	54	72	126
Abdomen	34	21	55	64	55	119
Nervous system	19	13	32	27	28	55
Disseminated*	1	24	25	3	7	10
Other/unknown	25	19	44	43	50	93
Total non-pulmonary**	387	385	772	820	773	1,593
Pulmonary only	1,014	2,299	3,313	796	1,062	1,858
Grand total	1,401	2,684	4,085	1,616	1,835	3,451
Percentage of cases with non-pulmonary lesions	28	14	19	51	42	46

*The high number of cases of disseminated tuberculosis in the European male population was due to HIV co-infection.
**Some patients with non-pulmonary lesions also had pulmonary tuberculosis.

The differences in the anatomical nature of tuberculosis between the majority and the ethnic minority populations has not been satisfactorily explained. Many patients of ISC origin are infected with the so-called Asian or South Indian variant of *M. tuberculosis*, a variant that differs from others in being attenuated in the guinea pig (Grange *et al.*, 1978). Nevertheless, the clinical nature of tuberculosis in these patients is indistinguishable from that of the disease caused by the more common variant that is virulent in the guinea pig. It therefore seems unlikely that the observed ethnic differences have a bacteriological cause.

The high incidence of tuberculosis in immigrant populations is usually attributed to a high risk of infection in their country of origin and therefore to a high risk of developing active disease in their adopted country. This is clearly of prime importance but other factors may make a significant contribution. In some reports it has been claimed that tuberculosis is most frequent in those recently arrived in the country and this has been attributed to the stress of immigration (see Davies, 1998). In this respect, it is important to distinguish between long-stay immigrants and short-term visitors such as students, otherwise the effect of recent arrival may be overestimated. Initial screening at the Port of Entry by the Port Medical Officer is at the discretion of the immigration officer who, though likely to refer arrivals from countries where tuberculosis is common, may nevertheless allow an unspecified number to slip through the net. Thus, though some cases of active tuberculosis may be found, it is essential that information on all new immigrants is passed to the Consultant in Communicable Disease Control (CCDC) who covers the intended destination address so that comprehensive screening can be arranged (Joint Tuberculosis Committee, 1994).

Other studies indicate that tuberculosis is most likely to develop several years after arrival in this country; a mean of 5.3 years was reported in London by Finch and colleagues (1991). In estimating the relationship between the time of arrival in a country and the subsequent development of active tuberculosis, it is important to consider visits by the patients to their country of origin. A study of tuberculosis among immigrants from the Indian subcontinent in the years 1976–1980 in the London Borough of Newham showed that about a third of the patients were infected before their initial arrival but a fifth had been infected during a subsequent visit to the Indian subcontinent (McCarthy, 1984).

Dietary factors may also play a role. Davies (1985) postulated that the high incidence of tuberculosis among Asian peoples in the UK resulted from deficiency of vitamin D, a vitamin known to be involved in protective immunity in this disease (Rook, 1988). In London, the incidence of tuberculosis is higher among Hindus than among Muslims and one explanation is that the former are usually vegetarians. Certainly, this group is prone to rickets and osteomalacia and the mean time of onset, five years after immigration, corresponds with that of tuberculosis (Finch et al., 1991).

A further important difference between tuberculosis in indigenous and immigrant populations is the prevalence of drug resistance. As a general rule, drug- and multidrug-resistant tuberculosis is relatively more common in developing nations and so it is not surprising that immigrants from such countries reflect this high prevalence (for further details see Chapter 1).

Tuberculosis Control in Ethnic Minority Groups

As the incidence of tuberculosis is usually much higher in ethnic minority populations than in the majority population, control measures focusing on these groups are required. Recommendations for tuberculosis control in such minorities have been made by a European Task Force (Rieder *et al.*, 1994). The five principal recommendations were:

(1) Establishment of notification systems based on physician and laboratory reports so that populations with a high incidence of tuberculosis can be identified.
(2) Screening procedures on entry to the country aimed at detecting those with active tuberculosis and infection with *M. tuberculosis* amenable, respectively, to curative and preventive therapy.
(3) Utilisation of existing governmental and non-governmental organisations to provide culturally and socially sensitive therapeutic interventions and long-term followup.
(4) Provision of comprehensive services for the prevention and treatment of tuberculosis.
(5) Evaluation of the effectiveness of screening procedures on an ongoing basis.

A survey of countries within the European Union and the European Free Trade Association showed that all had screening services based on radiography at or soon after entry, all utilised preventive chemotherapy, and all had mandatory notification systems. The Task Force noted that screening on entry only detects a minority of the cases of active tuberculosis that occur in immigrants in the first few years after arrival.

Follow up procedures are therefore indicated, but it was acknowledged that there are many barriers to the successful implementation of
these.

The Task Force concluded that screening of immigrants is best performed at the port of entry, before the immigrants are dispersed in
the country, but they concede that in some countries it is more efficient to delegate the screening to local health authorities (Rieder *et al.*,
1994). Whatever system is used, regular evaluations of the efficiency of
screening procedures are essential. To facilitate further action by health
authorities and physicians, a simplified scheme for reporting radiological
findings was proposed (Table 3).

Table 3. A simplified coding of radiographic findings for the implementation of
subsequent public health and medical action (as proposed by Rieder *et al.* (1994)).

Degree of urgency (for public health action)	
0	No urgency
1	Abnormality requiring further examination
2	Urgent evaluation needed
Radiographically most likely diagnosis (for medical action)	
N	Normal
A	Anomaly of a technical nature
P	Pathology other than tuberculosis
T	Abnormality compatible with tuberculosis

The Task Force also noted that, while radiography was the generally
preferred initial screening method, some countries also used tuberculin
testing but that the management of reactors varied from country to
country. There was general agreement that tuberculin-positive adults
known to be HIV positive or to have fibrotic pulmonary lesions seen
on radiography required preventive anti-tuberculosis therapy. Children
with large reactions likewise required preventive therapy. There was
less agreement over the management of asymptomatic adults with large

tuberculin reactions but with no present or past evidence of active tuberculosis.

In Canada, a relatively high prevalence of tuberculosis occurs in the non-Canadian-born segment of the community, but Enarson and his colleagues (1979) have noted that this segment is not homogeneous, but is comprised of several subgroups with widely different morbidity risks related to the prevalence of tuberculosis in their country of origin. These subgroups also differ in their relative incidence of drug-resistant disease. Since the second World War, immigrants to Canada have been required to have a chest radiograph before entry and this has worked well except in instances where there had been a sudden and unexpected flood of refugees (Gaudette and Ellis, 1993). Nevertheless, over 90% of cases of tuberculosis in non-Canadian-born persons occur in legal immigrants who were found, on screening, to be free of active disease on entry (Enarson *et al.*, 1979). This stresses the need for continued surveillance and, possibly, preventive therapy for all tuberculin reactors (Gaudette and Ellis, 1993).

Until 1990, miniature X-ray screening at the border was compulsory for all foreign workers and students on entry to Switzerland (Bonvin and Zellweger, 1992). Subsequently, screening has been limited to workers and students arriving for the first time from high-prevalence countries and has been conducted within one week of arrival in the canton (county) of residence in order to obtain a work or study permit. Since 1992, refugees and asylum seekers are screened in registration centres at the borders. Between 1988 and 1990, radiological screening of 50,784 immigrants entering the Vaud Canton of Switzerland revealed 674 abnormalities, leading to a diagnosis of tuberculosis in 256. It was noted that two thirds of those found to have tuberculosis requiring treatment appeared to be asymptomatic. This underdeclaration of symptoms was attributed to poor communication, cultural differences in the interpretation of signs and symptoms and a fear of being refused entry or a work permit.

In the UK, screening on arrival is undertaken at some ports of entry and the immigration authorities send the names and addresses of immigrants to the appropriate Consultants in Communicable Disease Control who arrange for suitably qualified nurses to visit the immigrants in their homes and, if indicated, to refer them to the local chest clinic for screening. Unfortunately, many addresses given by the immigrants are only temporary ones so that less than 50% of them are adequately screened (Davies, 1998).

Some immigrants are from countries or communities with a high incidence of HIV infection. In general, HIV testing does not form part of the screening of immigrants, although it is compulsory in some countries. Likewise, opinions differ as to the desirability of performing an HIV test in those found to have tuberculosis, even though this disease is a well-recognised complication of immunosuppression. As outlined in Chapter 1, there were, in December 1997, an estimated 30.6 million people infected with HIV and one in 100 sexually active adults worldwide were living with HIV (UNAIDS/WHO, 1997). It appears that, with better education and treatment, AIDS is declining in the industrialised world, but this is little consolation to those regions in sub-Saharan Africa and South and South-East Asia where the figures continue to rise.

It is vital that every effort should be made to encourage HIV testing of newly diagnosed cases of tuberculosis particularly as treatment for HIV infection is now available and the prognostic outlook has improved over the past decade. Physicians specialising in sexually transmitted diseases should liaise closely with colleagues in charge of contact-tracing in the event of dual diagnosis (HIV and tuberculosis) in the index case to ensure that all cases of tuberculosis are notified and that the possibility of HIV infection in contacts can be borne in mind (Festenstein, 1995).

Notification and Contact-Tracing

Contact-tracing is an important procedure in the control and prevention of tuberculosis throughout society, including ethnic minority communities. The objectives are threefold:

- To identify those who have been infected;

- To identify those who are at particular risk, e.g. infants, the young unvaccinated, and those who are immunologically compromised;
- To find, if at all possible, the source of infection of the index case, i.e. the case whose notification has initiated the contact procedure. A child, for example, who has a tuberculous neck gland is not infectious, but is a 'warning beacon' that someone somewhere is infectious and requires urgent treatment.

In the UK, the procedure of notification, i.e. completing the official Notification of Infectious Disease Certificate and despatching it to the Proper Officer, the Consultant in Communicable Disease Control (CCDC) or, in Scotland, the Consultant in Public Health Medicine, is a statutory duty imposed on all medical practitioners under the Public Health (Tuberculosis) Regulations of 1913 (see Keers, 1978). On receipt of the notification certificate, the CCDC sends a copy to the chest physician in charge of the chest clinic serving the patient's home address for appropriate action to be taken. The main purpose of notification is therefore to set in motion the machinery for tracing and examining contacts. Notification is also of statistical importance as the incidence of tuberculosis in any area may be assessed from the notification figures which are subsequently collected by the boroughs and sent to the Office of Population Censuses and Surveys (OPCS-Statistics and Research) for analysis.

Unfortunately, there are some doctors who are ignorant of the need for and the purpose of notification (Harvey, 1991; Sheldon *et al.*, 1992). Failure to notify a case of tuberculosis may be serious for two reasons. First, contact-tracing is impeded and new cases may be missed. Many of these contacts are children who are at risk of tuberculous meningitis and for whom early diagnosis and treatment of tuberculosis is particularly important. Secondly, the accuracy of the tuberculosis statistics is ultimately affected and, as future Government policy concerning tuberculosis control is influenced by changing tuberculosis rates, the consequences could be far-reaching.

Contact-tracing requires team work in which the tuberculosis health visitor/nurse plays a vital role, working in close liaison with the chest clinic, the CCDC and the general practitioner. The tuberculosis health visitors/nurses have an important educative role in their daily contact with the patients and their relatives. Their role in regular supervision of their patients' treatment or chemoprophylaxis is essential, in addition to the screening of contacts and new immigrants. If local health authorities ignore the need for maintaining satisfactory trained tuberculosis nurse staffing levels, they do so at their own peril (Coker and Miller, 1997). Education and training of young doctors and nurses in tuberculosis must receive special attention if the high level of vigilance that is essential for the control and prevention of tuberculosis is to be maintained.

Problems Encountered in the Management of Tuberculosis in Ethnic Minorities

Rubel and Garro (1992), in a study of the social and cultural factors requiring consideration in the successful control of tuberculosis, state that the reasons for long delays in seeking treatment, as well as subsequent patient non-compliance, have received little attention. This is despite the fact that the patients' understanding of their symptoms and their assessment of available health care resources are widely acknowledged to be crucial to tuberculosis control, as early case-finding is essential to breaking the chain of transmission. The authors describe the role of social and cultural factors in the paradox of the continuing importance of tuberculosis as a contributor to morbidity and death, given the availability of effective shortcourse chemotherapy. The patients' interpretation of symptoms that trigger the search for care may be influenced by their ethnic group and health culture, which is the understanding and information they have from family, friends and neighbours, as to the nature of the symptoms. In many cultures, the patient's problems are compounded by the social stigma of tuberculosis, the fear of which may contribute to a lengthy delay in seeking professional care and even abandonment of treatment. Thus, a knowledge of these social and cultural factors is a critical tool in tuberculosis control; but education of care workers, patients, and communities in tuberculosis is also vital to overcome the ignorance, fear and stigma which still continues to permeate society. In this context, women may suffer more from the social consequences of tuberculosis. A diagnosis of this disease may result in divorce, broken engagements and poor prospects of marriage (see Chapter 11). Accordingly, Liefooghe *et al.* (1995) have stated that all health care providers should act as 'destigmatisers'.

The importance of good communication

In a review of the health of British Asians, Ahmad and colleagues (1989) note that the research literature on this topic concentrates on the actual diseases, with very few reported studies on the quality of care and communication between patient and doctor. They also remark that most of the studies have been conducted by white professionals who lack background knowledge of the ethnic minority groups being studied and therefore oversimplify the complex and multifactorial factors that lead to differences in the nature of disease and its management in the various communities.

Many of the problems encountered in the management of tuberculosis in patients from the ethnic minorities are the result of poor communication. The first lesson any embryo doctor should learn at medical school is to listen to the patients and to respond sympathetically so that the latter are reassured that they have not only been heard but also understood. This lesson applies of course to all those who work with patients, but it presupposes that the following is taken into account and corrected accordingly:

(1) The patient has a hearing defect;
(2) The patient's hearing is satisfactory but he or she is too polite to point out that the interviewer is mumbling and is therefore inaudible;

(3) The patient is too anxious or frightened to be able to comprehend what the doctor is trying to explain to him or her.
(4) The patient does not understand the doctor who is talking in
unfamiliar technical terms.

It is self evident that listening and talking to the patient, which costs
nothing but time, yields high dividends in the achievement of empathy,
trust and mutual understanding (Neuwirth, 1997). Some, those who
are blessed with intuitive understanding of the human dimension, have
no difficulty with this concept, yet others, who may have an enviable
knowledge of differential calculus and Newton's Laws of Motion, need
time, guidance and patience before they acquire such skills. All this
assumes we are dealing with a common mother tongue. If the patient's
mother tongue is different from that of the health care providers, as in
the case of patients who come from multi-racial, multi-lingual communities, the problems of communication are compounded. This may, in
turn, seriously diminish the standard of health care that these patients
receive.

The bilingual consultation

In the UK, the health care problems of minority groups who speak little
or no English were highlighted by the House of Commons Home Affairs
Committee in their first report in December 1986 on Bangladeshis in
Britain (House of Commons, 1986): "Because of language difficulties
medical problems are not discovered quickly enough, diagnosis is ham-
pered and treatment instructions are not always understood. Family or
friends sometime act as interpreters, but this can be embarrassing for
the patient and is not always adequate." In the absence of a professional interpreter, the services of an appropriate member of the hospital
staff has at times been requested and in dire circumstances it has been
known for a fellow compatriot to offer his or her help as interpreter.

Ebden and colleagues (1988) discuss the problems in bilingual consultations, including the extra difficulties posed by a language barrier

when the interpreter is untrained as, for example, a family member who is not necessarily fluent in both languages. With their permission, bilingual interviews with four Gujarati speaking patients were recorded on videotape. The interview was recorded as if it were their first visit to an outpatients department. Each brought an interpreter — a family member — of their choice. The Gujarati sections of the videotapes were translated into English independently. Analysis of the transcripts were divided into three areas: the structure of the questions asked by the doctor, the translation of terminology, and aspects of the culture and sociology of the Gujarati family that may hamper communication.

As might have been expected, the simple questions in each interview caused the least difficulty but, even in the best case, 16% were mistranslated. With complex and serial questions which caused more difficulty, even the two best interpreters mistranslated, or did not translate, almost a quarter of all questions. Errors in translations of specific words were frequent; 80 words or phrases out of the 143 questions and answers were mistranslated, misunderstood, or not translated, by at least one interpreter. These included anatomical mistranslations which may be ascribed to the patient's unawareness of the name of that particular part of the body, or because, in Gujarati, the body is descriptively divided up into different parts. Technical terms were translated poorly: 'tuberculosis' was not understood, but 'TB' could be translated.

Other problems described by the authors were generated by the different perceptions which an Asian family may have concerning topics which may be discussed within the family. These may relate, in part, to the patriarchal nature of families in which the father is the arbiter of such matters. Where children were the translators, questions about menstruation or bowel function were found to be embarrassing and were therefore often ignored.

Accordingly, it was concluded that, although from the doctor's standpoint the interviews seemed to be reasonably satisfactory, they were in fact misleading for linguistic or cultural reasons, and the quality of information given in the history in each case would have made the initial diagnosis difficult (Ebden *et al.*, 1988). Further difficulties may be

introduced by the racial background and by the family relationship between the patient and the interpreter.

Ideally, the employment of official interpreters, link-workers or advocates, who have received basic training in the meaning and use of
medical terminology, should be mandatory in hospitals and healthcare
centres where there are migrant patients who are unable to communicate in the language of the host country. In this context, an interpreter
is a person whose task is to translate, as accurately as possible from one
language to another, a consultation between a doctor or other member
of the health team and the patient (Phelan and Parkman, 1995). An
advocate, on the other hand, is not only fluent in both languages, but
usually belongs to the same ethnic community as the patient. With
this additional advantage the advocate is able to use his or her knowledge of the patient's cultural and sociological background to enhance
the latter's understanding of the interview.

Although many health authorities, local authorities and voluntary
agencies working in predominantly multi-ethnic areas provide some form
of interpreting service, interpreters and other bilingual staff cannot respond to all the interpreting demands, particularly 24 hours a day.

Interpreting services

An additional solution is the telephone interpreting service called Language Line, founded in 1990 by Lord Young of Dartington, formerly
Michael Young, the founder of the Consumers Association (Young,
1990). This was initially used at The London Hospital and the London
Chest Hospital, both hospitals serving the Borough of Tower Hamlets
where there is a large Bangladeshi (Bengali or Sylheti speaking) community (Walker, 1990). Language line was the first telephone interpreting
service in Britain and was modelled on existing Australian and Dutch
services which had been working successfully since the 1970s. Since its
launch in 1990, the service has expanded to cover a wide range of languages and now has the advantage of being available 24 hours each day
throughout the National Health Service. This includes its use in the

community and in the patient's home during visits by the Tuberculosis Community Nurse or Health Visitor.

Generally, the conversation is a three-way one — between the doctor or other health care worker, the patient and the interpreter. A special handset with a built-in microphone may be used in the consulting room, thus allowing for a more relaxed 'hands-off' conversation. In open areas, such as public wards and outpatients departments, two handsets without a microphone are required for greater privacy.

Health Advocates and Community Link-Workers are now available in hospitals in the East End of London to facilitate the health screening and treatment, whenever necessary, of the increasing numbers of immigrants, refugees and asylum-seekers from Turkey, the former Yugoslavia and the war-torn areas of Africa, in addition to the earlier immigrants from the Indian subcontinent.

Privacy and confidentiality

Unfortunately, complete privacy, which should be the prerogative of any adult patient in dialogue with his or her doctor, cannot be achieved in the presence of a third party, as occurs in bilingual consultation. In the ensuing correspondence to the aforementioned article by Ebden and colleagues (1988), Samra and five colleagues who were fluent in Punjabi, Urdu and Hindi, emphasised the problems of bilingual consultation and made several recommendations regarding the standard of translation and the desirability of an official training programme for interpreters in which doctors from the appropriate ethnic community should participate (Samra *et al.*, 1988). Their final comment was of particular importance for patients of the ethnic minority communities who, the correspondents advised, should recognise that it is in their interest to be familiar with the language of the land in which they have taken residence. Samra and colleagues therefore stressed the need for the support and help of community leaders through, for example, temples or mosques; "After all, if they have language difficulties it is they who may get less-than-ideal care, and bilingual consultations can prove frustrating and unsatisfactory".

These sentiments were shared by one of us in subsequent correspondence (Festenstein, 1988). At the London Chest Hospital which serves the London Borough of Tower Hamlets, a review of medical outpatient bookings in the 1980s revealed that 21% of patients were of Asian origin, and 73% of these had been born in Bangladesh or born in the United Kingdom of Bangladeshi parents (Samra et al., 1988). Many of these patients spoke very little English and many of the women who had come to the United Kingdom since the early 1970s could neither write in their mother tongue nor speak English. As they lacked confidence to come to the hospital on their own, they were accompanied by their husbands or other male relatives or by their children who acted as chaperones and interpreters but who had to take time off work or school. In January 1984, a class in English as a second language was started as a pilot project one afternoon per week in the outpatients department, and a crèche was arranged for those with pre-school children.

Two English language teachers (one of whom spoke Bengali) and the crèche worker were funded by the Tower Hamlets Institute of Adult Education which supervised and monitored the students' progress. A minibus was hired from Tower Hamlets Community Transport and a woman driver was employed to transport the women and their children to and from the class. The aim was to give the women a basic understanding of English so that they could describe their symptoms to the doctor and understand medical advice and, in addition, to ensure greater safety when they were prescribed potentially dangerous drugs. Some of the women attained sufficient confidence and ability to transfer to an English language class in the community. Owing to lack of funding, the Tower Hamlets Adult Education Institute had to withdraw its support in 1989 but the class was continued for a further two years with support from the Workers Education Authority. Those of us who had worked with this project felt some disappointment and sadness at its closure but were assured that the classes had promoted goodwill between two large and equally important services, Education and Health, and between the hospital and the local Asian community.

Perceptions of disease and its treatment

In addition to overcoming the language barrier, an understanding of the patient's perception of disease is essential. Religious beliefs and values may be more important to some people than health considerations. Concepts of disease and its causation may be strongly affected by religious beliefs and a single disease process may carry several different names with quite different implications in the minds of the patients. Conversely, two diseases with quite different causations and prognosis may be known by the same name. For example, Ethiopian Jews who have settled in Israel use the same name, *Yesambe Nekeresa*, for tuberculosis and lung cancer, so the use of the Hebrew word *Shachefet* for tuberculosis is much preferred.

In the USA, a multidisciplinary team of clinicians, health educators and anthropologists undertook an investigation into the barriers to effective therapy among urban African American tuberculosis patients (Bock and Fishman, 1996). They concluded that the management of tuberculosis "requires a series of interpersonal encounters, where communication skills are the key resource". They then devised education programmes for health care providers based on video recordings of enacted encounters that went wrong and others that provide models for more effective communication.

Education of the patients is also of importance and a number of teaching aids have been devised. Those used at the London Chest Hospital are:

- A tape of a brief and simple description of tuberculosis and its treatment in the patient's own language, e.g. English, Bengali, Syhleti and Somali;
- A similar description in leaflet form;
- Teaching models of patients before and after treatment; these

are simple three-dimensional models initiated by Jean Gimpel, a leading historian of technology, who for many years had been using these models to teach people in rural societies about tuberculosis. With the resurgence of tuberculosis in the Western world he was convinced that this type of model could be as useful in the industrialised countries, as they had been in the developing countries. With the aid of the talented sculptor Katya Follett, appropriate models have since been made for the London Chest Hospital and for charitable organisations caring for homeless persons who are also at increased risk of tuberculosis.

It must also be borne in mind that immigrants may come from countries where concepts of rights and duties differ in certain respects from those of their new host country. The host country has an ethical duty to provide health care without discrimination and, in turn, minority groups have a duty to comply with treatment of an infectious disease in the interests of the health of the community. This duty must be stressed by ensuring that those with tuberculosis are aware that modern directly observed short course therapy is highly effective and will therefore cure the patient and prevent transmission of the disease to others. This may require careful explanation as the patients may come from regions where, because of poor health services, the disease is perceived as being an incurable one.

As well as a knowledge of the cultural, psychological and spiritual dimension of health and disease within a given ethnic group, a patient's personal history may seriously affect the provision of care. Tragically, torture is still prevalent in many countries and, unless a very careful explanation is given, simple diagnostic procedures such as radiology or venepuncture may elicit reactions of terror in refugees who have been tortured (Tala, 1994). In such cases, great sensitivity is required of hospital staff, which should not prove problematical if suitable training is given. Such training should be extended to secretarial, appointments and reception staff who, being the 'shop front' of the hospital, should be made aware of the important part they play as members of the hospital team.

For most people, referral to hospital does not arouse feelings of pleasurable anticipation. In addition to fear and anxiety concerning the diagnosis, once one becomes a 'patient' one no longer feels in full control: it is as if there has been a subtle change from being an adult to becoming a minor. Given these feelings in those who are members of the majority community and fluent in the language of the land, it must be very much worse for those of minority groups. It might improve the quality of care considerably if all health care workers, as part of their training, underwent the experience of being a patient in a hospital where they are unknown. Even the direct observation of therapy may engender a sense of oppressive control unless the supervisor is perceived as a friend and guide rather than as a commander (Sumartojo, 1993; Fox, 1997).

Conclusions

Throughout the world, ethnic minority groups, whether indigenous or immigrant, are particularly vulnerable to the ravages of tuberculosis. Many immigrants come from countries or regions with a high incidence of the disease and screening procedures are therefore desirable. The major barriers to effective management of tuberculosis in minority populations are, however, inadvertently erected by the health care providers themselves. For the effective resolution of this prevalent and important public health issue, numerous anthropological factors need to be taken into consideration and the trust and cooperation of communities and individual patients must be earned by patience, understanding and, above all, by clear and unambiguous communication.

References

Advisory Committee for Elimination of Tuberculosis (ACET) (1990) Tuberculosis among foreign-born persons entering the United States. *Morb. Mortal. Wkly. Rep.* **39**(RR-18), 1–21.

Ahmad, W. I. U., Kernohan, E. E. M. and Baker, M. R. (1989) Health of British Asians: A research review. *Commun. Med.* **11**, 49–56.

Bock, N. and Fishman, C. (1996) Improving adherence to TB treatment with participatory research and problem solving. *TB Notes* (Department of health and Human Services, CDC, Atlanta, GA) **3**, 21–22.

Bollini, P. and Siem, H. (1995) No real progress towards equity: Health of migrants and ethnic minorities on the eve of the year 2000. *Soc. Sci. Med.* **41**, 819–828.

Bonvin, L. and Zellweger, J. P. (1992) Mass miniature X-ray screening for tuberculosis among immigrants entering Switzerland. *Tubercle Lung Dis.* **73**, 322–325.

Broekmans, J. F. (1993) Evaluation of applied strategies in low-prevalence countries. In: Reichman, L. B., Hershfield, E. S., eds. *Tuberculosis — A Comprehensive International Approach* (Lung Biology in Health and Disease, vol. 66). New York: Marcel Dekker, pp. 641–667.

Bunce, C. (1996) Travellers are the unhealthiest people in Britain. *Br. Med. J.* **313**, p. 963.

Centers for Disease Control. (1989) Summary of notifiable diseases. United States. *Morb. Mortal. Wkly. Rep.* **38**, p. 45.

Coker, R. and Miller, R. (1997) HIV associated tuberculosis. *Br. Med. J.* **314**, p. 1847.

Davies, P. D. O. (1985) A possible link between vitamin D deficiency and impaired host defence to *Mycobacterium tuberculosis*. *Tubercle* **66**, 301–306.

Davies, P. D. O. (1998) Tuberculosis and migration. In: Davies, P. D. O., ed. *Clinical Tuberculosis*, 2nd ed. London: Chapman and Hall, pp. 365–381.

Ebden, P., Carey, O. J., Bhatt, A. and Harrison, B. (1988) The bilingual consultation. *Lancet* **1**, p. 347.

Enarson, D. A., Ashley, M. J. and Grzybowski, S. (1979) Tuberculosis in immigrants to Canada. *Am. Rev. Resp. Dis.* **119**, 11–18.

Enarson, D. A., Wade, J. P. and Embree, V. (1987) Risk of tuberculosis in Canada: Implications for priorities in programs directed at specific groups. *Can. J. Publ. Hlth.* **78**, 305–308.

Enarson, D. A., Wang, J. S. and Grzybowski, S. (1990) Case-finding in the elimination phase of tuberculosis: Tuberculosis in displaced persons. *Bull. Int. Union Tuberc. Lung Dis.* **65**(2–3), 71–72.

Finch, P. J., Millard, F. J. C. and Maxwell, J. D. (1991) Risk of tuberculosis in immigrant Asians: Culturally acquired immunodeficiency? *Thorax* **46**, 1–5.

Festenstein, F. (1988) Bilingual consultation. *Lancet* **1**, 888–889.

Festenstein, F. (1995) Control and prevention of tuberculosis in the UK. *Thorax* **50**, p. 1326.

Fox, R. (1997) Are you a commander or a guide? *J. R. Soc. Med.* **90**, 242–243.

Gaudette, L. A. and Ellis, E. (1993) Tuberculosis in Canada: A focal disease requiring distinct control strategies. *Tubercle Lung Dis.* **74**, 244–253.

Grange, J. M., Aber, V. R., Allen, B. W., Mitchison, D. A. and Goren, M. B. (1978) The correlation of bacteriophage types of *Mycobacterium tuberculosis* with guinea-pig virulence and *in vitro* indicators of virulence. *J. Gen. Microbiol.* **108**, 1–7.

Grange, J. M., Yates, M. D. and Ormerod, L. P. (1995) Factors determining ethnic differences in the incidence of bacteriologically confirmed genitourinary tuberculosis in South East England. *J. Infect.* **30**, 37–40.

Harvey, I. (1991) Infectious disease notification — A neglected legal requirement. *Hlth. Trends* **23**, 73–74.

House of Commons 96-1 (1986–87). (1986) *First Report: Bangladeshis in Britain.* Vol. 1. London: HM Stationery Office.

Johnson, P. (1987) *A History of the Jews.* London: Weidenfeld and Nicolson.

Joint Tuberculosis Committee of the British Thoracic Society. (1994) Control and prevention of tuberculosis in the United Kingdom: Code of practice 1994. *Thorax* **49**, 1193–1200.

Keers, R. Y. (1978) *Pulmonary Tuberculosis. A Journey Down the Centuries.* London: Ballière Tindall.

Kumar, C., Watson, J. M., Charlett, A., Nicholas, S. and Darbyshire, J. H. (1997) Tuberculosis in England and Wales in 1993: Results of a national survey. *Thorax* **52**, 1060–1067.

Liefooghe, R., Michiels, N., Habib, S., Moran, I. and De Muynck, A. (1995) Perceptions and social consequences of tuberculosis: A focus group study of tuberculosis patients in Sialkot, Pakistan. *Soc. Sci. Med.* **41**, 1685–1692.

McCarthy, O. R. (1984) Asian immigrant tuberculosis — The effect of visiting Asia. *Br. J. Dis. Chest.* **78**, 248–253.

Neuwirth, Z. E. (1997) Physician empathy — Should we care? *Lancet* **350**, p. 606.

Ormerod, L. P., McCarthy, O. R. and Paul, E. A. (1997) Changing pattern of respiratory tuberculosis in the UK in adult patients from the Indian subcontinent. *Thorax* **52**, 802–804.

Phelan, M. and Parkman, S. (1995) Working with an interpreter. *Br. Med. J.* **311**, 555–557.

Report. (1997) The health of indigenous peoples. *Contact* (A publication of CMC-Churches' Action for Health, World Council of Churches) **154**, 3–7.

Rieder, H. L. (1989) Tuberculosis among American Indians of the contiguous United States. *Publ. Hlth. Rep.* **104**, 653–657.

Rieder, H. L., Zellweger, J.-P., Raviglione, M. C., Keizer, S. T. and Migliori, G. B. (1994) Report of a European Task Force. Tuberculosis control in Europe and international migration. *Eur. Resp. J.* **7**, 1546–1554.

Rook, G. A. W. (1988) The role of vitamin D in tuberculosis. *Am. Rev. Resp. Dis.* **138**, 768–770.

Rubel, A. J. and Garro, L. C. (1992) Social and cultural factors in the successful control of tuberculosis. *Publ. Hlth. Rep.* **107**, 626–636.

Samra, J. S., *et al.* (1988) Bilingual consultation. *Lancet* **1**, 648.

Sheldon, C. D., King, K., Cock, H., Wilkinson, P. and Barnes, N. C. (1992) Notification of tuberculosis: How many cases are never reported? *Thorax* **47**, 1015–1018.

Sumartojo, E. (1993) When tuberculosis treatment fails. A social behavioural account of patient adherence. *Am. Rev. Resp. Dis.* **147**, 1311–1320.

Tala, E. (1989) Migration, ethnic minorities and tuberculosis. *Euro. Resp. J.* **2**, 492–493.

Tala, E. (1994) Tuberculosis care in foreigners: Ethical considerations. *Euro. Resp. J.* **7**, 1395–1396.

UNAIDS/WHO. (1997) *Fact Sheet: Report on the Global HIV/AIDS Epidemic, December 1997.* Geneva: World Health Organization. November 26th.

Walker, A. (1990) Language line. *Br. Med. J.* **300**, 1541.

Wang, J. S., Allen, E. A., Enarson, D. A. and Grzybowski, S. (1991) Tuberculosis in recent Asian immigrants to British Columbia, Canada: 1982–1985. *Tubercle* **72**, 277–283.

Young, M. (1990) As good as our words. *The Guardian*, June 1st, p. 25.

Zuber, P. L. F., Knowles, L. S., Binkin, N. J., Tipple, M. A. and Davidson, P. T. (1996) Tuberculosis among foreign-born persons in Los Angeles County, 1992–1994. *Tubercle Lung Dis.* **77**, 524–530.

CHAPTER 14

GENDER ISSUES IN THE DETECTION AND TREATMENT OF TUBERCULOSIS

Patricia Hudelson

Introduction

Most dictionaries define gender as a synonym for sex. The international health and development fields have, however, adopted the term to refer not only to physiological differences between the sexes, but also to the wide variety of behaviour, expectations and roles attributed by cultures and societies to women and men. In many countries, the socio-economic status and cultural position of women differ significantly from those of men, and these differences influence both the health risks that women face and the constraints and opportunities they experience in trying to resolve their health needs (Rathgeber and Vlassoff, 1993). A gender-sensitive approach to health and illness requires an understanding of the differential impact of disease on women and men within their social, economic and cultural contexts (Paolisso and Leslie, 1995).

This chapter reviews the information in the English-language literature on the role of socio-economic and cultural factors in the determination of gender differences that affect tuberculosis and its control. It is, however, important to note that there is little gender-sensitive research focused specifically on tuberculosis. While much has been written about the influence of socio-economic and cultural factors on adherence to tuberculosis treatment (Barnhoorn and Adriaanse, 1992), gender issues are rarely mentioned. Even less is known about gender-related aspects of infection rates, detection and treatment, treatment outcomes and the impact of tuberculosis on patients and their families. Many of the studies discussed in this chapter were not specifically designed to investigate gender issues, and it is therefore only possible to suggest certain issues and mechanisms that would benefit from more rigorous examination.

Gender and Tuberculosis

Tuberculosis is a major cause of death among women in the 15–44 year age group, causing about 10% of deaths globally (Murray and Lopez, 1997). The World Health Organization (WHO) has estimated that over 600 million women and girls world wide are already infected with the tubercle bacillus, and over six million are ill with tuberculosis at any given time (World Health Organization, 1996a). The World Bank estimates that tuberculosis leads to more deaths annually among women of reproductive age than all the causes of maternal mortality combined (World Bank, 1993).

Not much is known about the differential effect of tuberculosis on men and women. Cumulative experience of tuberculin skin test surveys in developed countries has shown that, in most situations, the prevalence of infection is higher in men than in women, beginning in adolescence. Although this implies a higher annual risk of infection in young men than in women, the incidence of clinical disease is often the same in each sex, suggesting a higher rate of progression of infection to disease in women.

It is also known that the male:female ratio of new tuberculosis case notifications shows wide variation both between and within countries. In the USA, the ratio is 2:1 (Centers for Disease Control, 1990), while in Nicaragua the ratio is nearly 1:1 (Cruz et al., 1994) and in Tanzania the ratio for new smear-positive cases is 1.9:1 (Chum et al., 1996). It seems unlikely that real incidence by sex would vary so widely between countries, suggesting that case-detection rates are unequal for men and women (Murray, 1991). Explanations for such gender differentials in tuberculosis and its control have, to date, been mainly speculative.

The presence of HIV infection has immensely complicated the global problem of tuberculosis control. In 1996, it was estimated that more than six million people were infected with both HIV and *M. tuberculosis* (World Health Organization, 1996b; see Chapter 1). In sub-Saharan Africa, where the prevalence of dual infections with both *M. tuberculosis* and HIV is the highest in the world, the recent upsurge in the number of cases of tuberculosis has overloaded the already scarce health care services and contributed to a serious shortage of hospital beds, drugs and personnel (Murray, 1991).

In countries affected by the HIV/AIDS epidemic, it is believed that women are at particularly high risk for both HIV and tuberculosis. In Nepal, for example, most people identified with AIDS so far have been female prostitutes returning from India, and almost all of these women have tuberculosis (Smith, 1994). Observations in some African countries indicate that tuberculosis has increased tremendously among 15–49-year old women, resulting in increased mortality among this age group. The HIV/AIDS epidemic accounts for a large part of this. Sichone (1993) reports that, in Zambia, some investigators have found a slightly higher rate of HIV infection in women than men. In HIV sentinel surveys conducted in 1990, 30% of mothers attending antenatal clinics were found to be HIV positive. In one urban clinic, women's seroprevalence doubled from 12% to 24.5% in just over two years. In Botswana, where the prevalence of HIV infection has doubled over the past five years, 43% of pregnant women in a major urban centre (Francistown) were found to be HIV positive. In Zimbabwe, where one in five adults are HIV positive, the percentage of pregnant women found to be HIV positive in a large city (Beit Bridge) rose from 32 in 1995 to 59 in 1996 and in an unnamed border town with a large population of migrant workers 70% of pregnant women were HIV positive (UNAIDS/WHO, 1997). In sub-Saharan Africa, heterosexual and mother-to-child transmission of HIV is common and therefore women and children are becoming infected at a faster rate relative to men. This means that women and children are increasingly becoming infected. It appears that women are more vulnerable to HIV infection than men; in part because the direction of sexual spread favours male-to-female transmission. Nevertheless, it is likely that socio-economic and cultural factors have a much more important role in terms of their effect on the level of exposure of women to HIV. The lower status of women in households and society mean that they often have no decision-making power on issues that determine their health and welfare, such as the use of condoms. The role of poverty in women's exposure to HIV during commercial sex exchanges has been discussed extensively in the literature (Schoepf, 1993; Bassett, 1991).

While the literature on gender issues in tuberculosis and its control in the context of the HIV/AIDS epidemic is scarce, it is clear that the combination of socio-economic and cultural factors that put women at risk for both HIV and tuberculosis create a potentially explosive situation. While the magnitude of the problem has yet to be fully described, attention to gender issues will be especially important for tuberculosis control in countries where the prevalence HIV infection is high.

Risk of Infection

Airborne transmission of the tubercle bacillus is facilitated by factors that favour the formation and persistence of infectious droplets (such as poor lighting and ventilation), factors that favour contact with infectious cases (occupational exposure, overcrowding), the frequency and duration of group activities, the frequency of casual contact (through travel or migration), and the number of infectious cases in the population (Smith, 1994). The presence or absence of such factors is related to socio-economic and cultural conditions which may be different for men and women, but few studies have looked at gender differentials in exposure to such risk factors.

A number of studies have, however, shown that in most situations the prevalence of infection is higher in men than women, beginning in adolescence (Styblo, 1991; Sutherland, 1976; Sutherland and Fayers, 1975). One hypothesis that has been suggested to explain this pattern is that as boys and girls take on increasingly differentiated social roles, their risk of infection also begins to differ. For example, it has been hypothesised that, in India, males are infected with tubercle bacilli more often due to the fact that they have a fairly large number of social contacts, in contrast to women who tend to stay at home or work in the fields (Barnhoorn and Adriaanse, 1992). While such social factors probably do play a role in determining exposure to infection, it is however unlikely that such social patterns occur in all of the countries and time periods in which tuberculin skin tests have shown gender-differences in prevalence data. Biological mechanisms may also play a role in determining gender differences in infection rates.

Development of Clinical Disease

Of those men and women infected, about 10% will develop clinical disease during their lifetime, usually within two years of infection (Smith, 1994). A number of studies have shown that in high-prevalence countries, women aged between 15 and 40 years have higher rates of progression to disease than men of the same age (Groth-Petersen *et al.*, 1959). There is some evidence that this may be due to the physiological changes associated with reproduction (Crombie, 1954), and some have speculated that rapid hormonal changes, post-partum descent of the diaphragm and expansion of the lungs, the nutritional strain of lactation, and stress associated with insufficient sleep may be responsible (Schaeffer, 1975; Snider, 1984).

Finch *et al.* (1991) studied 620 Asian (Hindu and Muslim) immigrants with tuberculosis in south London between 1973 and 1988. They found that, overall, more men than women had active tuberculosis, but that lymph node tuberculosis was more common among women of all groups and pulmonary tuberculosis was more common among Hindu women than Hindu men. Hindus were also at a significantly greater risk of tuberculosis at all sites than Muslims, and this excess of tuberculosis among Hindus was found in each of the 15 years studied. No firm conclusions can be drawn from this study, and the authors fail to discuss possible confounding factors such as age, socio-enconomic status or other factors that might have affected the care-seeking patterns of their study subjects. Nonetheless, the authors suggest that cultural factors may be relevant in explaining these findings, and that differences in Hindu and Muslim diets may play a role. Traditionally, Hindus are vegetarians, and previous studies have shown that at least half of Hindus living in the study area are vegetarians, compared to only 1% of Muslims. A study in northern London showed a prevalence of tuberculosis 2.8 times higher among strict vegetarians than among those taking a mixed diet, suggesting that dietary factors were of major importance in determining susceptibility to this disease (Chanarin and Stephenson, 1988).

Diagnosis

The WHO estimates that as many as half of all cases of active tuberculosis are never diagnosed (World Health Organization, 1991). Socioeconomic and cultural factors clearly play a role, although little is known about the effect of such factors on gender differences in case-finding. While there appear to be no studies that have specifically looked at reasons for gender differences in case-finding for tuberculosis, inferences may be made from gender-sensitive research on other diseases and from tuberculosis studies of active case-finding and patient reports of delayed care-seeking.

Studies carried out in developed countries have shown that women report more symptoms and use health services more than men (Mechanic, 1978). Women cannot, however, be taken as a homogeneous group. Some researchers found that mothers with pre-school children report fewer symptoms and use health services less than other women, and that employed women report less illness than housewives. Also, married women report fewer illnesses than women who are single, widowed or divorced. These studies suggest that women with more demanding roles may have less time to seek health care. Few studies have attempted to document and explain differential patterns of health service use among women and men in developing countries (Kutzin, 1993). Nonetheless, a few studies do suggest gender differentials.

In a study in Nepal of 297 new sputum-positive cases of tuberculosis, it was found that the mean reported duration of cough before diagnosis was 27 days for men and 49 for women (Smith, 1994). In a study comparing two methods of case-finding in eastern Nepal, Cassels *et al.* (1982) observed that active case-finding carried out by mobile teams identified a higher proportion of females, especially women over 45 years of age, than self-referral of patients to existing health services. The overall male:female ratio in active case-finding patients was 1.2:1 compared to 2.6:1 in the self-referral group. In another study in Nepal, it was found that mobile clinics had a much higher rate of females attending for sputum examinations than health posts and fixed clinics (Harper *et al.*, 1996). In an in-depth study of health post utilisation in the Lalitpur district, Nepal, men and women were compared and it was found that, in rural areas, men were more likely to use health posts while women tended to use traditional care more often. They also found that urban women used traditional care less than rural women. The authors suggest that these results reflect women's increased access to health posts in urban areas, as compared with rural areas.

Studies in Thailand and India suggest that care-seeking for women and children is affected by constraints on the women's time. In Thailand, women and children of all ages were under-represented in malaria clinics, based on sero-epidemiological findings. Village volunteers and rural health posts also reported detecting mainly male cases (Ettling *et al.*, 1989). In India, women between the ages of 20 and 49 and young children up to nine years of age were extremely under-represented, while there was over-representation of adult males. Furthermore, there was a strong correlation between the proportion of small children and of women aged 25–39 years, suggesting that mothers took advantage of consultations for their children to address their own health care needs (Beljaev, 1986). Reuben (1993) attributes such similarities across sites to the fact that underprivileged women are generally loaded with household chores and the care of young children, and so are less likely than men to seek care from health services far from home unless the illness becomes very serious. Although tuberculosis was not looked at specifically in these studies, one would assume that similar patterns of care-seeking would be found.

Cost concerns also have an important influence on care-seeking patterns, both in terms of the initial decision to seek care and subsequent adherence to prescribed treatment. User fees, drugs and laboratory costs, travel expenses, and opportunity costs are faced by all potential users of health services, not just women, but these costs appear to present more of a barrier for women because they tend to be poorer than men, are of lower status, are discriminated against, and possibly because the opportunity cost of their time is greater (Kutzin, 1993).

Time constraints vary seasonally, as do other variables such as income, availability of cash, and food supply, and affect the use of medical services. At harvest time, even though more cash is available, women have less time available for health-seeking (Cosminsky, 1987). Leslie (1991) suggests that opportunity costs pose greater obstacles to health service utilisation for women than for men. The need to give up a half day or full day's work to seek care may be too great a price to pay (Kutzin, 1993).

Adherence to Treatment

Poor adherence to drug therapy is the single most important cause of treatment failure in tuberculosis programmes. Unfortunately, health care providers and researchers have tended to see non adherence as a patient problem, ignoring environmental, structural and operational factors. But, in fact, those patients least likely to comply are those least *able* to comply — it would be necessary to ensure easy access to treatment for all persons before ascribing non adherence to patient-related shortcomings (Farmer, 1997; Chaulet, 1987).

A study in Ghana by van der Werf *et al.* (1990) revealed that non adherence to therapy was significantly more common among men than women although the authors do not provide any explanation for these findings. Financial barriers were reported by almost all defaulting patients, despite the fact that the hospital had been operating a poor and sick fund. Travel expenses could not be reimbursed and this was often a greater financial burden than the hospital charge. Cost may have been more of a barrier for men than women (since women in this part of Ghana are active traders and have control over their own income), or other factors may be responsible for observed gender differences in default rates.

Smith (1994) has suggested that the reason that several studies have shown that women are more compliant with tuberculosis treatment is that barriers to diagnosis of tuberculosis in women screen out those women most likely to default from treatment. Those who overcome diagnostic barriers are highly motivated, and thus most likely to comply with treatment. In their comparison of active case-finding and self-referral, Cassels *et al.* (1982) showed that patients detected by active case-finding defaulted from treatment more than self-referral patients, and older women were more likely to default than older men. Among the patients detected by active case-finding ranged over 44 years, 26 out of 29 (90%) of females compared to 18 out of 30 males (60%) had periods of default ($p < 0.025$). Interestingly, in the active case-finding group, proximity to a health facility appears not to influence the likelihood of default. Those patients detected by active case-finding were reluctant to seek treatment from any health facility, even though these facilities were easily accessible. Many patients refused to accept treatment and those that accepted often defaulted early.

In the Philippines, the reasons for default were quite different for men and women (Nichter, 1994). There was a high default rate among pregnant/lactating women because they feared the drugs would cause miscarriage, dry up their milk or harm the baby. In contrast, men reported stopping treatment once symptoms abated because they found it too hard to give up alcohol. Drinking plays an important social role and abstinence marks a man as seriously ill.

The Social Impact of Tuberculosis

Tuberculosis has its greatest impact on adults aged between 15 and 59 years. Because these are the most economically-productive people in society, and are also the parents on whom survival and development of children depend, the social and economic burden of tuberculosis must be great. Nonetheless, few studies have considered gender differentials in duration of incapacity from tuberculosis or the impact of tuberculosis on domestic work, social activities and personal life. Because women tend to be the poorest and most disadvantaged members of households, the impact of tuberculosis is likely to be greater on women than men.

Illness in women has consequences for both themselves and their families. A number of researchers have observed that when women are ill they wait longer than men before reporting their illness (Ettling et al., 1989; Cosminsky, 1987), and tend to disregard their own illness until it severely interferes with their daily activities (Bonilla et al., 1991). This has potentially serious consequences for other family members. A long-term study in Matlab, Bangladesh, revealed a strong correlation between maternal survival and child survival to age ten. A father's death was associated with an increase in child mortality of six per 1,000, irrespective of the child's gender, but a mother's death was associated with increases in child mortality of 50 per 1,000 in sons and 144 per 1,000 in daughters (Over et al., 1992).

There do not appear to be any studies that have specifically addressed the impact of tuberculosis in women on other household members. It has been suggested that children are more likely to be infected if their mother has tuberculosis than if their father has this disease. If this is true, it argues for an increased focus on detection and treatment of tuberculosis in women in order to reduce the risk of infection in children. Experience in tropical diseases reveals that women's illness has profound effects on the social and economic well-being of households (Watts *et al.*, 1989). There is no reason to think that the situation would be any different for tuberculosis, although the relative impact of tuberculosis as opposed to other diseases on women and their families is unknown.

The stigma associated with certain diseases appears to be greater for women than for men. In the case of schistosomiasis, for example, there is evidence that in several African countries it is thought to be associated with immoral sexual behaviour in women, but considered a sign of virility in men (Vlassoff and Bonilla, 1994). This means that women may be less inclined to admit illness and seek care. The social and economic consequences of disfiguring diseases such as leprosy are often devastating for women, and include ostracism and abandonment, job loss and divorce (Ulrich and Zulueta, 1993).

Very few studies have directly addressed gender differentials in stigma and tuberculosis. In one such study in Pakistan it was noted that the stigma of tuberculosis on women was particularly harsh. Women with tuberculosis were likely to be divorced, and husbands often took a second wife. Unmarried women with tuberculosis were likely to have more difficulty finding a marriage partner than those without tuberculosis (Liefooghe *et al.*, 1995).

Dinesh and colleagues (unpublished) conducted in-depth interviews with 16 tuberculosis patients who attended a tuberculosis clinic run by a non-governmental organisation in Bombay. They found that men worried more about loss of wages, financial difficulties, reduced capacity for work, poor job performance, and the consequences of long absences from work. Married women were concerned and anxious about rejection by husbands, harassment by in-laws, and unmarried women worried about their reduced chances of marriage, in addition to their concerns about dismissal from work. The wage-earning capacity of both men and women was affected, but women feared loss of employment (they were often hired as domestic help) whereas men, often being self-employed, lost income but not employment. Ten of 13 wage-earning respondents claimed that after the onset of illness their wages had decreased from Rs. 2500 to about Rs. 1000–1500 per month.

In addition, married men and single women perceived a greater level of family support for the initiation and completion of treatment (Dinesh *et al.*, 1995). Married women tried, often unsuccessfully, to hide their illness for fear of desertion, rejection or blame for bringing the disease into the household. The extent of family support to unmarried daughters is illustrated by one case in which a mother told others that it was she rather than her unmarried daughter who had tuberculosis, so as to protect her daughter from the stigma attached to visiting the tuberculosis clinic. Married women did not receive the same level of support as unmarried women: some were abandoned by their husbands and some were sent back to their natal homes until they were cured. The researchers also observed that male respondents expected and received care from their wives, while the reverse was seldom true.

Not only can women's illness effect their own and their families' lives, but illness of other household members can have important economic consequences for women. Women are usually responsible for caring for ill household members and for replacing the labour of the incapacitated person. Bonilla and colleagues (1991) found that when other household members were ill, women's work days lengthened, their work load became heavier and some of their own activities had to be deferred.

The effects on women of tuberculosis in other household members have not been studied but it is likely that, as with other diseases such as malaria, schistosomiasis and leprosy, women's workloads increase when other family members are ill. Women replace the labour of those who are sick, and may have to neglect domestic and child care duties. Furthermore, as with leprosy, the stigma of tuberculosis may affect all household members, not only the sick person. The consequences of the stigma of tuberculosis may be especially hard on unmarried women, even if they themselves do not have the disease, since even their close association with a tuberculosis patient may reduce their chances of finding a marriage partner.

Conclusion and Recommendations

Gender differentials are a potentially important source of inequity in tuberculosis control. The studies reviewed in this chapter suggest that socio-economic and cultural factors may be important in two ways: first, they may play a role in determining overall gender differences in rates of infection, progression to disease, treatment and the outcome of treatment; and second, even where male/female rates may not be different, gender-based differences may exist in terms of the barriers to detection and successful treatment of tuberculosis. Both have implications for successful tuberculosis control programmes and argue for increased efforts to identify and address gender differentials in the control of this disease.

Kutzin (1993) has discussed a number of approaches that health programmes might take in an effort to increase women's access to health services. These are all potentially relevant interventions for addressing gender differentials in tuberculosis control, but their effectiveness has not yet been evaluated:

- Reducing transport and time costs by bringing services closer to women, possibly through mobile or home-based outreach care.
- Promoting the integration of health services (Hellberg, 1995). Where specialised facilities or different schedules for 'clinics' within individual facilities exist, for example, for family planning, immunisations, and maternal care, women must make several trips if they need to use each of the services. An alternative model is employed by the Bangladesh Women's Health Coalition (BWHC) facilities, which offer a mix of curative and preventive services for women and their children, enabling clients to use a visit for more than a single purpose (Kay, 1991). Sichone (1993) suggests the use

of antenatal clinics to improve tuberculosis case-finding in Zambia.

- Integrating and supporting 'traditional' practitioners who provide health care services to women, and increasing the supply of female health care providers in the public health care system.

In addition, national tuberculosis control programmes could conduct routine reporting of case-finding and case-holding with analysis by age and sex. It would also be useful to collect information on the number and distribution of male and female health workers, by category of health worker. Such information would be useful both for developing appropriate interventions, and as a basis for monitoring the progress and effectiveness of control programmes. Awareness of gender issues could also be incorporated into the training of health workers.

Gender inequalities of health in developing countries must be examined and addressed as an integral part of the economic, social and cultural contexts in which they occur. Unequal access to health care is only one manifestation of more general gender inequity in society. This implies that strategies to reduce gender inequalities must include efforts to improve the status of women (Okojie, 1994). Factors such as access to income, legal rights, social status, and education may, in fact, prove far more important in determining women's access to health care than health care policies *per se* (Ojanuga, 1992). Unfortunately, the strategies likely to have the largest impact in terms of removing gender inequalities in health are beyond the means of most health programmes, since they involve major structural and social changes: improving socio-economic conditions, increasing education levels, reducing stigma and discrimination, and providing quality health care. The domain that disease control programmes have control over is much more limited. Nonetheless, it seems likely that tuberculosis control programmes that are responsive to the general constraints faced by women in seeking health care will have greater success in reducing sources of inequity in the detection and treatment of tuberculosis.

References

Barnhoorn, F. and Adriaanse, H. (1992) In search of factors responsible for noncompliance among tuberculosis patients in Wardha District, India. *Soc. Sci. Med.* **34**, 291–306.

Bassett, M. T. and Mhloyi, M. (1991) Women and AIDS in Zimbabwe: The making of an epidemic. *Int. J. Hlth. Serv.* **21**, 143–156.

Beljaev, A. E., Sharma, G. K., Brohult, J. A. and Haque, M. A. (1986) Studies on the detection of malaria at primary health centers. Part II. Age and sex composition of patients subjected to blood examination in passive case detection. *Ind. J. Malariol.* **23**, 19–25.

Bonilla, E., Kuratome, L. S., Rodriguez, P. and Rodriguez, A. (1991) *Salud y Desarrollo*. Bogota: Plaza and Janes.

Cassels, A., Heineman, E., LeClerq, S., Gurung, P. K. and Rahut, C. B. (1982) Tuberculosis case-finding in eastern Nepal. *Tubercle* **63**, 175–185.

Centers for Disease Control (1990) Summary of notifiable diseases, United States. *Morb. Mortal. Wkly. Rep.* **39**, 56–57.

Chanarin, I. and Stephenson, E. (1988) Vegetarian diet and cobalamin deficiency: Their association with tuberculosis. *J. Clin. Pathol.* **41**, 759–762.

Chaulet, P. (1987) Compliance with anti-tuberculosis chemotherapy in developing countries. *Tubercle* **68**(Suppl.): 19.

Chum, H. J., O'Brien, R. J., Chonde, T. M., Graf, P. and Rieder, H. L. (1996) An epidemiological study of tuberculosis and HIV infection in Tanzania, 1991–1993. *AIDS* **10**, 299–309.

Cosminsky, S. (1987) Women and health care on a Guatemalan plantation. *Soc. Sci. Med.* **25**, 1163–1173.

Crombie, J. B. (1954) Pregnancy and pulmonary tuberculosis. *Br. J. Tuberc.* **48**, 97–101.

Cruz, J. R., Heldal, E., Arnadottir, T., Juarez, I. and Enarson, D. A. (1994) Tuberculosis case-finding in Nicaragua: Evaluation of routine activities in the control programme. *Tubercle Lung Dis.* **75**, 417–422.

Ettling, M. B., Krongthong, T., Krachaklin, S. and Bualombai, P. (1989) Evaluation of malaria clinics Maesot, Thailand: Use of serology to assess coverage. *Trans. R. Soc. Trop. Med. Hyg.* **83**, 325–331.

Farmer, P. (1997) Social scientists and the new tuberculosis. *Soc. Sci. Med.* **44**, 347–358.

Finch, P. J., Millard, F. J. C. and Maxwell, J. D. (1991) Risk of tuberculosis in immigrant Asians: Culturally acquired immunodeficiency? *Thorax* **46**, 1–5.

Groth-Petersen, E., Knudsen, J. and Wilbek, E. (1959) Epidemiological basis of tuberculosis eradication in an advanced country. *Bull. Wld. Hlth. Org.* **21**, 45–49.

Harper, I., Fryatt, B. and White, A. (1996) Tuberculosis case-finding in remote mountainous areas — Are microscopy camps of any value? *Tubercle Lung Dis.* **77**, 384–388.

Hellberg, H. (1995) Tuberculosis prgrammes: Fragmentation or integration? *Tubercle Lung Dis.* **76**, 1–3.

Kay, B. J., Germain, A. and Bangser, M. (1991) *The Bangladesh Women's Health Coalition. Quality/Calidad/Qualité*, Number 3. New York: The Population Council.

Kutzin, J. (1993) (October) *Obstacles to Women's Access: Issues and Options for More Effective Interventions to Improve Women's Health.* Working Paper, Human Resources Development and Operations Policy. Washington: The World Bank.

Leslie, J. (1991) Women's nutrition: The key to improving family health in developing countries? *Hlth. Pol. Plann.* **6**, 1–19.

Liefooghe, R., Michiels, N., Habib, S., Moran, I. and De Muynck, A. (1995) Perceptions and social consequences of tuberculosis: A focus group study of tuberculosis patients in Sialkot, Pakistan. *Soc. Sci. Med.* **41**, 1685–1692.

Mechanic, D. (1978) Sex, illness, illness behaviour, and the use of health services. *Soc. Sci. Med.* **12B**, 207–214.

Murray, C. J. (1991) Social, economic and operational research on tuberculosis: Recent studies and some priority questions. *Bull. Int. Union Tuberc. Lung. Dis.* **66**, 149–156.

Murray, C. J. and Lopez, A. D. (1997) Mortality by cause for eight regions of the world: Global burden of disease study. *Lancet* **349**, 1269–1276.

Nichter, N. (1994) Illness semantics and international health: The weak lungs/TB complex in the Philippines. *Soc. Sci. Med.* **38**, 649–663.

Okojie, C. E. (1994) Gender inequalities of health in the third world. *Soc. Sci. Med.* **39**, 1237–1247.

Ojanuga, D. N. and Gilbert, C. (1992) Women's access to health care in developing countries. *Soc. Sci. Med.* **35**, 613–617.

Over, M., Ellis, R. P., Huber, J. H. and Solon, O. (1992) The consequences of adult ill-health. In: Feachem, R. G. A., Kjellstrom, T., Murray, C. J. L., Over, M. and Phillips, M. A., eds. *The Health of Adults in the Developing World.* Oxford: Oxford University Press.

Paolisso, M. and Leslie, J. (1995) Meeting the changing health needs of women in developing countries. *Soc. Sci. Med.* **40**, 55–65.

Rathgeber, E. M. and Vlassoff, C. (1993). Gender and tropical diseases: A new research focus. *Soc. Sci. Med.* **37**, 513–520.

Reuben, R. (1993) Women and malaria: Special risks and appropriate control strategy. *Soc. Sci. Med.* **37**, 473–480.

Schaeffer, G., Zervoudakis, I. A., Fuchs, F. F. and David, S. (1975) Pregnancy and tuberculosis. *Obst. Gynecol.* **46**, 706–715.

Schoepf, B. G. (1993) AIDS Action research with women in Kinshasa, Zaire. *Soc. Sci. Med.* **37**, 1401–1413.

Sichone, M. (1993) (May) *Tuberculosis and Gender in Zambia: The Burden on Women* (unpublished Master's thesis). Amsterdam: Royal Tropical Institute.

Smith, I. (1994) (August) *Women and Tuberculosis: Gender Issues and Tuberculosis Control in Nepal* (unpublished Masters thesis). Nuffield Institute for Health.

Snider, D. E. (1984) Pregnancy and tuberculosis. *Chest* **86**, 10S–13S.

Styblo, K. (1991) Epidemiology of tuberculosis. *Selected Papers Roy. Netherlands Tuberc. Assoc.* **24**.

Sutherland, I. and Fayers, P. M. (1975) The association of the risk of tuberculous infection with age. *Bull. Int. Union Tuberc.* **50**, 70–81.

Sutherland, I. (1976) Recent studies in the epidemiology of tuberculosis based on the risk of being infected with tercule bacilli. *Adv. Tuberc. Res.* **19**, 1–63.

Ulrich, M., *et al.* (1993) Leprosy in women: Characteristics and repercussions. *Soc. Sci. Med.* **37**, 445–456.

UNAIDS/WHO. (1997) *Report on the Global HIV/AIDS Epidemic — December 1997.* Geneva: World Health Organization.

van der Werf, T. S., Dade, G. K. and van der Mark, T. W. (1990) Patient compliance with tuberculosis treatment in Ghana: Factors influencing adherence to therapy in a rural service programme. *Tubercle* **71**, 247–252.

Vlassoff, C. and Bonilla, E. (1994) Gender-related differences in the impact of tropical diseases on women: What do we know? *J. Biosoc. Sci.* **26**, 37–53.

Watts, S. J., Brieger, W. R. and Yacoob, M. (1989) Guinea worm: An in-depth study of what happens to mothers, families and communities. *Soc. Sci. Med.* **29**, 1043–1049.

World Health Organization (1991) *Tuberculosis Research and Development.* Geneva: World Health Organization (WHO/TB/91.162).

World Health Organization (1996a) *Global Tuberculosis Programme. Groups at Risk: WHO Report on the Tuberculosis Epidemic in 1996.* Geneva: World Health Organization (WHO/TB/96.196).

World Health Organization (1996b) *Tuberculosis in the Era of HIV. A Deadly Partnership.* Geneva: World Health Organization (WHO/TB/ 6.204).

World Bank (1993) *World Bank World Development Report.* Washington: World Bank.

PART IV

ALTERNATIVE APPROACHES AND FUTURE DIRECTIONS

CHAPTER 15

THE WAY FORWARD: AN INTEGRATED APPROACH TO TUBERCULOSIS CONTROL

John Porter, Jessica A. Ogden and Paul Pronyk

Introduction

Tuberculosis control is usually perceived to be a public health strategy. It is one of the ways in which we endeavour to "address the public interest in health by applying scientific and technical knowledge to prevent disease" (Institute of Medicine, 1988). In a number of contributions to this book, however, it is argued that we need to make a shift in our understanding of public health, away from this prevention of disease perspective and towards a paradigm based on the creation/production of health (*pace* Kickbusch, 1997). Such a shift will have implications on how we understand, and therefore manage, the 'control' of tuberculosis.

Tuberculosis is also said to be a disease of development; a "barometer of social justice and equity" (Rangan *et al.*, 1997: p. 6). Although it affects all people in all countries, people in the poorest countries and amongst the poorest sections of communities suffer the most (e.g. Spence *et al.*, 1993; Rangan *et al.*, 1997). This, too, raises questions about the appropriateness of the current biomedically-orientated response, and suggests that a shift in perspective is due. Thus, it is an appropriate moment for those of us working in tuberculosis control to be brought up to date; to articulate with new knowledge and new perspectives on knowledge that has been around for a long time. Significantly, discussions about health research have begun to call for 'people centred health development' (Ramalingaswami, 1993; see also Antia and Bhatia, 1993). Ramalingaswami suggests that, for this to occur, the whole range of biomedical and clinical sciences on the one hand, and of social, economic and behavioural sciences on the other must engage in *interdisciplinary* studies. He suggests that this will require breaking out of the cloistered frames of existing organisational structures and current educational approaches. New partnerships will need to be fostered and new endpoints of programme implementation established with an eye toward fulfilling peoples' perceived needs (Ramalingaswami, 1993).

Changing Perceptions in Public Health

In recent years, public health professionals have been challenged to consider an approach to their work which takes seriously the important social dimensions of disease and it converse, well-being (e.g. Kickbusch, 1997; Mann, 1994). Such an orientation necessarily involves a fundamental re-evaluation of the way in which researchers, practitioners and policy makers perceive their work in relation to the communities they are ultimately hoping to benefit. It also requires a reconsideration of the ways in which these categories of health/public health professionals interact with each other. Fundamentally, a new approach to tuberculosis control will need to articulate with changes in the public health landscape and to take heed of new knowledge and new creativities.

A central core of a new approach to tuberculosis control will be qualitative research and social science perspectives. Indeed, it is apparent that public health experts are already looking more and more to social scientists to contribute to a new policy agenda in public health and infectious disease (Walker, 1995). Much of this awareness has grown out of the story of HIV/AIDS. While the history of the HIV/AIDS pandemic shows the strength of clinical and epidemiological research in the treatment and control of this infection, these disciplines were, for many years, held back by a lack of basic scientific information. Due to the absence of any effective biomedical interventions in the early years of the pandemic, social scientists were called upon to develop appropriate prevention strategies. Many of these researchers have played a key role in arguing for the need to take account of broader political, economic and social factors behind the HIV/AIDS pandemic.

Multidrug-resistant tuberculosis (MDRTB) is a biologically and socially complex development and, in order to be able to check it, we must understand the whole range of factors promoting and retarding its advance (Farmer, 1997). Anthropology and the other social sciences have several roles to play: first, to discern the precise mechanisms by which social forces (ranging from racism to violence) promote and retard transmission or recrudescence (Farmer, 1997). Second, ethnographic research will be important in identifying and ranking the barriers preventing those afflicted with MDRTB from having access to the best care available. Third, social scientists should become more engaged in multidisciplinary research and trials and to conduct research that exposes the precise mechanisms by which entrenched medical inequities are buttressed so that these inequities may be redressed.

'New' Knowledge about the Social Dimensions of Public Health

The association between income inequality and health

There is growing evidence that the *relative* distribution of income in a society matters in its own right for population health (Wilkinson, 1992, 1996). Studies have indicated that inequality of income predicts excess mortality within individual countries and this maldistribution of income is related not only to total mortality but also to infant mortality, homicides, deaths from neoplasms and cardiovascular disease (Judge, 1995; Kennedy *et al.*, 1996).

Income inequality induces 'spillover' effects on the quality of life, even for people not normally affected by material wants (Kawachi and Kennedy, 1997). Wide income disparities result in frustration, stress, and family disruption, which then increase the rates of crime, violence and homicide (Wilkinson, 1996). Wide income disparities tend to co-exist with under-investment in human capital, measured in a variety of ways including high school drop out rates, reduced public spending on education and lower literacy rates (Kaplan *et al.*, 1996).

Studies on inequality have led to a call for *social cohesion* and to the development of the concept of 'social capital'. Putnam (1993) indicates that the stock of social capital in a region can be measured, for example, by the extent of citizens' participation in community organisation. People living in regions characterised by high levels of social capital were more likely to trust their fellow citizens and to value solidarity, equality and mutual tolerance (Putnam, 1993). They are also likely to enjoy better quality of life and improved standards of health and well-being (Wilkinson, 1996).

Social vulnerability and the importance of social factors in disease transmission

As noted above, AIDS researchers have made important contributions to our understanding of the relations between social structural factors and disease. Parker (1996a) indicates that perhaps the single most important transformation in thinking about HIV/AIDS in the early to mid-1990s was the attempt to move beyond the distinctions commonly made by epidemiologists between 'risk groups' and 'the general population'. Parker (1996a) argues that the shift from the notion of individual risk to a new understanding of social vulnerability has been crucial not only to our understanding of the dynamics of the epidemic, but will be central to any strategy capable of slowing its progression.

This expanded understanding of the social factors that generate situations of vulnerability has created a perception of the ways in which social inequality and injustice, prejudice and discrimination, oppression, exploitation and violence continue to function in ways that have accelerated the spread of the HIV epidemic in countries around the world. It thus offers the possibility of enabling a reorientation and redirection of much of our research activity, to shift the object of study and the level of analysis in ways that can help us to more fully perceive the different historical and structural forces responsible for the degree to which some communities and individuals are more vulnerable to HIV/AIDS than others (Aggleton, 1996). As Mann and Tarantola (1995) state: "it is now clear that HIV/AIDS is as much about society as it is about a virus. This new understanding of the societal basis for vulnerability to HIV/AIDS has the potential to provide a strategic coherence to efforts in HIV/AIDS prevention and control". While this statement was clearly written about AIDS, it applies equally well to tuberculosis.

Health promotion and education

AIDS researchers have also led the way in the area of health promotion and education. HIV/AIDS interventions have demonstrated the limited effectiveness of behavioural interventions based solely on information and reasoned persuasion. Studies show that information in and of itself is insufficient to induce risk-reducing behavioural change. The relative limitations of individual psychology as the sole foundation for intervention and prevention programmes has also become increasingly clear (Aggleton, 1996; Parker, 1996b). The more effective interventions have engaged communities in the process of identifying the social obstacles to remaining HIV free, and developing locally meaningful ways of overcoming these problems (e.g. Welbourne, 1995). It is arguable that to be truly effective, HIV interventions must extend much more broadly to address the global factors which promote structural vulnerability.

Tuberculosis has a strong history of health promotion. The recognition of collective responsibility for tuberculosis impelled many activists to endorse a broader agenda of social reform. As M. V. Ball explained to the Warren, Pennsylvania, Academy of Science in 1909, "The fight against consumption is a fight against bad environment, in the home, in the city, in the workshop, and in the school". The elimination of tuberculosis became a powerful justification for strengthening municipal boards of public health, regulating tenement housing, inspecting sanitary conditions in factories, and providing school health services (Tomes, 1997). With the introduction of the DOTS tuberculosis control strategy, communities need to be intimately involved in articulating the social obstacles that prevent people with tuberculosis from receiving information and therefore treatment. A focus on those people who are most socially vulnerable will provide clues to improving the tuberculosis health care infrastructure overall.

In relation to AIDS programmes, Parker suggests that there needs to be a shift away from information-based education to a new set of models focusing on collective empowerment and community mobilisation (Parker, 1996a; cf. Welbourne, 1995). This shift, associated with the work of educators such as Paulo Freire, is from a 'banking model' of education practice to what might be more appropriately described as libertarian or dialogue-based education. In the former approach, education is little more than an act of depositing information, where knowledge is like a gift bestowed by those who consider themselves knowledgeable upon those whom they consider to know nothing. The latter model, on the other hand, aims to build up a critical perception of the social, cultural, political and economic forces that structure everyday life, and takes action against those forces that are oppressive (Parker, 1996a). This approach links well with Ramalingswami's concept of 'people centred development' (Ramalingaswami, 1993). For further details on aspects of education, see Chapter 21.

Increasing numbers of multidisciplinary and intersectoral collaborations

There is an increasing appreciation of the need for the different disciplines in public health to work together. For example, economists can work with political analysts to address health issues from a different and 'fuller' perspective (Lee and Zwi, 1996). Likewise, epidemiologists can begin to appreciate and accommodate social science methods and perspectives and *vice versa*. As Farmer (1996) has remarked, "a critical framework would not aspire to supplant the methods of the many disciplines, from virology to molecular epidemiology, which now concern themselves with emerging diseases". The aim is not to diminish the role of biomedicine, but to supplement it with perspectives from other disciplines: "The problem is not 'too much science', but too narrow a view of the sciences relevant to medicine" (from Eisenberg and Kleinman, 1981, cited in Farmer, 1996: p. 267).

Increasing international interest in ethics, human rights, and the broader meaning of 'health' within the context of globalisation

The increased interest in human rights and ethics can be seen in developments in academia: the Harvard School of Public Health has developed a discourse on the interaction between public health and human rights (Mann, 1995) and schools of public health are increasingly seeing ethics as a core component of their degree courses. Tuberculosis research methods have been put under scrutiny in several editorials in medical journals addressing ethics in international research and which question specific conditions around the use of placebos in tuberculosis and HIV studies in Africa (Angell, 1997; Halsey, *et al.*, 1997). These studies highlight the power imbalance present when researchers from well-financed institutions in western industrialised countries work with researchers in low-income countries.

Ethicsists are also beginning to develop a critique of policy. Brock (1995), for example, states that

> *"Policy issues are often more complex than clinical issues because they are concerned with complex issues of institutional design. To speak to them intelligently, one needs to understand the complexities of institutional design and how the institutions function. One needs to draw on work in political philosophy, not just ethics where bioethicists are more comfortable and better trained. There is a tendency to think that if one shifts one's attitude to policy,*

one is no longer doing ethics, but one's doing something else. I think it is a mistake to conceive of ethics narrowly in this way. We need to attend to these issues of policy".

Problems with the Tuberculosis Control Model

There are six elements which characterise tuberculosis and other infectious disease control programmes. They tend to (1) be disease specific, (2) be vertically-rather than horizontally-structured, (3) concentrate on product rather than process, (4) be standardised across country contexts, (5) have a short-term orientation, and (6) be viewed as 'health sector interventions'. Each of these six elements merit reconsideration in the creation of a new, more humane and ultimately more effective approach to tuberculosis control.

(1) Infectious disease control programmes are fundamentally disease-specific. The nature of their empirical underpinnings, organisational structure, financial support, and outcome measures reflect an emphasis on the control of single-disease entities (World Health Organization, 1996). Tuberculosis in the 1990s is no exception, although this has not always been the case. The idea of an integrated approach to tuberculosis control was present in the 1980s when there was a decision to incorporate tuberculosis control into Primary Health Care (World Health Organization, 1982, 1988), but it appears that the means and political will to achieve this goal were lacking. Consequently, when the incidence of tuberculosis rose in the early 1990s, the acute response was to re-establish a vertical tuberculosis control programme.

(2) Vertically-structured programmes have had a significant organisational role in the administration and implementation of infection control efforts (Pronyk, 1997). These structures have been favoured in eradication programmes such as those for polio,

Chagas' disease, malaria and dracunculiasis (Cairncross *et al.*, 1997). However, vertical programmes are rarely long-term interventions, and focus on the achievement of primary endpoints, rather than on sustainability of benefits. They emphasise 'product/outcome' rather than 'process'. For example, tuberculosis control stresses 'cure'. Ramalingaswami (1993: p. 107) addresses the problem of verticality by noting that "a strong movement is now needed to make the strengths of vertical programmes subserve broader, cohesive actions and to enhance autonomy and self determination on the part of communities in health development".

(3) Tuberculosis control stresses *product* (outcome-cure) over *process*. The success of the World Health Organization Smallpox Eradication Programme and the current programmes to eradicate polio have helped to frame this goal-orientation. The argument could go something like this: smallpox was eradicated with the right technology and therefore, given the right technology, other infectious diseases can likewise be eradicated. Today, the tuberculosis offices at the Centers for Disease Control and Prevention in Atlanta are still called the Bureau of Tuberculosis Elimination. It is worthwhile to note, however, that it took more than mere technology to eradicate smallpox: the campaign entailed a monumental global effort whereby experts and lay people, doctors and village children all worked together to achieve a common goal (see Ogden, undated).

(4) Infectious diseases, including tuberculosis, are generally thought to be best 'controlled' by standardisation of treatment and programming (World Health Organization, 1996). This concept grows out of the belief that quantitative epidemiology is objective, value-neutral and capable of uncovering *universal laws* about disease exposure and causation (Wing, 1994). The DOTS programme for tuberculosis control is an example (Kaye and Frieden, 1996). Although this strategy was developed and

successfully applied in New York City, it cannot be assumed that
it can be applied equally well, without significant adaptation,
elsewhere in the world, including developing world contexts,
despite the enormous social, economic, cultural and epidemiological differences between these contexts. Can epidemiology
explain why there needs to be a 'single best option'? Or why
tuberculosis control 'should' concentrate only on those people
who have sputum-positive disease? Indeed, why does tuberculosis control continue to focus on biomedical interventions alone
rather than include strategies from other sectors and disciplines?

(5) Tuberculosis control is short term. Major funding for disease
control is derived from outside sources with a competitive and
often fragmented system of grant allocation, favouring quan-
tifiable, disease-specific outcome measures (Pronyk, 1997). An
example of this is the Health for All by the Year 2000 strategy
which attempts to define explicit targets for health outcomes,
by which countries may measure the success of disease control
efforts (World Health Organization, 1996). In such an environment, there is an obvious difficulty in developing and maintaining an integrated, long-term agenda for population health.
Support for tuberculosis control and prevention must 'compete'
with endemic diseases such as HIV, malaria, and diarrhoeal diseases for a finite amount of financial aid (Gilks, 1997).

(6) Tuberculosis control is seen only as a health sector intervention. The underlying assumption is that diseases such as tuberculosis arise independently, are self-contained, have distinct
exposure patterns and risk-factors within populations, and have
little bearing on one another (Pronyk, 1997). The fundamental commitment to biomedical approaches assumes that the influence of non-health sector conditions have little measurable
impact on disease and are therefore beyond the scope of the
planning process (Wing, 1994). Although tuberculosis is associated with poverty there are few signs of health care providers
working with other sectors like agriculture, defence, eduction or

town planning. And yet, is an upstream approach not the most appropriate way to proceed? (See Chapter 20.)

The current model of tuberculosis control is biomedical and focuses on the individual and the notion of individual risk. Recent research has identified the shortcomings of this approach and the need to look at the social dimensions of diseases like tuberculosis and HIV (Mann *et al.*, 1992; Mann and Tarantola, 1996; Parker, 1996a; Farmer, 1997). As already mentioned, Parker (1996a) suggests shifting from the notion of individual risk to a new understanding of social vulnerability.

The History of Tuberculosis Control since Alma-Ata: What are the Lessons?

In the early 1960s, the concept of a comprehensive tuberculosis control programme implemented on a country-wide scale through the network of existing health services was formulated by the World Health Organization (WHO). This concept was outlined in the Eighth Report of the World Health Organization Expert Committee on Tuberculosis (World Health Organization, 1964) and reaffirmed in the Ninth Report a decade later (World Health Organization, 1974). The main principles were that a tuberculosis programme should be country wide, permanent, and adapted to the expressed demands of the population so as to be both acceptable and accessible to them.

Though there was only a small tuberculosis office at the WHO in the 1970s, there was an understanding of the close relationship between tuberculosis, socio-economic conditions and efficiency of programme implementation. In 1978, the WHO and the United Nations Children's Fund sponsored an International Conference on Primary Health Care at Alma-Ata in the former USSR. At that conference, a statement, subsequently known as the Alma-Ata Declaration, was formulated (World Health Organization, 1978). Reports from the WHO in the 1980s show the degree to which attempts were being made to *integrate* tuberculosis control into the primary health care structure advocated by Alma-Ata

(World Health Organization, 1982; 1988). There was also acceptance of the importance of economic development as a long-term solution to health problems and the strong influence of external donors on tuberculosis control policy (World Health Organization, 1982: p. 26). Since vertical programmes 'competed with each other for scarce resources' and were 'wasteful and relatively unproductive', attempts were being made to integrate tuberculosis control into Primary Health Care (World Health Organization, 1988: p. 7).

The notion of *integration*, however soundly based on empirical data and operational experience, did not realise its promise due mainly to a lack of political and financial commitment to primary care in many countries. In India, for example, it is clear that the under-performance of the National Tuberculosis Programme was directly related to its integration into a general health service which was diverting crucial resources away from primary care and towards intensive, high-profile vertical programmes such as the population control programme (Nagpaul, 1982). The tuberculosis programme struggled on despite the lack of drugs, personnel and diagnostic facilities. Thus, it appears that integration is not enough: horizontal programming for tuberculosis and other infectious diseases needs to be backed up by political commitment to the health services themselves (see Rangan et al., 1997). Current research in India indicates that however promising a tuberculosis programme may be, it will be held back by the population's mistrust of the public health services until such time as those services themselves are meeting the needs of the people more generally.

The Way Forward

It is evident from WHO literature after Alma-Ata, that the WHO's Tuberculosis Programme was committed to integrating tuberculosis control into primary health care. This, however, was unsuccessful and the consequences were that a strong vertical programme was created in the 1990s based on the DOTS strategy. With the effects of globalisation, an increased interest in health, healthy communities, people-centred development, and justice, those international figures in charge of tuberculosis control have an opportunity now to develop the DOTS programme into an intervention that is broader than biomedicine.

The way forward needs to include the suggestions in Chapter 5 on the use of the concepts of equity, civic engagement and intersectoral collaboration as a first step in developing a 'process' for *engagement and integration*. In this chapter, three major themes which can further assist in finding direction for the development of tuberculosis control policy are discussed: First, the increasing public health interest in 'the creation of health' rather than simply adopting a biomedical disease focus; second, the concept of 'people-centred health development' and the use of interdisciplinary studies in research; and third, the importance of 'social vulnerability', not only as a concept but also as a focus for the identification of problems in the public health system and as a nexus for solving these problems.

Creation of Health

One feature in 'creating health' will be to recognise the importance of general health to individuals and populations. Tuberculosis control alone will not serve this basic need, but should be part of a wider commitment to primary care. It is vital that appropriate diagnostic equipment and expertise be in place and that the requisite tuberculosis drugs are available and free to those in need. Tuberculosis is not the only condition from which people suffer, and if drugs and facilities are not available for other conditions we will still be failing to meet the people's need for and right to health.

A second feature will be the need to address the broader conditions of health so that communities and individuals are able to enjoy not only health in the biomedical sense, but also well-being. This will require a broad, multi-sectoral approach. The goals of tuberculosis programmes need to change from the control/elimination of disease to the creation of health in its widest sense. Current movements within public health support this shift and provide valuable insights and strategies with which those concerned more narrowly with tuberculosis will need to engage.

These two aspects require more than epistemological transition. Practical problems demand pragmatic solutions. Government commitment to the well-being of their communities is vital and tuberculosis control needs to be seen as part of a broader programme of decentralisation and devolution of decision-making powers from the centre to the periphery (cf. Rangan et al., 1997). As indicated in the Ninth Report of the World Health Organization Expert Committee on Tuberculosis (World Health Organization, 1974): "a tuberculosis programme should be adapted to the expressed demand of the population so as to be acceptable and accessible to them".

People-Centred Health Development and Research

Those of us engaged in tuberculosis research have a vital role to play in developing a way forward. The essential national health research process described by Ramalingaswami (1993) is "for countries to understand their own problems, to enhance the impact of limited resources, to improve health policy and management, to foster innovation and experimentation, and to provide the foundation for a stronger developing country voice in setting international priorities". This process involves interaction between communities, policy and decision makers, and researchers, as shown in Fig. 1.

A key part of this process is interdisciplinary study. We need to recognise and respect the value and range of disciplinary perspectives represented amongst our colleagues and begin to work together with more confidence and less fear. By working with different disciplines it will be easier to address the issues of poverty, inequality and justice and find ways of developing infectious disease policies which address them.

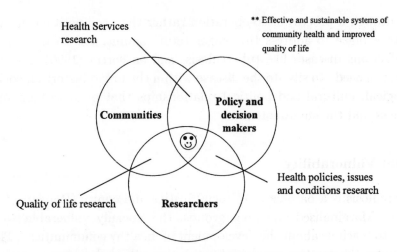

The essential national health research process

Fig. 1.   Essential National Health Research Process (adapted from Ramalingaswami, 1993).

The objectives include:

- Working with local researchers, practitioners and communities in identifying the key determinants of well-being.
- Defining the range of research questions which will help in the process of exploring these determinants.
- Carrying out the research in partnership with local research institutes and the local communities themselves, as well as making interdisciplinary and inter-sectoral linkages if and when appropriate.
- Engaging with policy makers in the creation of a meaningful process of policy development which will be responsive to change and be able to incorporate new data over time as community needs and priorities evolve.
- Disseminating the findings of the research widely through publication, teaching, training and media work in the participant country contexts as well as at home.

Through a process of co-operation rather than competition, we will create a place to address the longer term commitment to the control of infectious diseases like tuberculosis, and as Fortin (1990) has indicated the need "to situate the disease within the broad historical, social, ecological, cultural and political relationships that mediate humanity, sickness and the environment".

Social Vulnerability

Tuberculosis is a barometer of social justice and equity (Rangan *et al.*, 1997). Marginalised and poor groups, the 'socially vulnerable', have much to teach us about the development of 'healthy communities'. They encounter the greatest problems in accessing tuberculosis treatment and if we can understand and address their difficulties, we have a greater opportunity of creating an effective tuberculosis control strategy and structure. The socially vulnerable help to delineate 'what is wrong with our communities' and to identify the sites of breakdown of communication and understanding between individuals and community structures. In the current tuberculosis control strategy, the tip of the iceberg (pyramid) is targeted (i.e. only patients with sputum-positive tuberculosis), and little is known about the majority. If the pyramid is turned on its head and the issues of the socially vulnerable are targeted and addressed, the problems of the remainder (the majority) of tuberculosis patients will also be covered (Fig. 2).

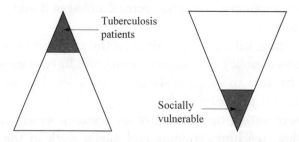

Fig. 2.   The inverted pyramid which looks at the socially vulnerable.

Ultimately, the socially vulnerable highlight the tension between the autonomy of the individual and the justice of the community structures in which they live. If tuberculosis control programmes can find ways of appropriately balancing this ethical dilemma then they can assist in developing 'the conditions in which people can be healthy'.

Conclusion

To prevent infectious diseases such as tuberculosis, there is a need to create healthy communities and societies (Kickbusch, 1997). While continuing to address the biomedical aspects of disease control and prevention, this requires a broader look at the non-medical factors that determine health: social life, the environment, human biology, and inequality in access to resources — globally as well as locally.

It is clear that a new approach to the control of tuberculosis cannot take place in the absence of a clearly articulated vision of what a community, a nation, a world without the preconditions under which tuberculosis thrives (e.g. social inequality and abject poverty) would look like. It may be useful to think of such a world as being 'healthier' — a world in which the well-being of more people is ensured. Thus 'health', in its widest definition, is at the centre of tuberculosis control.

References

Aggleton, P. (1996) Global priorities for HIV/AIDS intervention research. *Int. J. STS. AIDS.* **7**(Suppl. 2), 13–16.

Angell, M. (1997) The ethics of clinical research in the third world. *N. Engl. J. Med.* **337**, 847–849.

Antia, N. H. and Bhatia, K., eds. (1993) *People's Health in People's Hands: A Model for Panchayati Raj.* Mumbai: The Foundation for Research in Community Health.

Brock, D. (1995) The role of bioethics in health care policy. Broadening the bioethics agenda. In: Miles, S. ed. *The Role of Bioethics in Health Care Policy* (Conference Proceedings). Minneapolis: University of Minnesota.

Cairncross, S., Peries, H. and Cutts, F. (1997) Vertical health programmes. *Lancet* **349**(Suppl. 111), 20–22.

Farmer, P. (1996) Social inequalities and emerging infectious diseases. *Emerg. Infect. Dis.* **2**, 259–269.

Farmer, P. (1997) Social scientists and the new tuberculosis. *Soc. Sci. Med.* **44**, 347–358.

Fortin, A. (1990) AIDS development and the limitations of the African state. In: Misztat, B., Moss, D., eds. *Action on AIDS: National Policies in Comparative Perspective.* New York: Greenwood Press, p. 217.

Gilks, C. F. (1997) Tropical medicine in the HIV/AIDS era. *Lancet* **349**(Suppl. 111), 17–18.

Halsey, N. A., Sommer, A., Henderson, D. A. and Black, R. E. (1997) Ethics and international research. *Br. Med. J.* **315**, 965.

Institute of Medicine. (1988) *Future of Public Health.* Washington DC: National Academy Press, pp. 1–7.

Judge, K. (1995) Income distribution and life expectancy: A critical appraisal. *Br. Med. J.* **311**, 1282–1285.

Kaplan, G. A., Pamuk, E. R., Lynch, J. W., Cohen, R. D. and Balfour, J. L. (1996) Inequality in income and mortality in the United States: Analysis of mortality and potential pathways. *Br. Med. J.* **312**, 999–1003.

Kawachi, I. and Kennedy, B. (1997) Health and social cohesion: Why care about income inequality? *Br. Med. J.* **314**, 1037–1040.

Kaye, K. and Frieden, T. K. (1996) Tuberculosis control: The relevance of classic principles in an era of acquired immune deficiency syndrome and multidrug resistance. *Epidemiol. Rev.* **18**, 52–63.

Kennedy, B. P., Kawachi, I. and Prothrow-Smith, D. (1996) Income distribution and mortality: Cross sectional econological study of the Robin Hood Index in the United States. *Br. Med. J.* **312**, 1004–1007.

Kickbusch, I. (1997) New players for a new era: Responding to the global public health challenges. *J. Publ. Hlth. Med.* **19**, 171–178.

Lee, K. and Zwi, A. (1996) A global political economy approach to AIDS: Ideology, interests and implications. *New Political Economy* **1**, 355–373.

Mann, J. (1994) Human rights and the new public health. *Health and Human Rights* **1**, 229–233.

Mann, J., Tarantola, D. J. M. and Netter, T. W., eds. (1992) *AIDS in the World.* Cambridge, MA: Harvard University Press.

Mann, J. and Tarantola, D. J. M. (1995) Preventive medicine: A broader perspective to the AIDS crisis. *Harvard Int. Rev.* **17**, 469–487.

Mann, J. and Tarantola, D. J. M., eds. (1996) *AIDS in the World*, Vol. 2. Oxford: Oxford University Press.

Nagpaul, D. R. (1982) Why integrated tuberculosis programmes have not succeeded as per expectations in many developing countries — A collection of observations. *Ind. J. Tuberc.* **29**, 149.

Ogden, H. G., Undated. *CDC and the Smallpox Crusade.* US Department of Health and Human Services, Public Health Service. Atlanta: Centers for Disease Control.

Parker, R. G. (1996a) Empowerment, community mobilization and social change in the face of HIV/AIDS. *AIDS* **10**(Suppl. 3), S27–S31.

Parker, R. G. (1996b) Shifting paradigms in HIV/AIDS research and intervention: Behaviour, culture and politics. In: Poznansky, M., Gillies, P. A. and Coker, R., eds. *Advancing a New Agenda for AIDS Research.* London: Blackwell.

Pronyk, P. (1997) *The Control of Infectious Diseases: Re-examining Alma Ata* (MSc thesis), London School of Hygiene and Tropical Medicine.

Putnam, R. D. (1993) *Making a Democracy Work. Civic Traditions in Modern Italy.* Princeton, NJ: Princeton University Press.

Ramalingaswami, V. (1993) Health research, a key to equity in health development. *Soc. Sci. Med.* **36**, 103–108.

Rangan, S., *et al.* (1997) *Tuberculosis Control in India: A state-of-the-art review.* Delhi: Department for International Development (DFID).

Spence, D. P. S., Hotchkiss, J., Williams, C. S. D. and Davies, P. D. O. (1993). Tuberculosis and poverty. *Br. Med. J.* **307**, 759–761.

Tomes, N. (1997) Moralizing the microbe. The Germ Theory and the moral construction of behaviour in the late nineteenth century anti-tuberculosis movement. In: Brandt, A. M. and Rozin, P., eds. *Morality and Health.* New York and London: Routledge, p. 285.

Walker, B. (1995) A new agenda for AIDS research. *Br. Med. J.* **311**, 1448–1449.

Welbourne, A. (1995) *Stepping Stones — A Training Package on HIV/AIDS Communication and Relationship Skills.* London: Action Aid.

Wilkinson, R. G. (1992) Income distribution and life expectancy. *Br. Med. J.* **304**, 165–168.

Wilkinson, R. G. (1996) *Unhealthy Societies. The Afflictions of Inequality.* London: Routledge.

Wing, S. (1994) Limits of epidemiology. *Medicine and Global Survival* **1**, 74–86.

World Health Organization (1964) *Tuberculosis: Eighth Report of the WHO Expert Committee* (Technical Report No. 290). Geneva: World Health Organization.

World Health Organization (1974) *Tuberculosis: Ninth Report of the WHO Expert Committee* (Technical Report No. 552). Geneva: World Health Organization.

World Health Organization (1978) *Declaration of Alma-Ata. International Conference on Primary Health Care,* Alma-Ata, USSR, 6-12 September 1978. Geneva: World Health Organization.

World Health Organization (1982) *Tuberculosis control. Report of a joint IUAT/WHO Study Group* (Technical Report No. 571). Geneva: World Health Organization.

World Health Organization (1988) *Tuberculosis Control as an Integral Part of Primary Health Care.* 88/7778. Geneva: World Health Organization.
World Health Organization (1996) *World Health Report.* Geneva: World Health Organization.

CHAPTER 16

DEMYSTIFYING THE CONTROL OF
TUBERCULOSIS IN RURAL BANGLADESH

---

*A. M. R. Chowdhury, J. Patrick Vaughan, Sadia Chowdhury
and Fazle H. Abed*

Introduction

Tuberculosis remains a global public health problem. In many developed countries, tuberculosis was thought to have been virtually eradicated but is now staging a comeback, partly through its association with the Acquired Immuno Deficiency Syndrome (AIDS). In developing countries, however, tuberculosis remains a major public health problem despite the highly-effective treatment regimens available (Kochi, 1997). For instance, there are an estimated seven million new infections with tuberculosis each year in developing countries, and about two to three million deaths (Raviglione *et al.*, 1995; Wise, 1996). Despite the fact that tuberculosis disproportionately affects the poor and other neglected segments of the population, it has continued to have a low political priority (Murray *et al.*, 1990).

The assumption behind tuberculosis control programmes is that high rates of case detection and treatment will lead to a reduction in the incidence of new cases. However, the major challenge facing tuberculosis control programmes is how to screen the general population and detect a high proportion of the active cases, and then how to achieve successful compliance with effective treatment. In addition, tuberculosis is dreaded in countries like Bangladesh (Chowdhury and Kabir, 1988), and associated taboos and stigma, together with poor facilities and unfriendly health care providers, discourages patients from reporting to health centres (Chowdhury *et al.*, 1991). Another compromising factor is the long period for treatment (six to 12 months). Recognising the scale of tuberculosis as a public health problem, BRAC, a non-governmental organisation, began a community-based tuberculosis control programme in 1984 in one *thana* (sub-district) using village-based community health workers and directly observed therapy, short course (DOTS). In view of encouraging results, BRAC extended the programme to additional *thanas* in 1992 (Chowdhury *et al.*, 1991; 1992). In this chapter, the salient features of the BRAC programme and the lessons learnt in the subsequent scaling up process are presented.

The Tuberculosis Problem in Bangladesh

A chest radiology survey in 1964–1965 detected 3.2 million cases of pulmonary tuberculosis in Bangladesh (Islam, 1981) and it was estimated that 390,000 of these cases, or 0.5% of the population, were sputum positive. A national survey carried out in 1987–1988 showed that 0.87% of the population aged 15 years and over were sputum positive (Director General Health Services, 1989). Men were infected twice as often as women and the problem was more acute in urban areas (see Table 1).

Table 1.   Tuberculosis in adults 15 years and older as determined by the National Prevalence Survey on Tuberculosis in Bangladesh (1987–1988).

Population groups	% sputum positive
Total	0.87
Male	1.08
Female	0.60
Rural	0.80
Urban	1.61

Source: Ministry of Health and Family Welfare, Bangladesh.

In another survey carried out in 50 villages in the Manikganj district in 1984, 20% of the population aged 15 years and over had a history of chronic cough and examination of their sputum specimens revealed that 2.7% were positive for acid-fast bacilli and 3.1% had a positive culture for *M. tuberculosis.* Sixty three percent of smear-positive cases were also culture positive. Smear-positive rates in the community were estimated to be between 0.33% to 0.55% and culture-positive rates between 0.39% to 0.64%. Drug sensitivity tests indicated that 70% of the strains were sensitive to all 12 anti-tuberculosis drugs and the remainder were resistant to only one or two combinations of streptomycin, INH, thiacetazone and ethionamide (Islam *et al.*, 1986).

Tuberculosis Control Programmes in Bangladesh

Ishikawa (1985) identified three main types of tuberculosis control programmes in Bangladesh.

- Type A: Hospital- or clinic-based programmes, such as the government programmes, that had very limited or no links with the community;
- Type B: Hospital- or clinic-based programmes that had strong links with community health workers. These included most of the programmes run by non-governmental organisations; and
- Type C: Community-based programmes with little or no direct involvement with hospitals or clinics and where community health workers were the 'nucleus' of the programme activities. The BRAC programme described in this chapter falls into this category.

In addition to the above, many tuberculosis cases are treated by the large private and non-formal health providers and, in addition, anti-tuberculosis drugs are widely available for purchase from numerous small pharmacies. Most of these drugs are produced in Bangladesh and tests for quality control commissioned by the Leprosy Mission and carried out in Denmark found that these drugs were within acceptable standards (Chowdhury *et al.*, 1997).

The Bangladesh National Tuberculosis Programme

The Bangladesh National Tuberculosis Programme, which is reasonably typical of many such programmes in developing countries, is clinic-based and uses 57 hospitals and clinics with over 1,000 beds, all of which are located in urban areas. If the estimated number of active tuberculosis cases is correct, there are about 500 cases for each available bed. The government of Bangladesh has adopted directly observed therapy, short course (DOTS), and is implementing the programme with the active assistance of several non-governmental organisations, including BRAC. The government has recently intensified its programme with financial assistance from the World Bank and the government of the Netherlands (Government of Bangladesh, 1996).

Although integration of tuberculosis control into the health services has been an accepted policy of the government since 1976, much more needs to be done in this regard. Although a large number of government health workers are posted in primary care facilities (approximately 15 per 20,000 population), few of them until recently were actively involved in tuberculosis activities, apart from BCG vaccination given through the EPI programme. Health staff are not well trained in tuberculosis control and in the supervision of treatment compliance in hospitals or community facilities. Finally, as elsewhere in developing countries, tuberculosis control remains a low political priority despite increasing interest in recent years by donor agencies.

A recent review of the Bangladesh National Tuberculosis Programme, based on interviews with policy makers and programme staff, together with an analysis of official records, revealed a marked improvement in the performance of the programme in recent years. Since the introduction of DOTS in 1993, over 150,000 people with the disease have been treated, with an estimated success rate of 80%. In 1996, a total of 63,985 tuberculosis patients were registered by the National Tuberculosis Programme, which was about 21% of the estimated annual incidence (World Health Organization, 1997b). In addition, BCG vaccination coverage had improved from less than 2% in 1986 to about 80% in the 1990s for children under one year of age (Huq, 1991).

The Tuberculosis Control Programme of BRAC

BRAC is a large Bangladesh non-governmental organisation established in 1972. It is one of the largest and most influential development organisations in the world, with over 18,000 full-time staff and 35,000 part-time workers. BRAC operates in over 55,000 villages of Bangladesh and it has an annual budget of about US$100 million. The major focus of BRAC programmes are alleviation of poverty, empowerment of women, primary education and health. BRAC supports these programmes with separate training and research divisions (Lovell, 1992; Ahmed *et al.*, 1993; Chowdhury and Cash, 1996).

The core of BRAC poverty alleviation programmes at the village level are the women's groups, called village organisations, with membership from the poorest households. In each group, one woman is trained as a Shasthya Shebika (community health worker) who treats selected common illnesses in the village. She does not receive any salary but does receive a small mark-up on the sale of selected essential drugs. As a member of the village organisation she can also receive loans for her own income-generating activities. Each of the community health workers, who are mostly illiterate women with an average age of about 35 years, covers about 200 households, including members of her own village organisation.

These community health workers have been trained by BRAC in tuberculosis case-finding, treatment and follow up procedures. They communicate information about tuberculosis to the community, especially through village organisation meetings and posters, and detect cases of active pulmonary tuberculosis by following up individuals with chronic cough of four weeks or more duration, from whom they then collect two early-morning sputum samples. These samples are examined microscopically for acid-fast bacilli in a local BRAC laboratory, in which technicians have been trained by the National Tuberculosis Programme. Sputum-positive patients are contacted by their own community health worker and asked to register for treatment. The national programme also assists in maintaining quality control of diagnostic procedures.

Patients willing to participate in treatment are asked to pay a deposit of 200 Taka (about US$5), equivalent in rural areas to about two to four days wages, and to sign a written agreement as an incentive to complete their course of treatment. At the end of treatment, 100 Taka is returned to the patient and the rest is given as compensation to the community health worker for her work. If the patient is too poor to pay the deposit, this is often paid by the village organisation or other community members. The community health worker also receives 25 Taka for each new or relapsed positive patient whom she identifies. If patients do not complete their treatment, the whole deposit in forfeited and the community health worker gets her share while the remainder is retained by BRAC.

The BRAC tuberculosis programme was piloted and implemented between 1984 and 1991 in one *thana* (sub-district) and covered a population of 220,000 people. Results from this pilot programme (phase one), in which a standard 12-month DOTS treatment regimen was used, suggested that about two-thirds of patients completed the full course of treatment. The relapse rate was estimated to be about 10% for patients who had completed treatment four or more years previously. Between 1984 and 1994, the treatment regimen consisted of 30 streptomycin injections, given on alternate days for two months, and daily isoniazid (300 mg) and thioacetazone (150 mg) administration for 12 months. Drugs were provided free-of-charge to BRAC by the National Tuberculosis Programme and at no cost to the patients. Sputum specimens were examined for acid-fast bacilli at 1, 3, 6, 9, 12 and 13 months after treatment had started and patients with complications, or positive sputum at the end of their treatment, were referred to specialist clinics or hospitals. The second phase (1992–1994) expanded the BRAC programme to an additional nine *thanas*. In addition, from 1995 (the start of phase three) an eight-month regimen based on isoniazid, pyrazinamide, ethambutol and rifampicin daily for two months, followed by isoniazid and thiacetazone daily for a further six months, was used. Another eight *thanas* (making a total of 17) were also included in phase three.

Evaluation of the BRAC Programme

To evaluate the effectiveness of the programme, a cohort analysis of programme data for phases two and three was performed according to the outcome categories recommended by the World Health Organization (WHO) and the International Union Against Tuberculosis and Lung Disease. This analysis included assessment of the number of people with chronic cough who were identified as sputum positive for acid-fast bacilli, the proportion who accepted treatment and subsequent patient outcomes, including the proportion cured, died, failed treatment, defaulted and migrated. In order to assess the impact of the programme in the control of tuberculosis transmission, as measured by the prevalence of sputum smear-positive tuberculosis cases in the *thana* population, a cross-sectional household survey was carried out in 1995 in two programme *thanas*, one with low and the other with high tuberculosis detection rates. A third *thana*, socio-economically similar to the other two programme *thanas* but which had not had a BRAC programme, was selected for the comparison. Heads of households or their spouses in more than 3,000 randomly selected households in each *thana* were interviewed to identity individuals with a chronic cough of four weeks duration or longer. Each patient with a chronic cough was asked to give a sputum sample, which was examined for acid-fast bacilli by trained technicians using the Ziehl–Neelsen method in a local BRAC laboratory. Ninety-five percent of patients with chronic cough gave at least one sputum sample. For quality control, a random selection of the

slides were re-examined by technicians from the National Tuberculosis
Control Programme, who found the quality of staining, smearing and
microscopy to be well within acceptable standards. Before completion
of the household survey, however, an initial analysis of the laboratory
results showed that the proportion of patients who were smear positive
was lower than had been expected. Since this might have been the result
of poor case-detection and under-reporting of chronic cough, all survey
households in the three *thanas* were revisited and new information was
gathered by the same methods. The conclusion was that the survey
methods appeared to be sound since this second round only resulted in
one additional case of tuberculosis being detected.

This household survey also included the follow up of all tuberculosis
patients who had been previously diagnosed and treated by BRAC in
the two programme *thanas*. All previously treated patients were traced
and three sputum specimens were collected and examined as above. In
addition, tuberculosis patients under treatment, community members,
community health workers and local BRAC staff were all interviewed,
using both quantitative and qualitative methods, for their views about
the quality of care provided in the BRAC tuberculosis programme.

Results of the Evaluation Study

Between 1992 and 1994 (phase two), 3,886 tuberculosis patients were
identified in their villages by the BRAC community health workers.
Ninety percent of these had accepted the offered treatment and 81% of
these completed the full 12-month course. In 85% of those treated, the
sputum became negative for acid-fast bacilli by the start of the third
month. An outcome analysis of 3,497 patients in phase two who had
started treatment between April 1992 and December 1994 is shown in
Table 2. Although 81% were cured or completed the 12-month course,
9.6% had died, the drop-out or default rate was 3.1%, and the failure
rate was 1.5%. The overall successful cure rate was, therefore, at least
80% for patients who started treatment and 73% (81% of 90%) for all
the sputum-positive patients originally diagnosed.

Table 2. Treatment outcomes for acid-fast bacilli-positive patients treated with a 12-month regimen in 1992–1994 (phase two).

Outcome	Number of cases ($n = 3497$)
Cured/completed*	2833 (81.0)
Died	336 (9.6)
Failed treatment	51 (1.5)
Defaulted	109 (3.1)
Migrated/referred/transferred	168 (4.8)

*Cured-negative sputum at month 13; samples not available at month 13 for 402 patients who were, therefore, classified as completed. Source: Chowdhury *et al.* (1997).

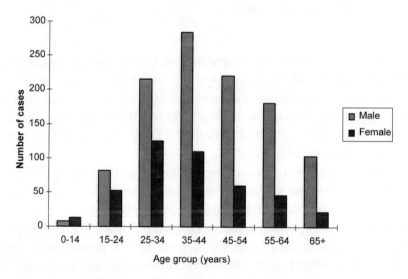

Fig. 1. The age-sex distribution of the smear positive patients for 1995.

Programme data were also analysed from phase three for all patients diagnosed and started on the eight-month regimen during 1995. A total of 1,741 patients (1,525 new cases and 216 patients previously treated) were confirmed to be sputum smear positive and all had accepted treatment. Figure 1 shows the age-sex distribution of the smear-positive

Table 3.   Treatment outcomes for acid-fast bacilli-positive patients treated with eight-month regimen in 1995 (phase three).

Outcome	Number of cases ($n = 1741$)		
	New ($n = 1525$)	Retreatment ($n = 216$)	Total ($n = 1741$)
Cured	2301 (85.3)	195 (90.3)	1496 (85.9)
Completed	1 (0.1)	2 (0.9)	3 (0.3)
Died	226 (8.2)	3 (3.2)	133 (7.6)
Failure	43 (2.8)	8 (3.7)	51 (2.9)
Defaulted	36 (2.4)	4 (1.9)	40 (2.3)
Migrated/ referred/transferred	23 (1.2)	—	18 (1.0)

Source: Chowdhury *et al.* (1977).

patients for 1995, which clearly shows that the greatest male-female differential was in the 35–44 years age group. At the end of the eight-month regimen more than 85% of new cases and 90% of relapsed patients were smear negative and were deemed to be cured. However, 8% of patients had died and about 2% had defaulted (Table 3). A similar pattern existed for all new cases for 1996.

Another approach to evaluating the health impact of the BRAC tuberculosis programme was a large-scale household cross-sectional survey to compare the sputum smear positive prevalence rates in programme *thanas* with a comparison *thana*. This survey included 44,505 people in sampled households (Table 4). A total of 795 people with chronic cough were identified, half were from the comparison *thana* and half from the two programme *thanas*. Two-thirds of all the symptomatic patients were men. For those with a symptomatic cough in the two programme *thanas*, 2.5% and 2.7% of sputum samples were smear positive, compared with 3.4% in the non-programme comparison *thana*. The apparent success of the BRAC programme is shown by the fact that the prevalence rates of smear-positive tuberculosis among people aged 15 years and older in the programme *thanas* was half that in the

Table 4. Prevalence of acid-fast bacilli-positive cases detected by household survey in programme and comparison *thanas*.

Thana	Total population 15 years or more	Number with chronic cough	Number acid-fast bacilli smear positive	Prevalence rate (per 1000)
A (Programme)	7146	181 (2.5)	5 (2.1)	0.07
B (Programme)	8639	236 (2.7)	6 (2.3)	0.07
C (Comparison)	8720	373 (4.3)	13 (3.4)	0.15

Source: Chowdhury *et al.* (1997).

non-programme comparison *thana*. However, a problematic finding was that the total number of patients identified by this survey was smaller than had been expected. For instance, in the sample of 8,720 people in the comparison *thana*, the total number of smear-positive patients should have been between 29 and 48 if the prevalence rates of 0.33% and 0.55% found in 1984 were still applicable in 1995. Because of the possibility that faulty household survey techniques had led to an under recording of positive cases, all households were in fact revisited but this only resulted in the detection of one new case. Three quarters of the smear-positive patients were men and all except one were over the age of 35.

During the household survey all previously treated tuberculosis patients were followed up and 90% of 483 patients who completed their treatment between 1992 and 1994 were successfully contacted. Eighteen patients were still sputum positive at the time of survey, nine each in the two programme *thanas* and, of these, 17 were found to have more than one fast bacillus per high-power field. The overall relapse rate was 4.1%, but when this was disaggregated for the time since treatment had been completed, the rate was 7.8% for two years or more, 3.3% for 12–23 months, and 4.5% for less than 12 months.

The evaluation also included studies of the perceptions of the patients and providers. The patients and other members of the community spoke highly of the care provided by BRAC through the community health workers. Even so, half of the interviewed patients complained of drug side effects such as loss of appetite, tingling sensations in their limbs, vomiting and skin rashes. They were satisfied, however, that the community health workers had provided prompt advice on how to deal with such side effects. Since the community health workers come from the same villages, patients had no problems in accessing them. The poorer patients did receive their drugs, which were supplied free of cost. The community health workers, on the other hand, did not encounter any problems in their work with tuberculosis patients. In their own words they "enjoyed the work" and tuberculosis control caused no disruption to their daily chores. About half of the tuberculosis patients mentioned that their family and villager neighbours had not shown any prejudices against them, while a quarter reported that they had been isolated from family members and the remaining quarter said the villagers both hated and were scared of them.

Discussion on the Evaluation Findings

Directly observed therapy, short course (DOTS) is now accepted as the treatment regimen of choice for tuberculosis in many developing and developed countries (Bayer et al., 1995; World Health Organization, 1997a). However, although the WHO has described this approach as a 'breakthrough strategy' for combating the global tuberculosis epidemic, only about 10% of the world's tuberculosis patients have access to it. Of the 13 countries in which 75% of the world's tuberculosis patients live, until recently only five, including Bangladesh, have adopted DOTS for their national strategy (World Health Organization, 1997a). In addition, international health policies for combating tuberculosis have given priority to establishing government national programmes and have paid little attention to the importance of community-based approaches.

    In countries such as Bangladesh, where the government health infrastructure is poorly developed, particularly in rural areas, non-governmental organisations like BRAC have a major role in tuberculosis control. The innovative BRAC programme has been built up from the 'bottom-up' by relying on community health workers and local-level supervision. This combination has been shown to be highly successful in identifying villagers with possible tuberculosis and then encouraging them to accept and comply with DOTS treatment in their own villages. In the BRAC tuberculosis control programme, treatment compliance and cure rates have progressively improved from the pilot phase to phase two and again in phase three, when the eight-month regimen was introduced.

The evaluation of the BRAC programme strongly suggested that it has managed to progressively improve tuberculosis case-detection and cure rates in a rural population in Bangladesh. The findings on the different approaches to evaluating the impact of the programme on health has produced similar and consistent results. At least 90% of diagnosed patients had accepted the 12-month regimen and this had risen to almost 100% for the eight-month course, with cure rates of at least 80% and 85% respectively for the 12-month and eight-month course. Even with an acceptance rate of 95% and a cure rate of 85%, it is nevertheless important to emphasise that the overall success is 81% for all diagnosed cases ($0.95 \times 0.85 \times 100$) and that the mortality rate was 8–10% and that relapses occurred in 3–4% of all patients given treatment. Such programme indicators are consistent with those achieved in other programmes that have relied on professionally trained health workers (Weis *et al.*, 1994; Wilkinson 1994, 1997; World Health Organization, 1997a; Kochi, 1997).

The fundamental assumption in tuberculosis control is that if a large but, at present, unknown proportion of all pulmonary tuberculosis patients are treated, transmission will be reduced and the annual incidence will gradually decline over time. This evaluation produced some evidence that is consistent with this assumption. The cross-sectional household survey, carried out in 1995 in *thanas* where BRAC had started the tuberculosis control programme in 1991, showed that the prevalence of smear-positive tuberculosis in these programme *thanas* was half that in the comparison *thana*, where only the normal government tuberculosis services were available. These rates, although lower than previous population estimates made in 1984, were based on sound epidemiological methods and the adequacy of the survey findings had been thoroughly checked by repeating the survey. The figures appear to be comparable, therefore, even if the survey had possibly underestimated the true prevalence. An alternative interpretation is that the true prevalence may have actually decreased during the previous two decades or so, possibly because of the wide availability of the BRAC services and cheap anti-tuberculosis drugs in Bangladesh which has had a progressive drug policy since 1982 (Reich, 1994; Chowdhury, 1996).

The evaluation findings also suggest that the BRAC programme was detecting about 50% of all the existing pulmonary tuberculosis patients in the total population. When this detection rate is combined with the treatment results from phase three, however, only about 40% of all existing cases are successfully treated, calculated as follows: acceptance of 0.95 × cure rate of 0.85 × overall detection rate of 0.50 = 0.40. It is not known whether or not this proportion is sufficient to reduce the transmission of tuberculosis.

The key to tuberculosis control is, therefore, in raising the overall detection rate for all active cases of pulmonary tuberculosis in the population. BRAC believes that this situation can be significantly improved by placing a greater emphasis on social mobilisation and the introduction of the shorter regimen. In addition, the National Tuberculosis Programme is working more closely with private providers, such as BRAC, that have an important role in tuberculosis control. A close working relationship between the government and BRAC programmes in the same *thanas* is likely to improve the credibility of community health workers by enhancing their performance.

The important factors that may have contributed to the success of the BRAC programme have already been commented on and can be summarised as follows (Grange and Zumla, 1997):

Learning from pilot projects. BRAC gives importance to a prolonged organisational learning phase, with pilot projects in a few *thanas* before expanding to a much larger programme. BRAC is a learning organisation which believes that monitoring and evaluation enables it to learn from its own experiences (Lovell, 1992). BRAC maintains an independent and active research evaluation division that is always closely involved in evaluating new 'pilot' initiatives before they are expanded. Even during scaling up, operations research and evaluation activities continue as an integral part of all of BRAC's programmes, thus providing BRAC with an opportunity to continue to be a learning organisation.

Involvement of community health workers. These health workers are the backbone of the BRAC programme. On a house-by-house basis they identify the patients with chronic cough, collect sputum specimens, provide treatment at the door-step and maintain follow up and tracing of contacts. They live in the community they serve and are well respected for their services. They also enjoy their work and receive monetary incentives for identifying patients and ensuring that treatment is completed successfully. Since community health workers are women they are also well placed to assist female patients. Unfortunately, the government's national programme does not have similar community health workers involved in tuberculosis control.

Patient's bond money. The bond money that a patient pays to BRAC for their treatment is probably the single most crucial factor in achieving the high treatment completion rate. The bond acts as incentive to both the patient and their community for the regular intake of drugs. In a previous mass programme for oral rehydration therapy (ORT), BRAC also successfully used an incentive salary system for front-line programme workers (Chowdhury and Cash, 1996).

Treatment at the door-step. Since tuberculosis is a dreaded illness and cultural taboos lead to patients being stigmatised, there is a low attendance at government health facilities (Chowdhury and Kabir, 1988).

In addition, health workers are seen as unfriendly and their behaviour also dissuades patients from seeking health care. In contrast, BRAC health workers actively seek out possible cases of tuberculosis and provide counseling and treatment services at the patient's door-step.

Provision of free drugs. The national programme supplies free anti-tuberculosis drugs to BRAC and these are passed on free to the patients by the community health workers. The government tuberculosis programme also provides free drugs but frequent drug shortages and embezzlement have led to a lack of confidence in the government services.

Programme management. BRAC is a non-governmental organisation that is well known for its innovative approaches to social development and its ability to manage its programmes both effectively and efficiently. BRAC also places much emphasis on team work, in service training and staff supervision. Although BRAC has evolved into one of the world's largest non-governmental organisations, it has a firm belief in the practices of good management.

Availability of external technical assistance and financial resources. BRAC has developed good collaborative relationships with many external agencies. For instance, much needed technical support has come from the Research Institute for Tuberculosis in Tokyo, Japan, and the National Anti-Tuberculosis Association of Bangladesh (NATAB). Financial support has come from UNICEF, Swedish SIDA, Swiss Development Cooperation, and the United Kingdom's Department for International Development. In addition, the Government of Bangladesh has extended its full cooperation to BRAC, including technical support, free drug supplies and quality control of the diagnostic laboratories for sputum testing. As a partner to the Government of Bangladesh, BRAC now runs its tuberculosis control programme in 39 *thanas* and will add a further 11 in 1998.

Acknowledgement

We thank N. Ishikawa and colleagues at the Research Institute of Tuberculosis in Tokyo, Japan, for their long-standing support. The BRAC Tuberculosis Programme is supported by the Government of Bangladesh, the National Tuberculosis Association of Bangladesh, the Department for International Development of the United Kingdom, SIDA, Swiss Development Cooperation, and UNICEF. Other BRAC research contributors include Kaoser Afsana, Jalaluddin Ahmed, Aminul Alam, Akramul Islam, S. N. Mahmud and B. Roy.

References

Ahmed, M., *et al.* (1993) *Primary Education for All: Learning from the BRAC Experience.* Washington DC: Academy for Educational Development.

Bayer, R. and Wilkinson, D. (1995) Directly observed therapy for tuberculosis: History of an idea. *Lancet* **345**, 1545–1548.

Chowdhury, A. M. R. and Kabir, Z. N. (1988) *Perceptions About the Six Immunisable Diseases and Vaccinations in Two Areas of Rural Bangladesh.* Dhaka: BRAC (unpublished document).

Chowdhury, A. M. R. (1990) *A Tale of Two Wings: Health and Family Planning Programmes in an Upazila in Northern Bangladesh.* Dhaka: BRAC.

Chowdhury, A. M. R., *et al.* (1991) Controlling a forgotten disease : Using voluntary health workers for tuberculosis control in rural Bangladesh. IUATLD *Newsletter*, December.

Chowdhury, A. M. R., Mahmood, M. and Abed, F. H. (1991) Impact of rural credit for the rural poor: The case of BRAC in Bangladesh. *Small Enterprise Development* **2**, 4–13.

Chowdhury, A. M. R., Alam, A., Chowdhury, S. A. and Ahmed, J. (1992) Tuberculosis control in Bangladesh. *Lancet* **339**, 1181–1182.

Chowdhury, A. M. R. and Cash, R. A. (1996) *A Simple Solution: Teaching Millions to Treat Diarrhoea at Home.* Dhaka: University Press Ltd.

Chowdhury, A. M. R., Chowdhury, S. A., Islam, M. N., Islam, A. and Vaughan, J. P. (1997) Control of tuberculosis through community health workers in Bangladesh. *Lancet* **350**, 160–172.

Chowdhury, Z. (1996) *The Politics of Essential Drugs.* Dhaka: University Press Ltd.

Connolly, M. A. and Raviglione, M. C. (1996) *Assessment of Tuberculosis: Management in Community Case Projects in India.* Geneva: World Health Organization.

Director General of Health Service (DGHS) (1989) *Report on the National Prevalence Survey on Tuberculosis in Bangladesh 1987–88.* Dhaka: Mininstry of Health and Family Welfare.

Government of Bangladesh. (1996) *National Guidelines for Tuberculosis Control.* Dhaka: Ministry of Health and Family Welfare.

Grange, J. M. and Zumla, A. (1997) Making DOTS succeed. *Lancet* **350**, p. 157.

Huq, M., ed. (1991) *The Near Miracle.* Dhaka: University Press Ltd.

Ishikawa, N. (1985) Promotion of the community based tuberculosis programme in Bangladesh. *Proceeding of the XIV Eastern Regional Tuberculosis Conference, Kathmandu.*

Ishikawa, N. (1995) DOTS as a way to secure the cure. *Newsletter from Kiyose, Tokyo*, No. 9, (September).

Islam, I. (1981) National tuberculosis control programme in Bangladesh. *Proceedings of the XIIth Eastern Regional IUATLD Conference, Dhaka.* Paris: IUATLD

Islam, M. S., Koseki, Y. and Ishikawa, N. (1986) Epidemiological study of tuberculosis in a rural area in Bangladesh. *Proceedings of the World Conference of IUATLD, Singapore.* Paris: IUATLD

Kochi, A. (1997) Tuberculosis control — Is DOTS the health break through of the 1990s? *World Health Forum* **18**, 225–247.

Lovell, C. H. (1992) *Breaking the Cycle of Poverty.* Hartford: Kumarian Press.

Murray, C. J. L., Styblo, K. and Rouillon, A. (1990) Tuberculosis in developing countries: Burden, intervention and cost. *Bull. Wld. Hlth. Org.* **64**, 2–20.

Raviglione, M. C., Snider, D. E. and Kochi, A. (1995) Global epidemiology of tuberculosis; morbidity and mortality of a world wide epidemic. *J. Am. Med. Assoc.* **273**, 220–226.

Reich, M. (1994) Bangladesh pharmaceutical policy and politics. *Hlth. Pol. Plann.* **9**, 130–139.

Wilkinson, D. (1994) High compliance tuberculosis treatment programme in a rural community. *Lancet* **343**, 647–648.

Wilkinson, D. (1997) Managing tuberculosis case-loads in African countries. *Lancet* **349**, p. 882.

Weis, S. E. *et al.* (1994) The effect of directly observed therapy on the rates of drug resistance and relapse in tuberculosis. *N. Engl. J. Med.* **330**, 1179–1184.

Wise, R. (1996) Global paradox. *Lancet.* **343**, p. 282.

World Health Organization (1997a) *Report on the Tuberculosis Epidemic 1997.* Geneva: World Health Organization.

World Health Organization (1997b) *Review of the National Tuberculosis Control Programme of Bangladesh.* Dhaka: World Health Organization.

CHAPTER 17

A RESPONSE BY NURSES TO THE CHALLENGE OF TUBERCULOSIS IN THE UNITED KINGDOM AND RUSSIA

Virginia Gleissberg

Introduction

Following the introduction of effective chemotherapy in the 1950s, a sharp decline in the incidence and mortality of tuberculosis was seen globally and it was generally assumed that the persistent scourge of the previous centuries was finally under control. In both the UK and Russia, service provision and vigilance have declined and the incidence of tuberculosis has increased (Fig. 1) but for arguably different reasons.

United Kingdom

In the UK, as in other Western countries where tuberculosis rates were falling dramatically and were expected to continue to do so, services were scaled down, expertise in the management of tuberculosis diminished and there was a general complacency surrounding what was considered to be a conquered disease. The rise in incidence of the disease in the early 1990s, particularly in areas such as inner London (Fig. 1), together with the increasing number of drug-resistant cases, began to alarm the medical establishment and tuberculosis once again became the focus of significant attention. The increase has been attributed to a number of factors including the reduction in services, large numbers

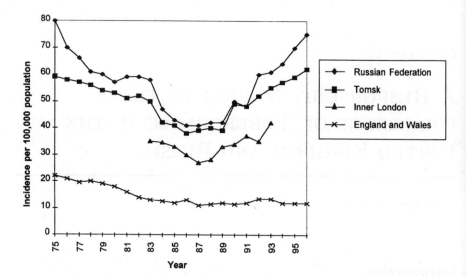

Fig. 1.   Incidence of tuberculosis per 100,000 population in the Russian Federation, England, and Wales, 1975–1996. Sources: Russian Federation: Central Tuberculosis Training and Research Institute (1997); Tomsk: Tomsk Oblast Tuberculosis Services data (1997); Inner London: Office of Population Censuses and Surveys (OPCS) Notification data (1994); England and Wales: Communicable Diseases Surveillance Centre, Colindale (1997).

of refugees arriving from high-incidence countries, and increasing levels of poverty and homelessness. Although the advent of HIV had a significant impact in other countries, such as Africa and the USA, this was not the case in the UK although the reluctance of physicians to notify HIV patients who developed active tuberculosis may well have masked the true extent of the overlap in the UK (Darbyshire, 1995; McEvoy and Maguire 1995).

Russia

In Russia, the circumstances were somewhat different. Following 'Perestroika' in 1989 and the economic chaos which has arisen from the move towards capitalism, the extensive services and provisions, which were made available for the care of tuberculosis patients during the

Communist era, could no longer be supported. The health of the population is deteriorating, particularly amongst men (according to the statistics of the Ministry of Health, Russian Federation (1997), life expectancy for the average Russian male fell from 63.8 in 1990 to 59.6 in 1996), the consumption of both tobacco and alcohol is increasing (Leon *et al.*, 1997), and a growing number of Russian people are facing poverty, with inflation spiralling out of control as their salaries and pensions stay at the same level, and are frequently unpaid (Bank Austria, 1997). All this has provided the ideal setting for tuberculosis to exploit an ever more vulnerable population.

Nurses

Tuberculosis nurses in the two countries have also been affected by recent developments. Since the early part of this century nurses in both the UK and Russia have played an important part in providing care for those suffering from this disease. Tuberculosis patients in both countries commonly experience fear, stigma and vulnerability and, although the response they receive from both their health service and the local community may vary, they all require care and support if they are to have any hope of recovery. This chapter will focus on the role of nurses in the fight against tuberculosis, the challenges currently facing nurses both in the UK and in the Russian Federation, and attempts to develop nursing services to meet those challenges, illustrated by accounts of the author's experience of working in both countries.

The Role of the Nurse in the Care of Tuberculosis Patients

The early days prior to effective treatment

Nurses have a long history of working in the field of tuberculosis and as the profession evolves so too do the skills which nurses have to offer to the patients. The role of the nurse in this field arose from the need to educate patients and the general public about how to prevent the spread of the disease and to care for themselves should they develop it. According to reports cited by Robbins (1997) the early tuberculosis nurse was a formidable creature. At the beginning of the century in America, independent, educated, ambitious women became tuberculosis visiting nurses and instilled a strict sanatorium-style regime into the households of patients who could not afford to go away and 'take the cure'. They were ardent public health campaigners and exposed the appalling conditions in which many urban dwellers were living. They had a lot of success and were often a poor family's only hope if tuberculosis did strike. In the UK, although sanatoria were more accessible to all classes, beds were often scarce and not all patients stayed for the full course of their 'treatment'. Health visitors were employed, like their counterparts in America, by tuberculosis dispensaries to visit patients at home in order to educate them and their families, monitor progress and identify any additional potential cases of the disease within the household (Bryder, 1988).

Tuberculosis nurses in those days were, however, not always popular. Patients often felt exposed and stigmatised as a result of their attention and the strict regime they had to follow such as keeping windows open in the middle of winter inevitably signalled to their neighbours that there was tuberculosis in the household. Physicians also had varied opinions about them. While some felt that the work these nurses did with the patients in their own homes was the most effective tool available at the time to treat tuberculosis (Sachs, 1908) others did not appreciate what they saw as 'interference' with their patients (Robbins, 1997).

The introduction of effective chemotherapy

With the continuing reduction in the incidence of the disease, tuberculosis nurses branched out into other areas of respiratory medicine and became specialists in conditions such as asthma and chronic obstructive airways disease. By the late 1980s tuberculosis was so uncommon that it was rarely, if ever, featured on a school of nursing syllabus. Therefore, the level of knowledge among UK nurses in general with regard to this disease often mirrored that of the lay person together with commonly held myths and misconceptions. Specialist posts did still exist but were restricted to areas, mainly poorer urban areas, with a higher than the national average incidence of tuberculosis.

The recent upturn in the incidence of tuberculosis has led to a much greater interest, which is reflected by new modular courses on the disease which have become available in a number of universities in the last few years, and by the increasing coverage in the nursing literature. In some areas, services have been expanded with an increase in tuberculosis nursing posts although many areas remain under-staffed. The British Thoracic Society has recommended in the national guidelines for the control and management of the disease that there should be appropriate numbers of tuberculosis nurses available according to the number of notifications in a given area of the UK (British Thoracic Society, 1994, 1998).

Specialist nurses, health visitors and chest clinic sisters based either in chest clinics or community health centres are responsible, to a greater or lesser extent, for treatment monitoring, contact-tracing, new entrant screening, BCG vaccination programmes, and health education. Much of their work continues to take place in the patients' homes although there is often contact with the patient in hospital as well as in outpatient clinics. Tuberculosis nursing services in different areas vary according to local demand and resources, but there is now great potential to address poor staffing and facilities at a time when the disease is the focus of much attention. The move towards creating more specialist posts within the nursing profession, offering more autonomy and decision-making powers, attracts highly-qualified individuals to tuberculosis nursing posts. Ideally, a close working relationship is built up between the physician who essentially makes the diagnosis and prescribes treatment and the nurse who plans and implements the appropriate care for each individual patient and their contacts to ensure the best possible outcome. This requires a wide variety of skills and experience (as described below) which is why specialist nurses and health visitors are recommended.

Education

Education continues to be a vital part of the work of tuberculosis nurses. The incidence of, and mortality due to, this disease was on the decline well before the introduction of effective chemotherapy and although it is difficult to determine specific reasons for this it has been attributed to public health measures such as improved sanitation (Shaw, 1995); the role of public health nurses in America (Zilm and Warbink, 1995) and health visitors in the UK in educating tuberculosis patients and their families as to how to care for themselves and control the spread of the disease; and improved after-care for patients including modest financial support and dispensary monitoring (Bryder, 1988). This has particular significance today as we come to terms with the emergence of multidrug resistance resulting in a growing number of patients with potentially incurable disease. Patients with multidrug-resistant tuberculosis nowadays have the same uncertain prognoses and face similar long periods of physical as well as mental isolation as people who had the disease before effective chemotherapy was available. They are therefore in need of a great deal of support and understanding as well as advice on how best to care for themselves and protect others.

Patients respond to a diagnosis of tuberculosis in many different ways and nurses will use their listening skills to identify the fears and concerns of each individual in order to provide appropriate information and build up a relationship based on trust and understanding. It cannot be assumed that all patients will want the same information as their circumstances often vary a great deal as do their priorities.

Counselling

The nurse will also act as a counsellor to provide the necessary support and reassurance during the prolonged and often isolating treatment period. Following the discovery of effective chemotherapy, nursing support has been shown to significantly enhance the patient's chance of completing treatment (Snutsk-Torbec, 1987). It is well-documented that tuberculosis patients belong to the more vulnerable groups in society (Bhatti *et al.*, 1995) and that many of them do not regard health as their main priority. This, together with the extended course of treatment required often long after symptoms have subsided, requires a sensitive and resolved approach to their care.

Clinical skills

Nurses with specialised knowledge and skills can discuss concerns that the patient may have, monitor their progress and recognise any adverse reactions to treatment. Such nurses, employed on a permanent basis and providing care for patients throughout their treatment, can help to maintain a consistent approach to the care of patients and avoid confusion and mistrust arising from conflicting information and advice. This is particularly valuable in health care settings where a rotational system is in operation, such as the UK and the USA, and where medical personnel change frequently (Snutsk-Torbec, 1987).

Supervision and support

The alarming rise in the incidence in tuberculosis in many areas of the world has led to a serious rethink about how policies and services can best be developed to meet the growing demands. Since declaring the tuberculosis situation a global emergency in 1993 the World Health Organization (WHO) has recommended that National Tuberculosis Programmes (NTP) around the world adopt a strategy called Directly Observed Therapy, Short Course (DOTS) as the most effective and affordable method of controlling the disease (World Health Organization, 1997a). The DOTS strategy consists of several key factors including political commitment, diagnosis by bacteriology, treatment by closely supervised short course chemotherapy, and effective data collection and monitoring systems. Due to stretched resources it is very difficult to organise supervised treatment for all patients though, by developing close working relationships with patients, nurses are in a good position to assess how best to provide appropriate levels of monitoring and support on an individual basis. This may include full or partly observed therapy, support for others involved in supervision such as members of the family or hostel workers, or regular review in a clinic or in the patient's home.

Community care and accessibility

The emphasis is on ambulatory as opposed to inpatient care for tuberculosis patients and nurses have an increasing role to play in the treatment, support and supervision of patients in the community. With the vulnerable and sometimes difficult nature of the client group it is important for patients to be met with acceptance, tolerance and understanding. Everything possible must be done to encourage tuberculosis patients and those vulnerable to the disease to use the available services for investigation, contact-screening, routine follow up and other services. As well as a sympathetic attitude, this requires a reasonable degree of flexibility to make services as accessible as possible and specialist nurses can offer a wider choice to patients with regard to clinic times and home visiting. Although treatment is essentially standardised, a nursing emphasis on providing individualised patient-centred care lends itself to offer the levels of support that the patients invariably need. Teamwork is essential and the greatest success can be achieved when the physician, nurse and patient work closely together.

United Kingdom

The current situation

By the mid 1980s tuberculosis was considered to be largely under control with below 6,000 cases a year and only occasional deaths. Tuberculosis services were incorporated into general hospitals and usually managed by chest physicians on an outpatient basis. Patients with nonpulmonary forms of the disease were sometimes managed by surgeons or other specialists according to the site of the lesion although it was recommended that a chest physician should be informed of every case of tuberculosis as they are considered to have most experience of its treatment (Byrd *et al.*, 1977; British Thoracic Society, 1994). All cases of tuberculosis still have to be statutorily notified.

St Mary's Hospital, Paddington, London — An Operational Example

Background

St. Mary's Hospital in Paddington is a large teaching hospital in central London in an area where a significant proportion of the population are homeless, immigrants and refugees. As in the rest of the UK the huge drop in the incidence of tuberculosis led to a reduction in services offered and by 1993 the Chest Clinic Sister was the only nurse who had any involvement in the care of patients with this disease. There was an average of 100 notifications of tuberculosis a year from St. Mary's Hospital but the decline had slowed and the number was beginning to rise again by the beginning of the 1990s.

By 1993 the consultant chest physicians at St Mary's Hospital were becoming concerned about the increase which was showing no signs of slowing. The Chest Clinic Sister had meanwhile retired and it was decided that her replacement should look at developing the tuberculosis service across the hospital in response to the growing demand.

Description of tuberculosis services in 1993

Patients with suspected tuberculosis were mostly referred by general practitioners and usually received urgent appointments. Some patients were referred from other departments within the hospital and others were identified in contact or new entrant screening clinics. Children were usually seen in the paediatric department, apart from those referred from school screening sessions or who had missed BCG vaccination. If a case of sputum smear-positive tuberculosis was found the patient was admitted for two weeks in isolation (usually in a side room of a medical ward) although not all suspected pulmonary cases were isolated. Patients were usually notified to the public health authorities by the doctor (not always a chest physician) who diagnosed and commenced them on treatment for tuberculosis but the chest team was not always informed if the patient had non-pulmonary disease. Bacteriology reports of acid-fast bacilli seen on smear microscopy or *M. tuberculosis* isolated by culture were routinely sent to the chest clinic for the chest physicians' information but they themselves rarely had time to chase these up. St Mary's Hospital also has a large treatment centre for those infected by HIV and are suffering from AIDS. Physicians in this department were often reluctant to notify their patients if they developed tuberculosis, mainly because they were concerned about confidentiality. The chest clinic was also rarely informed of these patients so their contacts were often neglected and their adherence to treatment was not always monitored.

A draft protocol had been written by one of the chest physicians and he was keen that it should be expanded for hospital-wide use as guidance for the control and management of tuberculosis. This would be especially useful as the rotation of house doctors and registrars often led to inconsistent management of patients suspected of and suffering from tuberculosis and confusing messages being given to both patients and nursing staff.

Local nursing issues

The Chest Clinic Sister was also known as the tuberculosis health visitor and her role with regard to this disease focused on contact-tracing, patient support, Heaf testing, BCG vaccination and new entrant screening. The level of knowledge with regard to tuberculosis among general hospital nurses appeared to be quite poor and there were many requests for updating. Little information regarding tuberculosis patients and those

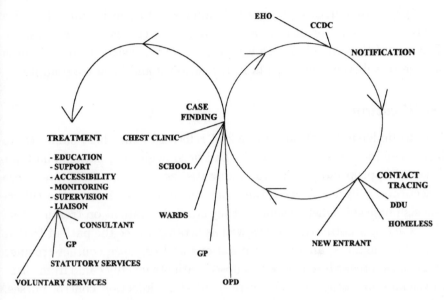

Fig. 2.   A model programme focusing on the four main components of tuberculosis management — notification, contact-tracing, case-finding and treatment.

using the screening services available at the chest clinic (contacts or new entrants) was formally documented and nursing records were brief.

Addressing the problems

The protocol for the control and management of tuberculosis at St Mary's Hospital evolved from discussions among physicians from all departments, ward staff, infection control nurses, occupational health advisors, laboratory personnel, and management representatives led by the tuberculosis nurse specialist in order to promote a wide ownership and maximise adherence. The service was developed along British Thoracic Society guidelines with appropriate adaptations for the local client group (British Thoracic Society, 1994). A model was also developed based on the protocol and focusing on what were considered to be the four main components of tuberculosis management (see Fig. 2), i.e. notification, contact-tracing, case-finding and treatment. Teaching sessions were given to nurses and junior doctors within the hospital to raise awareness about the disease and to publicise changes to the system. The aim of this model of care was to provide a consistent and seamless service to tuberculosis patients in the hospital and local community.

Notification

Due to under notification and lack of referral to the chest clinic, there have been incidents when contacts had been neglected, patients had not received appropriate follow up, and statistics regarding case rates were inaccurate. Physicians were therefore encouraged to inform the tuberculosis nurse specialist as soon as they started a patient on treatment so that she could notify the case as well as arrange to see the patient to discuss the diagnosis, answer any questions and organise contact-tracing. Information regarding newly diagnosed patients usually came from chest physicians but other sources were ward staff, infection control nurses, laboratory personnel and physicians from other specialities.

Contact-tracing

There were two screening clinics per week run by the tuberculosis nurse specialist in the chest clinic for contacts and other vulnerable groups such as new entrants and the homeless. The clinics were run on a drop-in basis to maximise accessibility and links were built up with community organisations working with vulnerable groups to provide information regarding the disease and the screening services available at St Mary's Hospital.

Case-finding

Priority appointments were given to anyone referred to the chest clinic with suspected tuberculosis. Information regarding the available services were circulated to local general practitioners and throughout the hospital to raise awareness generally and encourage the prompt referral of potential cases.

Treatment

A nurse-led clinic was set up to run alongside the weekly consultant out-patient tuberculosis clinic in order to monitor treatment and progress, offer support and pick up any problems promptly. If a clinical problem arose the patient could be referred immediately to the consultant and, likewise, if the consultant diagnosed a new case the patient could be seen immediately by the tuberculosis nurse specialist. Once on treatment, patients were seen at least once a month either in the clinic, at home or some other mutually acceptable place. Many patients were seen more frequently, some as often as three times a week for supervised treatment and the intervals between follow up appointments often varied throughout the treatment period according to the needs of the individual patient. All patients were invited to phone the tuberculosis nurse specialist directly if they had any concerns.

Results

In 1995, audit showed that all known cases of tuberculosis among HIV-positive patients were being notified (Pym *et al.*, 1995). The annual rate of tuberculosis in this group was so high that a new post was created for a HIV/tuberculosis nurse specialist. New documentation had been introduced for all those attending the tuberculosis clinic and data were available on the outcomes of all screening and treatment administered. Every patient on treatment was seen at least once a month and less than 3% of patients were lost to follow up (by 1996 there were on average 140 patients a year). All patients with suspected pulmonary tuberculosis were isolated until shown to be smear negative on three sputum specimens and there were regular training sessions held on wards where patients were most commonly admitted. Health education material had been developed for both staff and patients and the tuberculosis nurse was often used as a resource by both hospital and community staff.

Russia

Tuberculosis services in Russia before the revolution in 1917 developed along much the same lines as in the UK. There was a realisation that tuberculosis mainly affected the poor and also that rest and good food often enhanced the chances of recovery. When the Communists came to power they abolished the Anti-Tuberculosis League which, like many charities at the time, was considered to be bourgeois, but were soon to recognise the importance of having a specialist body focusing on this disease and incorporated a tuberculosis control section within the People's Health Care Committee which was established in 1918. Sanatoria, specialist hospitals, dispensaries and tuberculosis research centres were built all over the Soviet Union and, apart from priority funding from the government, huge publicity campaigns encouraged the general public to donate money to tuberculosis services (Lygoshina, 1998).

Despite the growth of tuberculosis institutions and the development of various surgical treatments, the disease remained a common one and it was particularly prolific following the Second World War. Mass BCG vaccination and screening programmes were introduced, increasing numbers of staff were trained, and more institutions were built until there was a network of specialist services covering the whole of the Soviet Union. The size of the government's investment demanded justification and elaborate systems for data collection were developed. The serious penalties faced by those who did not produce satisfactory results is thought to have led to a certain amount of falsification of statistics presented to the Ministry of Health (Lygoshina, 1998).

By the mid-1980s annual incidence rates had fallen significantly and were steady at just above 30 per 100,000 population, but by 1996 the rate was estimated at 67.5 per 100,000 (Gessen, 1997). This resurgence of tuberculosis has been attributed to a general health care crisis arising from economic difficulties and subsequent reductions in funding (Field 1996; Barr and Field, 1996).

Tomsk, Siberia — An Operational Example

Background

Tomsk Oblast (Province) is about twice the size of England with just under one million inhabitants. It lies on the Western Siberian basin in the middle of the Russian Federation. Just over half of its inhabitants live in the town of Tomsk and the rest are spread out in villages and small towns throughout the Oblast. Access to health care for those living in remote villages is difficult due to extreme weather conditions and various geographical factors. Many roads are impassable during the seven month-long winter and freezing prevents travel by waterways. Conversely, in the more swampy areas, villages can only be reached once winter has arrived.

In 1994, MERLIN (Medical Emergency Relief International), a British relief agency, established a collaborative project in the Tomsk Oblast. The project had involved donations of essential drugs and equipment and a clinical trial to compare Russian tuberculosis treatments with those recommended by the WHO (World Health Organization, 1997a). Initially, the Russians were sceptical about the efficacy of the WHO's methods but the results of the trial convinced them that it would be safe to implement a pilot WHO-style Tuberculosis Control Programme (TBCP). I arrived in Tomsk in September 1996 to review nursing practices, assess training needs and implement training in preparation for the TBCP which was planned for January 1997.

Description of tuberculosis services in 1996

Tuberculosis services in the Tomsk Oblast are centralised and the major institutions are in the town of Tomsk. These consist of a polyclinic, a day hospital and a hospital that provides specialised tuberculosis services to people from all over the Oblast and are independent from the general medical services. The regional hospital (Fig. 3) is based on a site 5 km outside the town in the middle of a forest. The Tuberculosis Polyclinic (Fig. 4) receives referrals from the general medical services

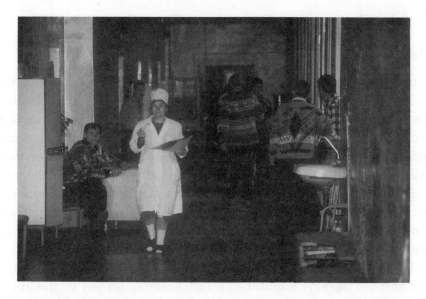

Fig. 3.   The Tomsk Regional Tuberculosis Hospital (by courtesy of MERLIN).

within the town as well as from the rural tuberculosis doctors, one of whom is based in each of the 19 rayons (administrative areas) which make up Tomsk Oblast. Patients are then investigated in the polyclinic and referred to the appropriate institution for treatment. There are also separate facilities in Tomsk for children and psychiatric patients with the disease and a tuberculosis prison colony receives referrals from prisons throughout the Oblast.

One of the major problems for the Tomsk tuberculosis services was the expensive far-reaching system that had developed throughout Russia to manage the disease (Drobniewski *et al.*, 1995). Prolonged inpatient care, radiological diagnosis, mass screening, individualised and often prolonged treatment regimens, adjunct therapies, and surgical interventions all added to the cost of care. The strategy that the MERLIN team were advocating required the concentration of scarce resources on finding and giving short course chemotherapy to the most infectious cases by implementing the WHO DOTS recommendations, reducing

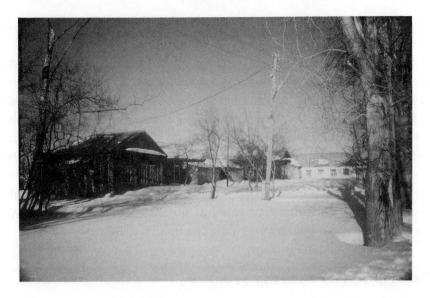

Fig. 4.   Bakchar Polyclinic, 250 km east of Tomsk town.

the length of inpatient stay and introducing structural and economic reforms to make the best use of available resources.

Local nursing issues

Russian nurses faced daunting problems both personally and professionally. The number of patients increased even as the supply of drugs, equipment and their salaries diminished. Apart from extensive health services, the Communist regime provided a lot of social support for people with tuberculosis including accommodation, food coupons and pensions. Staff working in the tuberculosis services also received benefits including extra payment and food coupons. Due to the present difficult economic situation these things are no longer available. Accordingly, the living conditions for the nurses and their patients also deteriorated as social care and incentives disappeared for both. The staff work under considerable pressure, are very poorly paid (they often receive only a proportion of their salaries months in arrears) and have a very low status. Recruitment is difficult especially into the tuberculosis services, especially since incentives are no longer provided.

Nurse training takes three years for those who leave school at the age of sixteen and two years for those who leave at eighteen. Nurses in all institutions are not encouraged to show initiative and are expected to follow the doctor's instructions as well as ensure that they complete the work demanded by Prikaz (decree from the local or central government). There was a lack of in-service training and access to up-to-date information regarding advances in tuberculosis treatment and control. On the whole, the nurses in the Tomsk tuberculosis services felt professionally undervalued and frustrated at not being able to provide what they considered to be adequate care for their patients.

Description of nursing practice

The nurses' knowledge regarding the Russian approach to tuberculosis care was good, but they had little or no information about WHO recommendations. Levels of practice varied according to the attitude of the particular nurse. Whereas some would do the bare minimum of what was required others would stretch themselves to the limit.

Community nurses based in the polyclinic had the most demanding workloads, undertook the greatest variety of activities and were the only nurses involved in home visiting. Most of the community nurses were frustrated at being unable to care adequately for patients, in part due to the enormous workloads which were seen to be increasing with the changes being implemented in the tuberculosis services. There was a lack of prioritisation of activities which was particularly evident in the organisation of home visiting: nurses would spend as much time and effort trying to find someone who had not attended their compulsory annual check up as they would to locate a patient who had defaulted from treatment. Treatment for alcoholic patients was particularly difficult to manage and, although there were no specific figures available, nurses felt that alcoholism was a growing problem. Transport was difficult for both patients using the tuberculosis services and nurses visiting patients at home.

Nurses working in the day hospital were mainly involved with administering adjunct and complementary therapies to patients who usually attended daily for treatment. One nurse organised daily and intermittent supervised therapy (Fig. 5). Any non-attenders were discussed with the doctors and if the patient did not return they were usually referred back to the polyclinic although there was no formal system for doing so. The day hospital was a popular facility among the patients because they could obtain free meals and rest in one of the two wards which were available to them. Hospital nurses essentially provided nursing care to inpatients with tuberculosis. As a group they were most threatened by the planned changes as the move was towards ambulatory care which would result from a strengthening of the day hospital and polyclinic facilities with a corresponding reduction in inpatient care.

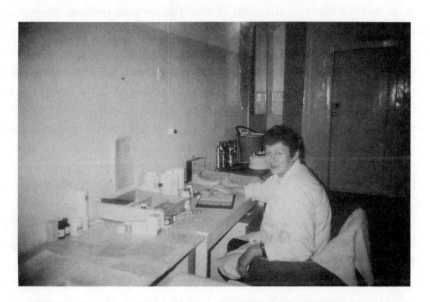

Fig. 5. Nina, the DOT nurse at the Day Hospital in Tomsk town.

Postal systems between central and district services were slow and under-resourced. There were few phone lines available within the tuberculosis services (usually only one or two in even the biggest institutions). Information regarding those who had been discharged for follow up in the community as well as those who had left the hospital of their own accord would therefore reach the appropriate outlying services sometimes weeks later. This created difficulties in maintaining contact with patients, thus resulting in significant breaks in treatment.

Addressing the problems

That some patients (i.e. sputum smear-positive patients) should take priority over others is a completely alien idea but one which is vital in order to reduce the transmission of the disease and prevent drug resistance. A nursing protocol was written and teaching sessions were set up. These were based on the existing system but stressed the need for prioritisation and offered comprehensive guidance for the follow up of non-attenders. The aim was to improve communication between the tuberculosis institutions in Tomsk to speed up the transfer of information about non-attenders and discharged patients in order to reduce gaps in treatment. Training was also needed with regard to the new treatment cards that were being introduced as a part of the programme.

Particular attention was paid to community nurses throughout as the emphasis was on developing ambulatory care. The main concern of the community nurses was the potential increase in their workload, so it was important to outline how they could use the proposed changes to define priorities and make their workloads more manageable. Stress was placed on the important role that all the nurses working within the Tomsk Oblast tuberculosis services had to play in the implementation of the programme, particularly in relation to communication, treatment monitoring, documentation and health education.

Implementation of training

Training was offered to all nurses working in the regional Tuberculosis Polyclinic, day hospital, hospital and tuberculosis prison colony and those working in or around Acino (110 km northwest of Tomsk) or Khozhevniko (150 km southeast). These areas were chosen as they were accessible to nurses from a number of outlying areas and had been identified as having significantly higher numbers of tuberculosis patients than other areas. Time restraints prevented more than two such sessions and teaching on the new documentation and the Tuberculosis Control Programme had to be combined. The training sessions were organised by the head nurses of each institution who also encouraged their staff to attend. It was necessary to organise three sessions at the regional tuberculosis hospital in order to include as many nurses as possible, taking into account the fact that they worked irregular hours. The training sessions were well attended although enthusiasm and active participation in discussion varied a great deal. The most active group were the nurses from the tuberculosis prison colony which was the only institution where in-service training was organised on a regular basis.

Evaluation

I returned to Tomsk three months after the beginning of the TBCP to evaluate the nurses' progress. They reported better compliance which they believed was due to improved health education as well as the regular supply of medication. A total of 165 tuberculosis cases were notified in Tomsk Oblast between January and March 1997, 53 of whom were started on DOTS on an ambulatory basis. Of the 24 new patients being treated at the polyclinic on an outpatient basis, five had missed appointments, all of whom had been followed up and had resumed treatment within a few days (range two to five days). Only one treatment card had been filled out incorrectly. No new patients had been lost to follow up from the tuberculosis hospital and, of the 30 treatment cards seen there, 27 were filled in correctly by the nurses although there was some confusion with regard to how they should record treatment given during weekend leave. Nursing activities in the day hospital were more difficult to assess as the treatment cards for the new patients were not kept separately from those of chronic patients and people receiving chemoprophylaxis. The nurse who was responsible for administering directly observed therapy was seeing around 150 patients a day (including 55 new patients) and felt overwhelmed by the paperwork she was expected to complete. The WHO-style treatment cards had to be completed in addition to the service's old treatment cards and much of the information was duplicated. Of the 20 treatment cards seen, only five of them were up-to-date, although all of them were attached to the old treatment cards which were fully complete and contained the information which was missing from the new cards.

Communication had improved between the hospital and the polyclinic as the head nurses had organised twice weekly meetings to discuss referrals and discharges. Previously, there had been no set pattern to meetings and reliance had been placed on the poor postal and telephone links. There was, however, still a delay in the completion of discharge documentation by some medical staff. Non-attenders from the day hospital were not always reported to the nursing staff but were discussed between the doctors alone, so little information was available to assess their subsequent follow up. The non-attenders that were reported were recorded by the head nurses and followed up by the appropriate polyclinic nurse.

When questioned, nurses working within the Tomsk tuberculosis services were generally able to describe various aspects of the nursing protocol and demonstrated a clear understanding of their role within the tuberculosis control programme. Most were enthusiastic about implementing the nursing protocol but their efforts were frustrated by some doctors who remained reluctant to follow the short course treatment regimens or who were simply unaware of any changes to the role that nurses played in caring for the patients.

In November 1997, I returned to Tomsk as the Programme Coordinator. By June 1998 a number of developments had occurred. The

Moscow-based Central Training and Research Institute, which has been working with the WHO for a number of years and was the official Russian monitor of the Tomsk tuberculosis Control Programme, reported to the Federal Government that the Programme had been successfully initiated. The default rate for 1997 was 7.4% (53 defaulted out of 716 new cases identified).

Four new community tuberculosis nurses had been recruited to the regional Tuberculosis Polyclinic and two new posts were created for nurses who would concentrate on administering DOT in patient's homes in Tomsk town and following up defaulters. There is now a system in place for the management of defaulters which both nurses and doctors follow. Communications improved after six new phone lines were installed in the regional Tuberculosis Polyclinic and discharge information was being entered into a central database also at the polyclinic. There continued to be frustrations, particularly with transport and erratic payment of salaries, but the head nurse of the ambulatory services reported improved morale, particularly due to improved staffing levels and the identification of priorities which had both led to more realistic workloads for the nurses. Morale among staff at the tuberculosis hospital was lower than that among community staff as wider reforms include plans to reduce inpatient care and bed numbers at the Regional Tuberculosis Hospital which are destined to be cut by half by the end of 1998. The medical staff were increasingly prescribing the recommended short course regimens and nurses reported that the new treatment cards had helped to improve patient monitoring.

Conclusion

There is no doubt that the resurgence of tuberculosis is presenting many countries with difficult challenges. Nurses and physicians alike have begun to adapt their practice accordingly but this is by no means a universal trend for a number of reasons. In many areas, through either poor political commitment or straightforward financial constraints, there continues to be a huge lack of resources available to address the problem (World Health Organization, 1997b), information is not always available to the relevant health care providers (Uplekar *et al.*, 1998), and traditional beliefs among both health care providers and their patients often lead to mistrust and scepticism with regard to changing treatment practices (Brouwer *et al.*, 1998).

In Russia, there are other considerations which should be taken into account. Although I have had three years' experience working as a tuberculosis nurse specialist in central London, relating the tuberculosis situation and services available to those in the UK to the nurses in Tomsk was a difficult task. The historical relationship between the East and the West during the Cold War could not be ignored and had to be approached with a great deal of sensitivity. The Russians tend to be proud of their background and, although it was difficult during Communist times, the concept then had been that the Soviet Union was very advanced and dominated the world in many fields. The difficulties which Russia encountered following 'Perestroika' has left many people bewildered and disillusioned. It was not surprising that the nurses and other members of the tuberculosis services found it difficult to accept help from the West. As far as many of tuberculosis nurses were concerned their service had been just fine before the financial problems had started and could be again as soon as the necessary funding was provided.

Although often met with scepticism, there were useful comparisons to be made between the UK and Russia particularly in relation to working with homeless and alcoholic patients. The nurses in Tomsk found it difficult to believe, for instance, that a British nurse could understand the hopelessness which they encountered in some of their alcoholic patients. In terms of the organisation of services I could also share my experience of frustration at having to constantly fight for resources to provide adequate care for tuberculosis patients and those vulnerable to tuberculosis in the area in which I had been working.

My experience has been that nurses play an extremely important part in caring as well as organising appropriate care for tuberculosis patients and those vulnerable to this disease. The nature of their role and skills makes them well-placed to offer what is needed by this vulnerable group and can make an important contribution to any tuberculosis control programme.

References

Bank Austria. (1997) Eastern Europe: An overview. *East-West* **7**, 16–17.

Barr, D. A. and Field, M. G. (1996) The current state of health care in the Former Soviet Union: Implications for health care policy and reform. *Am. J. Publ. Hlth.* **86**, 307–312.

Bhatti, N., Law, M. R., Morris, J. K., Halliday, R. and Moore-Gillon, J. (1995) Increasing incidence of TB in England and Wales: A study of likely causes. *Br. Med. J.* **310**, 967–969.

British Thoracic Society: Joint Tuberculosis Committee. (1994) Control and prevention of tuberculosis in the United Kingdom: Code of practice 1994. *Thorax* **49**, 1193–1200.

British Thoracic Society: Joint Tuberculosis Committee. (1998) Chemotherapy and management of tuberculosis in the United Kingdom: Recommendations 1998. *Thorax* **53**, 536–548.

Brouwer, J. A., Boeree, M. J., Kager, P., Varkevisser, C. M. and Harries, A. D. (1998) Traditional healers and pulmonary tuberculosis in Malawi. *Int. J. Tuberc. Lung Dis.* **2**, 231–234.

Bryder, L. (1988) *Below the Magic Mountain: A Social History of Tuberculosis in Twentieth Century Britain*. Oxford: Clarendon Press.

Byrd, R. B., Horn, B. R., Solomon, D., Griggs, G. A. and Wilder, N. J. (1977) Treatment of tuberculosis by the nonpulmonary physician. *Ann. Int. Med.* **86**, 799–802.

Darbyshire, J. H. (1995) Tuberculosis: Old reasons for a new increase. *Br. Med. J.* **310**, 954–955.

Drobniewski, F., *et al.* (1996) Tuberculosis in Siberia: 2. Diagnosis, chemoprophylaxis and treatment. *Tubercle Lung Dis.* **77**, 297–301.

Field, M. G. (1996) The health crisis in the Former Soviet Union: A report from the "post-war" zone. *Soc. Sci. Med.* **41**, 1469–1478.

Gessen, M. (1997) TB: The triumphant march of a once-defeated scourge. *Itogi*, September 16.

Leon, A. D., *et al.* (1997) Huge variation in Russian mortality rates 1984–94: Artefact, alcohol or what? *Lancet* **350**, 383–388.

Lygoshina, T. V. (1998) Russia. In: Davies PDO, ed. *Clinical Tuberculosis*. 2nd ed. London: Chapman and Hall.

McEvoy, M. and Maguire, H. (1995). Tuberculosis in London: A review, and an account of the work of the London Consultants in Communicable Disease Control Group Working Party. *J. Hosp. Infect.* **30** (Supplement), 296–305.

Ministry of Health, Russian Federation (1997) Official statistics 1996. Moscow: Ministry of Health, Russian Federation.

Office of Population Censuses and Surveys. *Infectious Diseases Quarterly: OPCS Monitor Series 1983–1994*; MB2 83/1 – 94/4. London: HM Government Statistical Service.

Pym, A., Churcill, D., Coker, R. and Gleissberg, V. (1995) Audit suggests that undernotification is common. *Br. Med. J.* **311**, p. 570.

Robbins, J. M. (1997) Class struggles in the tubercular world: Nurses, patients, and physicians. *Bull. Hist. Med.* **71**, 412–434.

Sachs, T. B. (1908) The tuberculosis nurse. *Am. J. Nursing* **8**, 597–598.

Shaw, T. (1995) The resurgence of tuberculosis: Current issues for nursing. *Nursing Times* **91**(40), 35–37

Snutsk-Torbec, K. G. (1987) Treatment of tuberculosis in a nurse managed clinic. *Heart and Lung* **16**, 30–33.

Uplekar, M., Juvekar, S., Morankar, S., Rangan, S. and Nunn, P. (1998) Tuberculosis patients and practitioners in private clinics in India. *Int. J. Tuberc Lung Dis.* **2**, 324–329.

World Health Organization (1997a) Treatment of tuberculosis: Guidelines for National Programmes, 2nd edn. Geneva: World Health Organization.

World Health Organization (1997b) Report on the Tuberculosis Epidemic. Geneva: World Health Organization.

Zilm, G. and Warbinek, E. (1995) Early tuberculosis nursing in British Columbia (History of TB nursing from 1895–1920) *Can. J. Nursing Res.* **27**, 65–81.

CHAPTER 18

TUBERCULOSIS AND HEALTH SECTOR REFORM

Elizabeth Tayler

> *"Health sector reform is a sustained process of funda-*
> *mental change in policy and institutional arrangements,*
> *guided by government, designed to improve the function-*
> *ing and performance of the health sector, and ultimately*
> *the health status of the population".* (Cassels, 1995)

Introduction

Health sector reform is occurring in developed and developing countries
in all continents of the world. Major changes in the organisation and
financing of health services have already commenced and these are going
to have a significant impact upon the way in which tuberculosis control
is organised.

Tuberculosis control is a part of the general health services, thus the
quality of tuberculosis services is to a large extent reliant upon what is
going on within the health service as a whole. The current weakness
and poor performance of the health sector is an important constraint
to achieving effective control of the disease. There are exceptions to
this; good tuberculosis programmes have developed much more rapidly

than other services in countries such as Tanzania (Styblo and Chum, 1986), Cambodia (Norval, 1998), and Nicaragua (Cruz, 1994) where there has been extensive external technical and financial input. This heavy reliance on external support means that replicating and sustaining this type of approach is difficult.

Patients with tuberculosis usually present with a cough. Whether they are diagnosed at all, and the delays involved if they are, will depend upon the accessibility and quality of the health provider that they first visit. Any initiatives such as decentralisation which are designed to improve first contact services should therefore improve tuberculosis control by reducing the period over which patients are transmitting disease.

There are, however, major risks for disease-specific programmes in the reorganisations that are being planned. The impetus for reform is often political and there is little evidence as yet that the strategies which are being so widely advocated; decentralisation, integration, restructuring ministries of health, increasing the involvement of the non-government sector in health care provision and exploring alternative sources of financing, will achieve the stated objectives of improving health system performance and the health status of the population (Korat Statement, 1997). Disease-specific programmes have achieved notable public health successes and effective ways of working, including adherence to standard clinical protocols, quality control, supervision and monitoring activities and outcomes. Integrating these functions with the general services, without compromising quality and effectiveness, will be a major challenge. In particular it will be important to ensure that any impairment in the performance of essential public health functions is transitory and not sustained. This is particularly true in tuberculosis control where, from a public health perspective, because of the risks of propagating drug resistance, bad control is probably worse than no control at all.

This chapter begins by examining where pressures for reform are coming from and will look at the objectives of reform, and the debates as to the optimal way of achieving these objectives. It will then look at how tuberculosis control programmes have developed and examine the tensions that occur between the categorical programme approach and one which seeks to develop the health sector as a whole in a more integrated and decentralised manner. It will then explore the impact that reforms are having, or could potentially have, upon tuberculosis control programmes, and conclude by identifying areas of particular importance for 'health reformers' if the quality of service currently offered by categorical programmes is to be maintained and areas where those concerned with tuberculosis control may need to amend their strategy.

Why Reform the Health Sector?

Health systems in many countries function poorly. As a result, people with tuberculosis are mismanaged and die. Even in those countries where tuberculosis control programmes run well, they may be an isolated pillar of excellence, reliant upon extensive external support, while in general health services there is an all too familiar range of problems:

- Scarce resources are used inefficiently, on inappropriate and cost-ineffective services, with disproportionate spending on tertiary rather than on primary levels.
- The infrastructure is weak, staff salaries are low and they may not be paid regularly, facilities are dilapidated, and the supply of drugs is unreliable.
- People cannot access the care that they need — the barriers preventing this may be the physical distances involved, the costs of seeking care, cultural factors or on the basis of their age or sex.
- The services provided do not respond to what people want: people face unmotivated and poorly trained staff, long waiting times, inconvenient clinic hours and a lack of confidentiality and privacy (Cassels, 1995).

There is apparent frustration among governments and donor agencies supporting health care that, after decades of effort, there has been

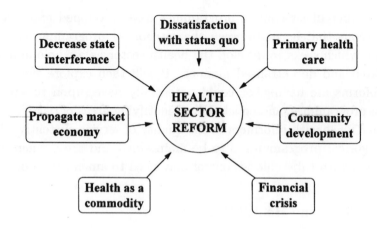

Fig. 1.   Factors promoting health care reform.

little progress in developing services which can operate without the need
for continued extensive external support. This is one of the major motivating forces for reform; other factors, as shown in Fig. 1, are important
in many countries.

Advocates of primary health care continue to stress the importance
of developing health services in an integrated fashion, with extensive involvement of the community that they are designed to serve. Additional
factors which seem to have triggered the pandemic of reforms seem to
have come from shifts in political thinking over the last decade and an
ongoing financial crisis.

In the 1970s and 1980s, health was widely accepted as a fundamental right, and with that went the obligation of governments to provide
health services. Optimism about the prospects for ongoing financial
growth led to expectations that this would become feasible. In many
circles, this paradigm is now shifting towards a perception that health
care is more of a commodity to be purchased in the market. In addition, the neoliberal notion that state intervention and control results
in inefficiencies has resulted in a reassessment of the role of the state
as a provider of health care and the role of the 'market in health care'
(Musgrove, 1996).

The other major pressure for change is the financial crisis; the realisation that currently, in almost all countries, insufficient resources are allocated to health to meet the aspirations and needs of the whole population, and that this position is unlikely to improve. There is therefore a need for rationing and a change in the organisation of service delivery to increase the efficiency, effectiveness and equity of what is being provided. This is true in countries of the OECD, and even more the case in many developing countries. Fourteen of the 123 countries for whom information on the amount spent on health care was available in the 1997 World Bank sector strategy were spending US$10 or less per capita on health (World Bank, 1997). In many of these countries, a significant proportion of this figure comes from overseas development assistance, and yet this too is currently decreasing. In 1986, the OECD countries spent an average of 0.33% on overseas development assistance, by 1995 this had shrunk to 0.27%, and this trend is likely to continue (Kirker, 1997; Development Assistance Committee, 1997).

Tuberculosis Control Programmes

Until the 1950s most patients with tuberculosis were treated in sanatoria and separate institutions, with their own staff and funding systems. Since then there has been a shift towards incorporating service delivery within general health services in most countries, although the former model still persists in countries of the former Soviet Union. Figure 2 shows schematically how tuberculosis services have been organised relative to general services in the past.

Although, in most countries, service delivery itself is integrated, other components may not be. Thus, patients receive treatment at a general health service facility from staff who are also carrying out a wide range of other functions. The supply of these drugs, the recording and reporting system and arrangements for training and supervision may, however, be specific for tuberculosis (see Fig. 2). These components are all crucial for effective disease control, so that where the supply of

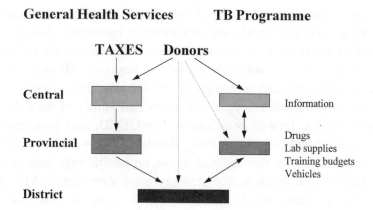

Fig. 2. Schematic representation of how tuberculosis services have been organised relative to general services in the past.

drugs has been erratic, training and supervision of staff poor, and collection and interpretation of data ineffective, the tuberculosis programmes themselves have developed their own systems. This has been popular with donors as separate systems can be rapidly developed, implemented and show tangible results. External aid specifically for tuberculosis programmes increased from US$16 million in 1990 to US$60 million in 1995 (Kochi, 1997).

In many countries, this approach works well for tuberculosis or any other disease control programme. Patients who present with the particular disease are likely to receive effective treatment, and demonstrable results are provided for governments and donors. If, however, separate and incompatible systems for every programme are allowed to proliferate, the co-ordination of the health sector as a whole becomes more difficult. There will be duplication and, where resources in terms of staff, vehicles and money are scarce, the externally funded programmes are likely to receive a disproportionate share. Ministries of Health complain that they do not have the capacity to co-ordinate multiple programmes, with different donors demanding different systems of reporting and accounting. The challenge therefore seems to be how to maintain the technical excellence which some tuberculosis programmes have achieved, whilst operating in a more co-ordinated fashion which supports the more sustained development of the health service in general.

The key elements of the World Health Organization (WHO) DOTS framework for tuberculosis control are:

(1) The need for political commitment to tuberculosis control.

(2) Effective diagnosis of patients who present with symptoms.

(3) Treatment with an effective drug regimen according to standardised protocols.

(4) A reliable supply of drugs.

(5) A recording and reporting system to monitor the control measures (World Health Organization, 1994).

As such, it is flexible and has been adapted to a very wide range of settings. The risk is that it will be imposed unthinkingly and with no adaptation, and strategies which may have been effective in one place will be uncritically replicated in other very different situations.

Where there is a well organised drug supply system, an effective information system, a functioning network of laboratories, and where staff are being trained and supervised within the general health services, the need for separate programmes to manage these elements decreases. In tuberculosis as well as in other conditions there is, however, a perceived risk that attention to detail will decrease within a general system, and therefore quality will be compromised. Even if the programme is not directly managing everything, some co-ordination between epidemiological data, drug supplies, commissioning of services and policies for treatment in all relevant facilities of the health sector is likely to be necessary. This is particularly true in the period in which major changes are occurring, and key factors such as quality control and supervision may be overlooked. Reconciling the need for co-ordination of activities to control a specific disease with a desire for greater co-ordination between the services for different diseases, and within the sector as a whole, is an ongoing challenge. It is particularly difficult where financial and managerial capacity is limited and attempts are being made to decrease staffing levels in the Ministry of Health.

Approaches to Reform

The need for reform in the health sector is widely accepted, as are the objectives of increasing the efficiency, accessibility and equity of health services, and ultimately the health of populations. There is less agreement on the process by which these objectives should be attained. The essence of the debate centres upon whether the first priority is to sort out what is done by the health service, or how it is to be organised and financed. Protagonists of allocative efficiency, 'the Whats', argue that scarce resources are being wasted upon ineffective therapies and that concentrating resources upon the provision of cost-effective services, which address the greatest avertible burden of disease, will be the best way to achieve maximal health gain.

Protagonists of the systems approach, 'the Hows', argue that unless there are trained staff, effective financial flows, acceptable accessible facilities and a functioning drug supply system, health services cannot be effective. These services ought to respond to the demands for health care from the community which they serve, even when they do not fit into a predetermined package of cost-effective interventions.

The middle ground between these approaches seems elusive. Evaluating changes in the organisation of health services is difficult, and in most countries reforms are only at their planning, or early implementation, stages and evidence of the feasibility or effectiveness of either approach is lacking. At this stage this may be inevitable. It is, however, important that processes, whether decentralisation or burden of disease assessment, should not become aims in themselves, irrespective of their impact on the effectiveness of health services.

This debate is characterised by the differing positions which can exist even within the same institution such as the World Bank. The 1993 World Development Report focused upon burden of disease and identified tuberculosis as a high priority (World Bank, 1993), while the health sector strategy paper concentrates upon systems issues and gives scant reference to any particular disease (World Bank, 1997).

There have been gains in terms of improved service efficiency and accessibility in many countries in tuberculosis control and other important areas such as child health, immunisation and leprosy care. It would be counterproductive if all these gains were sacrificed, particularly if the efficacy of the system that replaces them does not turn out to be any better.

What is Health Sector Reform?

Although there is no one package which comprises 'Health Sector Reform' certain broad themes characterise the changes that are occurring in the management and financing of health services in most countries. How these themes develop in practice will depend upon the size, development and pre-existing organisation of health services within the country, as well as the predominant driving forces within the reform process. Extensive reforms are occurring in Africa, South America, parts of Asia, certain OECD countries, and the former Soviet Union. While the basic principles and certain lessons are generalisable, other details will be context-specific. The processes by which reforms are occurring are likely to be more context-specific than the contents of these reforms. For this reason process is likely to be crucial, and this section will therefore concentrate upon the contents of the reforms. This discussion draws mainly upon experiences in sub-Saharan Africa, but many aspects will be applicable to other situations and circumstances. In broad terms, the following types of process seem to be the dominant components of reform.

Decentralisation

In essence, decentralisation is the process whereby functions, resources and authority are transferred from the centre to the periphery. Associated with this 'geographic' shift, there may be a transfer of control from central administrative structures, such as the Ministry of Health, to other agencies such as local government and semi-autonomous or private bodies. The aim of developing local control is to increase responsiveness and accountability. The decentralisation of health services is often politically motivated and may be part of a larger process. In 'health systems parlance' decentralisation generally implies a transfer of managerial or financial authority, whilst in technical programmes such as tuberculosis control the term is used to imply that patients are being treated in more peripheral settings.

Integration

This is a term which is widely used, often to describe different facets of health service delivery, which can be a source of confusion and misunderstanding. There are certain key themes:

(1) Integration of services and tasks, e.g. multipurpose clinics, multipurpose staff functions, and the co-ordination of primary and secondary care services.
(2) Integration of management and support functions, e.g. planning, budgetary and information systems, also the co-ordination of supervision and research activities.
(3) Integration of organisational components, e.g. incorporating hospitals within the overall health planning in a district, working with different providers (public, private for profit and private not for profit) and intersectoral working (World Health Organization, 1996).

These processes are occurring at all levels from the peripheral health posts to the Ministry of Health.

In addition, there is growing interest amongst donors in pooling their resources with those of government in a 'Sector Wide Approach' towards health service development. The concept behind this is that government and donors agree upon priorities and systems for managing and monitoring progress, rather than relying on separate programmes with their own systems of implementation, accounting and information flows. It is envisaged that this may result in more efficient and coherent management of the health sector as a whole, and better co-ordination between government and donor activities (Cassells, 1997).

Alternative funding mechanisms

Health services have always been constrained by limited resources and unrealisable demands for health care. Over the last few years this has been exacerbated by cuts in public spending.

In low-income countries, there is often not enough money to provide even basic services, in middle- and higher-income countries there is not enough to provide universal comprehensive care in line with all advances in medical technology. Alternatives to government finance for health care are therefore being sought. By 1993 almost all countries in sub-Saharan Africa either operated some form of cost recovery or were about to introduce systems for it (Nolan and Tarbut, 1995). This is in line with an increasingly prevalent ideological impetus to shift the burden of responsibility for some health services from the state to the individual. Various strategies are being advocated:

User charges. Patients attending public services have to pay for part of their care. Practical details of how much, for what, and what the money is used for vary. Where these fees are locally retained they can be used to protect the drug supply, pay staff incentives, maintain facilities, or support other interventions which improve the quality of services (McPake *et al.*, 1993). In some settings, the costs of collecting and accounting for the fees can, however, be greater than the amounts recovered. Most studies have revealed that, while in many instances there is an improvement in quality, introduction of user fees is associated with decreased utilisation (Waddington and Enyimayew, 1990; Yoder, 1989), particularly by the poorest people in the community. The actual proportion of costs that are recovered through such schemes are low — usually 5–10% (Creese and Kutzin, 1995). In China, however, the drive is towards more ambitious cost recovery with patients bearing the full costs of their treatment (Yu, 1992).

Insurance schemes. These may be local private schemes often related to employment, or social insurance schemes organised at a local or, more rarely, national level. Such schemes do result in the clear identification of resources to be used for health and may result in improved quality. On the other hand, the administration costs are high and there is a major risk that the prices charged by hospitals and physicians will be inflated as a result of the scheme. Insurance schemes are difficult to introduce, and are unlikely to have a major impact in countries where there is only a small formal employment sector, or when taxes are already high (Kutzin, 1994). Coverage of the poor is likely to be particularly low.

Community Financing. This usually evolves as a means of financing community development schemes. Payments may be in kind — work for health schemes, or the submission of agricultural produce by participating families at the beginning of the year. Experience with most such initiatives suggest that they are localised, coverage of the very poor is not good, and cost recovery is only about 5–10% (Creese and Bennett, 1997).

Changing role of the Ministry of Health

The Ministry of Health has traditionally been a part of the civil service. In many countries, staffing levels were high and salaries low, with control of activities through direct management and bureaucratic control. Very often the units of organisation have been 'programmes' — concerned with direct management of all the aspects of their particular condition.

While the details of reorganisation will obviously vary widely, key themes include a decrease in the number of staff employed, a change of focus away from direct management towards policy development, setting norms and guidelines, and control through contracts. In some cases, the separation of the policy making and executive functions extends to a physical separation, with the creation of a parastatal organisation outside the ministry and the civil service, to implement policy and manage the service. Within this organisation there is a shift away from rogrammes towards more integrated functions such as departments of uman resources, monitoring and evaluation.

In some countries such as Zimbabwe one of the key elements of the lecentralisation process has been to shift power to the regions. In others, uch as Zambia, Tanzania and the UK the focus has been upon the listrict, and the regional level is losing its separate status and becoming management 'outpost' of the central level.

Plurality of providers

n the 1970's and 1980's, the role of government was seen to be financing nd providing health care. In practice, however, many people sought are from private practitioners, mission hospitals, non-governmental or-anisations and a range of other providers. Explicit recognition of the vider range of providers, and a shift towards contractual rather than ureaucratic control, has led to interest in a new model of care, wherein overnment funding is being used to finance provision of services by on-governmental providers. In addition, there is a recognition that hese other providers do have a crucial role in health care provision, nd that government needs to explore innovative ways of working with hem and influencing practice.

Impact of Health Sector Reform upon Tuberculosis Services

The prerequisites for good tuberculosis control are broadly the same as or most other diseases, although the risks of developing drug resistance nean that it is better to do nothing than to do it badly. In addition, he protracted treatment period and the benefits of treatment to the ommunity as a whole — in terms of preventing transmission of disease — mean that certain elements such as the drug supply and the mech-nisms for financing treatment will need special consideration in any nove to integrate services.

In many countries, the success of the tuberculosis programme can be ascribed to the development of a DOTS 'management system' which co-ordinates and controls inputs, process and outputs. Sustaining such a system as an entity may be difficult, and may even be contrary to the spirit of the reform, meaning that integrating the management of successful tuberculosis programmes with the broader health service may be more of a challenge than integrating other disease control activities. The impact of reforms can be considered in terms of the effects on resource management — financing, prioritisation and quality maintenance, as well as the practical aspects of how a patient is managed. In some countries, a significant part of the reform process is concerned with community development and intersectoral working. This analysis, however, will concentrate upon health service issues.

Resource Management

Health financing issues

In nearly all countries provision of tuberculosis services is still officially free even though informal charging certainly exists (Gilson, 1988). In certain notable exceptions such as a large proportion of China, patients are being expected to pay the full costs of their treatment, elsewhere the 'free government services' are so inaccessible, or poor, that most people resort to the private sector. In many countries, the resources available for health care are inadequate and governments are starting to explore alternative ways of financing services.

(1) In almost all countries there are good practical and theoretical reasons why the responsibility for funding tuberculosis is likely to remain with the government.

(2) From an equity and an efficiency point of view, government spending on public health services, such as tuberculosis control is likely to result in greater gains, than private spending of an equivalent amount of money.

(3) Good tuberculosis treatment is a very cost-effective intervention which benefits not only the recipients of treatment but also the community.

(4) Tuberculosis patients are disproportionately poor and unlikely to be insured.

(5) The costs of collecting user fees, if they were set at an affordable level, would consume a large proportion of the revenue generated (Bennet and Banda, 1994). Although they may seek treatment in the private sector, most patients can only pay for the initial relief of symptoms, rather than treatment to cure — a scenario which is associated with high risks of propagating drug resistance.

Priority setting. Tuberculosis has received considerable funding from donors and through loans from development banks. If the shift towards more integrated funding occurs, with government and donors sharing priorities as opposed to dedicated project funding, it may decrease the amounts specifically available for tuberculosis control. Although it is a cost-effective intervention that contributes significantly to the relief of the burden of disease in most communities, funding a quality service for tuberculosis may not be a high priority for policy makers, who may be more interested in political expediency and meeting their populations' demands for acute care. Even in high-prevalence areas there will only be one or two new cases of tuberculosis per thousand population each year, and there is an understandable desire to address more common albeit less serious conditions.

Priority setting at any level is difficult, decentralising these decisions to those with minimal training will potentially create problems, particularly when these resource allocation decisions are not confined to health, but encompass all local government spending, as is occurring in countries such as the Philippines. Given that resources are so limited and that facilities are increasingly accountable for their budgets, the incentives to develop popular revenue-generating activities at the expense of public health functions is strong.

Thus, within a decentralised system an adequate central allocation to tuberculosis is not enough. Where resource allocation decisions are taken at the periphery, some form of 'earmarking' is probably necessary to preserve the funding and functioning of essential services, even where there may be an ideological incentive to encourage local autonomy.

Maintaining service quality

A high-quality service is reliant upon motivated people who accept responsibility for developing and maintaining the tuberculosis control strategy, who are trained to implement it, and who ensure that it is being done properly.

Ownership. One of the key constraints to the maintenance and expansion of tuberculosis programmes has been perceived to be a 'lack of ownership' by national and local authorities. One of the risks of external consultants designing and funding programmes, with minimal local input into their design or flexibility in their implementation, is that local directors of health services or other policy makers will not develop commitment to ensuring that the project continues to function and develop. Separate supply and information systems may mean that directors of general health services have little involvement in, or commitment to, tuberculosis control.

If a tuberculosis control service is fully integrated into the general health services, the performance of the service should become the responsibility of the director of health services. It is, however, but one of many priorities and there is a risk that without dedicated attention standards will slip. An identified individual, accountable to the director of health services, who takes day to day responsibility for the performance of the service, is still likely to be necessary. Actual service delivery is undertaken by the general health staff. Within such a system lines of accountability and responsibility are horizontal — the quality of the programme is the responsibility of the district itself, even if higher levels are used as a resource for supplies and technical assistance.

Human Resource Development. Training and supervision are rarely seen as a high priority in health services that are short of resources. It is much more likely that money will be spent on drugs rather than training staff how to use them. In Indonesia, only 0.2% of the spending on tuberculosis goes on training and supervision (Sawert H, personal communication concerning unpublished cost study in Indonesia, 1997). In the context of tuberculosis, this creates ideal conditions for the development of drug resistance. One of the strengths of vertical programmes has been their flexibility to spend money on good training. One of the weaknesses has been that this has distorted priorities, with resources being concentrated upon training for specific programmes and very little left for general health service provision. Directors of health facilities are also concerned about the disruption of service provision through frequent health worker absences for 'workshops'.

In most countries, training for tuberculosis care is fairly protracted and is reliant upon specialised modules, centrally arranged courses and daily training allowances. In future, it is envisaged that training courses will be driven more by demand (from the district) than supply (from the central programme). Districts are therefore likely to demand briefer training courses which are more tailored to the needs and pre-existing skills of their workforce and a more coherent approach between diseases.

While tuberculosis control is not 'complicated' there are certain basic principles that need to be learnt well, particularly in a decentralised system where disease-specific control and supervision is likely to be less intense. The move away from specialist workers to teams, and use of 'multipurpose workers', means that more staff will have to be trained. This therefore represents a considerable 'training burden' which may be difficult to accommodate when tuberculosis is one of the many priorities and resources have to be spread more thinly. Refining and simplifying training materials and courses will be a major challenge.

Supervision is another crucial area that is vulnerable to cuts when savings have to be made. There may be less need for managerial and financial vertical linkages in a decentralised system, but in most developing countries technical knowledge and capacity is limited and there is still need for support in these areas from higher levels. Supervision is essential for identifying and addressing problems in the facilities visited, and also in validating the data that they supply. If the proposed shift towards contracting for services, and relating outputs to financial remuneration occurs, the temptation to distort data grows and the need for checks increases. Without dedicated vehicles and adequate fuel, routine separate supervision is unlikely to be possible. Therefore, innovative solutions and new models of operating, such as sharing vehicles, recruiting 'non-tuberculosis workers' to perform simple focused checks, and enlisting the assistance of non-governmental organisations and other agencies, are going to become important.

Uniformity

One of the strengths of a national programme is the potential consistency in policies and strategies between districts and regions. The greater autonomy associated with decentralisation is likely to diminish this. Even where districts are obliged to supply basic tuberculosis services, higher levels will have fewer sanctions to ensure that national policies and guidelines are actually adhered to. Local variations in the priority afforded to tuberculosis, and the knowledge and capacity of staff, are likely to increase the disparities in quality of service provision. This is likely to be significant in those countries where there is extensive internal migration.

Operational efficiency

One of the implications of decentralised priority setting and the trend towards funding a facility, rather than programmes of activities, is that the financial flexibility to shift resources between activities and levels of the tuberculosis service may be lost. In practice, this has always been difficult, and has only happened to a limited extent. It is, for example, well known that ambulatory care can be a better option for both the patient and the health service, but ensuring that money follows the patient when they are transferred into primary care is difficult. Under the new system, getting the money to follow the tuberculosis patient is likely to be even more difficult.

Drug supply

Even in decentralised systems the potential economies of scale and importance of proper quality control mean that centralised procurement of TB drugs should normally be retained, even if delivery systems within the country are integrated. The effects of increasing district control over drug budgets and the ordering of supplies is likely to be highly dependent upon the organisation capacity and training of individual districts. Although treating tuberculosis as a special case may conflict with the ideological desire for total integration, there are good reasons why it needs separate consideration. These include the relatively high costs of a full course of treatment, the risks of developing drug resistance if there is not good adherence to the standard regimen by the patient, physician and pharmacist, and the protracted treatment period which increases the vulnerability of all these participants to errors and non-compliance. Thus, although cost recovery systems and rotating drugs funds do seem to allow districts to maintain better drug stock levels, they are probably not applicable for tuberculosis.

Patient Management

The factors outlined above may have a very significant effect upon the tuberculosis programme, but the bottom line by which any service must be judged is how it addresses the needs of the patients. What might the impact of reforms be upon the management of the individual patient with tuberculosis?

Case-finding

If reforms in the health service do achieve their aims of increasing the accessibility and quality of primary health services, then the identification and diagnosis of symptomatic patients is likely to improve. Involving more general workers in tuberculosis control is likely to increase awareness and may decrease the stigmatisation and isolation felt by some 'tuberculosis workers'.

It is, however, likely that widespread introduction of user fees will dissuade many patients from seeking diagnosis and treatment. It is known that the introduction or increase of user fees results in sharp and sustained falls in utilisation, particularly amongst rural populations and the poor (Creese and Kutzin, 1995). In most contexts, exemptions do not seem to work well, as there is confusion over who is exempted, and informal charging occurs anyway (Gilson, 1994). As tuberculosis patients present with cough and may not be aware that they have the disease, many patients will be dissuaded from seeking care irrespective of any exemptions policy.

Where user fees are used to enhance the quality of health services there is a risk that such improvements will be confined to fee-generating services, and public health functions such as tuberculosis which are provided 'free' will be further marginalised.

Diagnosis

The impact of user fees on diagnostic services has not been reported, but is likely to be an important issue. As with other incentive issues, the details are likely to be crucial and context-specific. It is necessary to balance the disincentive to patients of paying for an investigation against the impact that this extra revenue may have upon the sustainability of the service and laboratory staff morale. Getting such details right is an important issue for systems in transition, and one which may be overlooked. Whatever position is adopted, a clear policy should be made to avoid confusion.

Developing and maintaining a system of quality control in the laboratory is always difficult. Laboratory services are rarely a high-priority area for policy makers and, although the consequences of laboratory error can be grave, systems of quality control are sometimes almost seen as a luxury. Considerable technical expertise is required to supervise laboratory services well (Collins *et al.*, 1997), and these skills are not possessed or rapidly acquired by other health staff. This is one of the clearest examples of the need to preserve some vertical linkages to ensure the maintenance of technical standards, although it may be that within an integrated system all the functions of the laboratory should be supervised together.

Treatment

Although national programmes may be using a standardised regimen, there may be a plethora of other regimens used in the private sector, and even within government hospitals, which in many countries may be treating a larger proportion of patients than the national programme itself. If reforms do achieve their aims of increasing involvement with, and influence over, such providers, this may increase the adherence to national policies and compliance with effective regimens. Similarly, the emphasis on improving primary care and community-based services should allow many more patients to be treated in their communities, thus avoiding the costs and disruption of hospitalisation.

There is a major risk that training will be inadequate for the maintenance of a quality service, and ensuring patients are properly supervised as they take their treatment will be seen to be too difficult and time consuming. Strategies for influencing private practitioner behaviour remain elusive and while new initiatives such as contracting are interesting it is by no means clear that either directly observed therapy or supervision from higher levels will be feasible and affordable under such systems.

Recording and reporting

Within a decentralised health system, particularly one in which fi-
nances are being generated locally, there may be little incentive to notify
cases or to report treatment outcomes to higher levels. Tuberculosis is
unusual amongst medical conditions in its use of case-by-case recording of treatment outcomes. Ensuring that this is properly done may
be more difficult in a decentralised system, even though it is widely
accepted that monitoring of outcomes is important, particularly during
periods of transition.

Incorporating the various information systems which different disease
control programmes have developed into a more coherent and unified
form is likely to be difficult. Doing it effectively will have important
implications for monitoring the performance of health services and the
impact of reforms as well as preserving the quality of separate disease
control activities. If it is to happen, health system planners will have
to acknowledge that information on specific disease control activities
is crucial to the maintenance of effective services, and those concerned
with disease control will have to acknowledge the risks of information
overload, and refine and simplify their systems. The risk is that general intransigence, and a reluctance amongst tuberculosis specialists to
change even the less essential elements of the tuberculosis recording and
reporting system, will result in the system being lost in its entirety.

One of the challenges will be to refine and simplify such systems to
ensure that they generate data which is useful to policy makers. Recording of other information, such as age and sex, or sub-classifications of
retreatment cases, is likely to divert scarce resources from the basic
elements, and runs the risk of the system being perceived as 'too complicated', thereby jeopardising its continuation.

Conclusions

Reforms are occurring in countries across the world, and the impact
upon tuberculosis control will be considerable. Changes are going to

occur irrespective of the wishes of those charged with control of a particular disease such as tuberculosis.

Maintaining Quality — Issues for Reformers

Certain key challenges are common to most disease-specific programmes, and a more common approach by the categorical programmes may be of benefit. In many countries such issues seem to be:

(1) Ensuring adequate funding for essential public health programmes, and effective financial flows that ensure that funds are appropriately spent at the peripheral level.

(2) Ensuring that there is effective technical supervision between levels of service, to identify problems, to assist and retrain staff, and to validate their performance.

(3) Ensuring that even where services are primarily co-ordinated according to function rather than programme, some co-ordination and accountability for performance of specialised services and disease control activities is retained.

(4) Ensuring that the strengths of the information systems of categorical programmes and their measurement of outcomes is not lost in the shift towards a more integrated system.

Improving sustainability — accepting inevitability. Issues for programme managers

For those involved in the design and implementation of tuberculosis programmes there may be a need for significant changes in the ways that services are organised and delivered, with fewer dedicated resources for tuberculosis *per se*. Variations in the situations of countries and the nature of their reforms, mean that global generalisations are not always helpful. Effective solutions are likely to be country- and context-specific, and in many situations it will be attention to details which determines the effectiveness of any reform process. Particularly during periods of rapid transition there is a risk that key elements may be overlooked. The following areas seem to be particularly likely to require reorganisation, refinement or simplification.

(1) Training and supervision;
(2) Recording and reporting;
(3) Supplies of drugs and diagnostic equipment.

Equally important are likely to be the shifts towards more collaborative ways of working, with a focus upon tuberculosis within the context of the broader health service. This will mean acknowledging the importance of other partners and stakeholders, those concerned with management of other diseases, policy makers, the private sector and the community as a whole. It will not be easy, and the prospect of such changes may be threatening to those involved in disease control, who will need to be politically adept and may have to develop new skills of communication, collaboration and advocacy. There is, however, no 'do nothing' alternative. Although the risks of responding proactively to reforms may be considerable and starting to collaborate with other participants may be a painful process, ignoring the developments in the broader health service, not being involved in the planning process, and simply reacting to an unsatisfactory situation once it is a *fait accompli* is more likely to jeopardise effective tuberculosis control in the long term.

References

Bennett, S. and Banda, E. N. (1994) *Public and Private Roles in Health A Review of Analysis and Experience in sub-Saharan Africa.* Current Concerns SHS Paper. 6. Geneva: World Health Organization (WHO/SHS/CC/94.1).

Cassells, A. (1995) Health sector reforming less developed countries. *J. Int. Dev.* **7**, 329–347.

Cassells, A. (1997) *Sector-Wide Approaches/A Stake Holders Guide.* London: Department for International Development.

Collins, C. H., Grange, J. M. and Yates, M. D. (1997) *Tuberculosis Bacteriology. Organization and Practice.* 2nd edn. Oxford: Butterworth Heinemann.

Creese, A. and Kutzin, J. (1995) *Lessons from Cost Recovery in Health.* Forum on Health Sector Reform. Discussion Paper 2. Geneva: World Health Organization (WHO/SHS/NHP/95.5).

Creese, A. and Bennett, S. (1997) *Rural Risk Strategies and Health. Presentation and Initiatives in Health Care Financing Conference.* Washington: World Bank.

Cruz, J. R., Heldal, E., Arnadottir, T., Juarez, I. and Enarson, D. (1994) Tuberculosis case finding in Nicaragua. Evaluation of routine activities in the control programme. *Tubercle Lung Dis.* **75**, 417–422.

Development Assistance Committee (1997) *Development Co-operation. 1996 Report.* OECD A7-A8.

Gilson, L. (1988) *Government Health Care Charges. Is Equity Being Abandoned?* EPC Publication No. 15. London School of Hygiene and Tropical Medicine.

Kirker, M. (1997) *Presentation on Tuberculosis from a Donor Perspective.* IUATLD Conference. Paris.

Kochi, A. (1997) *Global Tuberculosis Programme Report. Presentation to CARG.* Geneva: World Health Organization (WHO/GTB/CARG/797.03).

Korat Statement. (1997) Towards evidence based health care reform. In: Nitayarumphong S., ed. *Health Care Reform at the Frontier Of Research And Policy Discussions.* Thailand: Office of Health Care Reform Ministry of Public Health (ISBN 974 7767 76.7).

Kutzin, J. (1994) *Experience with Organisational and Financing Reform of the Health Sector.* SHS Paper No 8.

McPake, B., Hanson, K. and Mills, A. (1993) Community financing of health care in Africa: An evaluation of the Bamako initiative. *Soc. Sci. Med.* **36**, 1383–1395.

Musgrove, P. (1996) *Public and Private Roles in Health Theory and Financing Patterns.* Washington DC: World Bank.

Nolan, B. and Tarbut, V. (1995) *Cost Recovery in Public Health Services in sub-Saharan Africa.* Washington DC: World Bank Economic Development Institute.

Norval, P. Y., *et al.* (1998) DOTS in Cambodia. *Int. J. Tuberc. Lung Disease* **2**, 44–51.

Styblo, K. and Chum, H. J. (1987) Treatment results of smear positive tuberculosis in the Tanzania national tuberculosis and leprosy programme. *Proceedings of the 25th World Conference on Tuberculosis and Respiratory Disease, Singapore 1986.* Singapore: Professional Postgraduate Services, pp. 122–126.

Waddington, C. J. and Enyimayew, K. A. (1990) *Patient Surveys at Niamey National Hospital. Results and Implications for Reform of Hospital Fees.* Prepared under USAID Project 683–0254. Bethesda, Maryland: Abt Associates.

World Health Organization (1994) *Framework for Essential Tuberculosis Control.* Geneva: World Health Organization.

World Health Organization (1996) *Integration of Health Care Delivery.* WHO Technical Report Series 861. Geneva: World Health Organization.

World Bank (1993) *World Development Report.* Washington DC: World Bank.

World Bank (1997) *Health Nutrition and Population Sector Strategy 1997.* Washington DC: World Bank.

Yoder, R. A. (1989) Are people willing and able to pay for health services. *Soc. Sci. Med.* **29**, 35–42.

Yu, D. Z. (1992) Changes in health care financing and health status: The case of China in the 1980s. Innocenti Occasional Papers. Economic Policy Series No. 34.

CHAPTER 19

APPLYING HUMAN RIGHTS TO
TUBERCULOSIS CONTROL

David Nyheim

> *"The adoption of the human rights paradigm has the po-
> tential to revolutionise the health field. The human right
> principle that 'all human beings are born free and equal
> in dignity and rights' is a powerful concept despite of
> its simplicity. By applying the principle of equality to
> health, we have no choice but to examine the relation-
> ship between the individual and all those who have power
> to affect his or her health".* (Nahid F. Toubia, 1994)

Introduction

A consideration of human rights can influence how we understand, and
choose to make an impact on, the determinants of health. Whereas
human rights issues clearly call for 'upstream' political action, little
attention has been given to its relevance to more 'downstream' practical
implications for health care interventions.

Three propositions can be made linking human rights and health.
These propositions all relate to the axiom that the right to life (Article 3

in the United Nations Declaration of Human Rights) is inextricably
linked to the right to be healthy.

- Ill health is often linked to an abuse of human rights.
- Human rights are deprived as a consequence of ill health.
- Health care interventions affect human rights.

These propositions are supported by research, particularly in the field
of tuberculosis, although the quantitative tools at our disposal make it
difficult to define, for example, the exact causal associations of socio-
economic factors to disease. Also, it is uncommon for the effects of
health interventions on the outcome of disease to be reported in other
than biomedical terms. There is only limited understanding, therefore,
as to how one can (or, indeed, if one should) consider human rights in
health care interventions.

The issue of human rights has remained, as such, a peripheral concern
to health policy makers and planners. The notion of human rights has
at best been an 'add on' to health programme development, seen as
something to be 'kept in mind' but not to be actively considered and
applied.

This chapter will seek to contribute to the debate on the role of human rights considerations in health policy and planning. Emphasis will
be placed on providing examples and perspectives on the relevance of
human rights to infectious disease control, with a focus on tuberculosis.
The argument is simple: human rights should be viewed as an analytical tool which may shed light on the rights implications, socio-economic
causes and consequences of tuberculosis, as well as the outcomes of tuberculosis control programmes.

The chapter is divided into two sections. First, a conceptual framework will be drawn, looking at approaches to defining human rights
and tuberculosis. Secondly, perspectives will be offered on the operational value of human rights as a tool for the analysis of disease control
programmes and policy.

Conceptual Framework

Definition of human rights

Human rights is defined as presented in the 30 Articles of the Universal Declaration of Human Rights (see boxes). The various Articles of the Declaration will be referred to throughout this chapter. For purposes of simplification and clarity, the Articles of the Declaration are grouped together under six headings, as shown in Fig. 1.

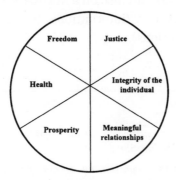

Fig. 1.   Classification of the Universal Declaration of Human Rights.*

Two key issues need to be kept in mind when considering human rights: the need to balance individual or group rights against the need of the community (Commonwealth Human Rights Initiative, 1991) and the need to balance cultural relativism with the 'universality' of human rights. Rights take on different meanings and degrees of importance in distinct cultural contexts (Toubia, 1994).

Human rights analysis should not be viewed as single-handedly shedding light on the socio-economic causes and consequences of disease, or even on the broader impact of control activities. Rather, it should be

*Articles 1, 3, 4, 13, 14, 18, 19, 20, 21, and 27 fall under 'freedom'; articles 2, 6, 7, 8, 9, 10, 11, 15, 28, and 30 fall under 'justice'; articles 3, 5, 12, 18, 19, and 26 fall under 'integrity of the individual'; articles 12, 16, 27, and 29 fall under 'meaningful relationships'; articles 17, 22, 23, 24, 25, and 26 fall under "prosperity" and articles 3, 5, 22, 23, 24, 25, and 26 fall under 'health'.

applied alongside other tools, such as gender and equity analysis, and considered complementary to these. Indeed, human rights are integral to both gender and equity analysis.

The human rights discourse encourages scrutiny of rights violations on a number of levels: sub-national, national, and international (Commonwealth Human Rights Initiative, 1991). It is necessary to look for the application of human rights analysis not only on a micro- or sub-national level (e.g. looking at local human rights violations and their impact on the individual), but also on a macro- or national/international level (e.g. looking at national/international human rights violations and their impact on populations).

The right to justice

Article 2:   *Everyone is entitled to all the rights and freedoms set forth in the [. . .] Declaration*

Article 6:   *The right to recognition everywhere as a person before the law*

Article 7:   *All are equal before the law*

Article 8:   *The right to effective remedy by the competent national tribunals for acts violating [. . .] fundamental rights*

Article 9:   *No one shall be subject to arbitrary arrest, detention, or exile*

Article 10:   *The right to fair and public hearing by an independent and impartial tribunal*

Article 11:   *The right to be presumed innocent until proved guilty according to law*

Article 15:   *The right to a nationality*

Article 28:   *The right to a social and international order in which the rights and freedoms set forth in this Declaration can be fully realised*

Article 30:   *Nothing in this Declaration may be interpreted [as the right] to perform any act aimed at the destruction of the rights and freedoms set forth herein*

Tuberculosis: definitions and levels of analysis

Tuberculosis has been defined in a number of ways in this book. Here, attention will simply be drawn to some issues relating to how tuberculosis can be viewed. Two basic observations can be made. First, disease is often defined by some combination of its causes, expression/manifestation and consequences. In this chapter, tuberculosis will be considered in an integrated way, covering all three definition facets. Secondly, disease is most frequently defined in biomedical terms (Evans *et al.*, 1994). In this chapter, tuberculosis will be defined in terms of its rights and related socio-economic context. Tuberculosis, therefore, is defined in this chapter as a disease with a number of rights and socio-economic causes, manifestations, and consequences.

This kind of 'problem-definition' also provides perspectives on how one can chose to see responses ('solution-definition') to disease, and define health policy. Consequently, health policy should be broadly defined and discussed, with an expansion beyond a health care focus to a consideration of other factors that have an impact on health status.

Application of Human Rights

Perspectives on applying human rights analysis in tuberculosis control will be provided in relation to three propositions on the links between health and rights: (a) ill health is often linked to an abuse of human rights; (b) human rights are deprived as a consequence of ill health; and (c) health care interventions affect human rights.

A recurring argument will be that human rights analysis offers a useful framework for understanding the rights and socio-economic context of tuberculosis. As a 'lens' (see Fig. 2), it facilitates a better understanding of the causes of disease and the broader implications of disease for the individual, as well as the broader impact of health interventions on the individual.

The information derived from this analysis has clear implications for disease control policy and planning.

The right to freedom

Article 1:   All human beings are born free and equal in dignity and human
               rights

Article 3:   The right to life, liberty and the security of person

Article 4:   No one shall be held in slavery or servitude

Article 13: The right to freedom of movement and residence within the bor-
               ders of each state

Article 14: The right to seek and enjoy in other countries asylum from
               persecution

Article 18: The right to freedom of thought, conscience and religion

Article 19: The right to freedom of opinion and expression

Article 20: The right to freedom of peaceful assembly and association

Article 21: The right to take part in government of his country

Article 27: The right freely to participate in the cultural life of the
               community

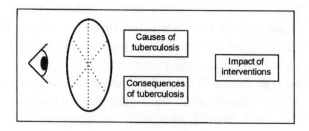

Fig. 2.   Human rights analysis as a 'lens'.

Proposition 1: Ill health is often linked to an abuse of human rights

A number of authors have illustrated how the abuse of human rights, particularly those relating to prosperity and health, are part of the causes of the global emergency of tuberculosis. Many reports reveal that tuberculosis is inextricably linked to poor socio-economic conditions.

The relationship between prosperity, adequate living standards (Article 25), and tuberculosis has been studied both on a macro and micro level. For example, McKeown *et al.* (1975) have demonstrated the link between the improvement of socio-economic conditions and the reduction in the incidence of tuberculosis. Nair *et al.* (1997) showed how the links between poverty and tuberculosis are interpreted on a micro-level. In their qualitative study of perceptions of tuberculosis in Bombay, a number of respondents stated that worry as well as germs cause the disease. Worries include family disharmony, marital problems and financial difficulties, such as 'being pestered by money-lenders'.

The right to prosperity

Article 17: The right to own property

Article 22: The right to social security

Article 23: The right to work

Article 24: The right to rest and leisure

Article 25: The right to a standard of living adequate for [...] health and well-being

Article 26: The right to education

Inherent in Article 25 is the concept of access to certain basic items, including health care. Human rights are affected by both the lesser or greater ability of the individual to benefit from health care.

The right to health
Article 3:   *Right to life, liberty and the security of person*
Article 5:   *No one shall be subjected to torture or to cruel, inhuman or degrading treatment*
Article 22: *The right to social security*
Article 23: *The right to work*
Article 24: *The right to rest and leisure*
Article 25: *The right to a standard of living adequate for [. . .] health and well-being*
Article 26: *The right to education*

It is a truism that when access to basic items, such as health care, are denied to the individual, his or her rights are violated. Individuals may live a long distance from health services and may therefore not be able to benefit from them, or there may be other barriers to access. In Ghana, for example, access to treatment of tuberculosis has been shown to be negatively affected by the cost of transport to the clinic (Twumasi, 1996), while in Vietnam the cost of anti-tuberculosis drugs prevented a number of patients from completing treatment (Johansson *et al.*, 1996).

Other cost-related factors which serve as barriers to access to health care include loss of income due to the absence of two earning family members: patient and accompanying relative (Basu, 1995). Other barriers to access, such as stigma, are outlined under Proposition 2 below.

On a macro-level, there is only limited documentation on the link between different international (non-health) policies (e.g. economic restructuring programmes) and their impact on the causes of tuberculosis and access to health care. While chronic national underdevelopment and indebtedness undoubtedly have an adverse impact on the prevalence of disease and access to health services (Porter and Ogden, 1997), these factors are not usually considered in discussions on the management of disease.

There are, however, some very visible examples of more hostile policies that have adversely affected both health and human rights. These include the international embargo on Iraq and the embargo of the USA on Cuba.

The above examples provide perspectives on the 'causes' of tuberculosis. By specifying, for example, what is meant by 'prosperity' (property, social security, work), the human rights framework provides a concrete and dynamic basis for exploring the meaning of concepts such as 'poverty' and 'poor socio-economic conditions'. On a programmatic level, such perspectives may facilitate the identification of vulnerable groups that should be helped to obtain greater access to treatment facilities (Toubia, 1994).

On a macro-level, greater scrutiny is required in order to encourage action for health in non-health domains. Human rights analysis in this broad context cannot shed light on what particular steps need to be taken, nor on how they can be taken. Instead, its contribution lies in its ability to raise awareness of the macro-level causes of disease, as well as calling for greater attention to the impact of non-health care policies on disease.

Proposition 2: Human Rights are Deprived as a Consequence of Ill health

The human rights violated by tuberculosis are numerous, with the most obvious one being the right to health. The impact of tuberculosis on health has been covered elsewhere in this book. Here, attention will be given to other human rights violated by this disease, including the right to prosperity and to engage in meaningful relationships.

The crippling economic effects of tuberculosis, and its impact on the right to prosperity, have been illustrated by a number of authors. For example, in the Haitian context, Farmer (1997, p. 349) illustrates how

458   D. Nyheim

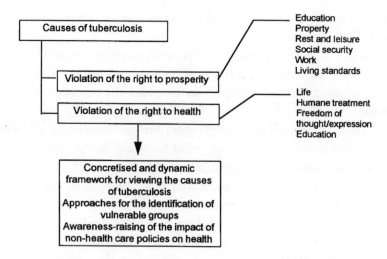

Fig. 3.   Summary illustration: ill health is often linked to an abuse of human rights.

"families living in poverty... lived in fear of tuberculosis, in part because
of its high mortality, in part because of its tendency to leave survivors
— or surviving kin — saddled with unpayable debt".

Narayan and Srikantaramu (1987) show how families of tuberculosis
patients in India see the ensuing economic problems as critically important. Nair et al. (1997) found that most patients report a 40–60%
reduction in income due to illness. Wage earners in the informal sector,
especially women, were also vulnerable to dismissal and unemployment.
The reduced income due to tuberculosis has a broader impact as it leads
to reduced opportunities for the education of children, more malnutrition and less sanitation (Narayan and Srikantaramu 1987).

The impact of tuberculosis on the individual in relation to his/her
broader social environment (family and community) has received considerable attention. For example, Uplekar and Rangan (1996) show how,
in Pune, local perceptions of the transmission of tuberculosis have led to
the physical isolation of patients. In Pakistan, Liefooghe et al. (1995)
found that divorce and broken engagements occur frequently among
tuberculosis patients. Female patients were more vulnerable to this

> **The right to engage in meaningful relationships**
>
> *Article 12:* *No one shall be subjected to arbitrary interference with [...] privacy, family, home or correspondence, nor to attacks upon [...] honour and reputation*
>
> *Article 18:* *The right to freedom of thought, conscience and religion*
>
> *Article 27:* *The right freely to participate in the cultural life of the community*
>
> *Article 29:* *Everyone has duties to the community in which alone [...] free and full development [...] is possible*

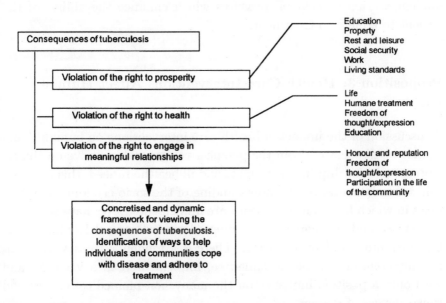

Fig. 4. Summary illustration: Human rights are deprived as a consequence of ill health.

outcome. In addition, women with tuberculosis have experienced rejection by their husbands and in-laws, reduced marriage opportunities, and unemployment due to their condition (Nair *et al.* 1997). For further details on gender-related human rights issues see Chapter 14.

These examples of the consequences of tuberculosis provide a rights-related picture (the right to prosperity and the right to engage in meaningful relationships) of what 'ill health' can mean for the individual. It is clear that ill health means more than the biomedical manifestations of disease, and that it has significant and important implications for the ability of the individual to function in society.

In terms of disease control programmes, this perspective on ill health provides ground for advocating measures that not only contain disease, but supply the necessary support enabling patients to cope with their disease. In addition, an understanding of the broad implications of ill health for the patient should encourage more appropriate planning and implementation of control measures which enhance the ability of the patient to adhere to treatment.

Proposition 3: Health Care Interventions Affect Human Rights

A discussion of the impact of health care interventions on human rights cannot be dissociated from the perspectives generated above on the reciprocal relationship between rights and ill health. Indeed, this relationship is fundamental to an understanding of the socio-economic environment in which health interventions are implemented. We have seen that the causes and consequences of tuberculosis are not solely biomedical, but have numerous other facets. There is a tendency to view biomedical interventions as being value-free, implemented in a vacuum, and with only a positive influence on the many non-biomedical causes and consequences of disease.

Infectious disease control interventions, particularly those required for the control of tuberculosis, have been criticised on account of their infringement on human rights. This critical analysis has largely focused on the balance between the rights of the individual and the community (see, for example, Bayer and Depuis, 1995). Attention here will be given to the impact of the general treatment of individuals on human rights,

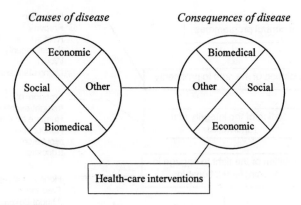

Fig. 5. Putting health interventions into context: Multiple and diverse causes and consequences of disease.

The integrity of the individual

Article 3: *The right to life, liberty and the security of person*

Article 5: *No one shall be subjected to torture or to cruel, inhuman or degrading treatment*

Article 12: *No one shall be subjected to arbitrary interference with [...] privacy, family, home or correspondence, nor to attacks upon [...] honour and reputation*

Article 18: *The right to freedom of thought, conscience and religion*

Article 19: *The right to freedom of opinion and expression*

Article 26: *The right to education*

---

particularly the rights to prosperity, health, engagement in meaningful relationships, and the integrity of the individual.

The treatment of tuberculosis involves a number of costs for patients and their families. Some of these costs have been illustrated above in the discussion on access to health care. A study by Rangan (1995) in Bombay, for example, showed that a third of patients interviewed spend 9% of their income solely on travel to the clinic to collect drugs.

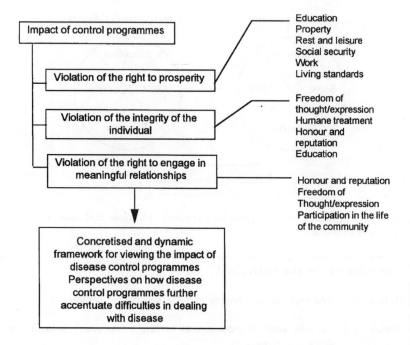

Fig. 6.   Summary illustration: Health care interventions may affect human rights.

Tuberculosis and its treatment often carry a significant stigma, with implications for the patient in respect of lost dignity and exclusion from the family and community. A number of examples have been given above. Other examples of how patients have been forcefully isolated (violation of the integrity of the individual) have also been given.

A study of hospitalised patients in Mexico City revealed that 15% of patients expected to be rejected by their families upon completion of treatment. In fact, 52% were not welcomed at home upon discharge (Rubel and Garro, 1992).

In societies where tuberculosis is a highly stigmatising condition, the observed treatment embodied in the DOTS strategy is also likely to compromise the right of individuals to engage in meaningful relationships. Furthermore, in relation to DOTS, the notion of the right to health calls for attention to the treatment of sputum-positive cases only.

Persons with sputum smear-negative tuberculosis are often not treated until their disease has advanced enough for sputum smear examinations to be positive.

These examples, and those given in previous sections, on the impact of disease control measures on the socio-economic status and rights of the individual, show how disease control programmes affect more than just the incidence of disease. It is clear therefore that tuberculosis control interventions not only have an impact on disease, but may violate individual human rights. These violations may also accentuate the deprivation of rights that follow from having the disease in the first place.

Conclusions: Emerging Operational Perspectives

This chapter has provided some perspectives on the operational value of human rights as an analytical tool for formulating disease control programmes and policies. Although some effort has been made systematically to explore and concretise the relationship between human rights, health and disease control programmes and policies, it is clear that the three propositions raised and explored in this chapter are valid:

- Ill health is often linked to an abuse of human rights.
- Human rights are deprived as a consequence of ill health.
- Health care interventions affect human rights.

The human rights framework is an important lens through which to view and gain perspectives on disease and to facilitate the making of decisions in the way that disease is managed. It is not, however, an 'exclusive' tool but one that needs to be applied with other methods of analysis that address issues such as gender and equity.

Disease control programmes need to be planned with an understanding of the broad causes (and causal webs), manifestations, and consequences of tuberculosis. The human rights framework calls for a problem-orientated definition of the disease that extends beyond the purely biomedical to a consideration of socio-economic and other factors.

The way in which responses to disease control measures are ascertained is equally important as health is clearly affected by activities outside the health sector.

As has been illustrated in this chapter, human rights analysis provides a concrete and dynamic framework within which a better understanding of the rights implications and socio-economic causes and consequences of disease, as well as the impact of disease control programmes, may be achieved. Programmatic perspectives raised include:

- the potential for using the human rights framework to identify groups vulnerable to tuberculosis, and who are likely to suffer the most due to this disease;
- the need for attention to the impact of non-health care sector policies on disease;
- the need for a broad-based support of individuals and communities in coping with the disease, as well as facilitating adherence to treatment; and
- the need for attention to the human rights violated, not only by the disease but also by the measures used to control it.

It is clear, however, that more systematic research is required in order to fully explore the links between human rights and health, and particularly the implications of the human rights framework for disease control programmes. There are a number of gaps in the evidence provided to support the three propositions presented in this chapter:

- the discussion on the causal relationship between the abuse of rights and ill health did not include perspectives on the dimensions and consequences of the lack of freedom, justice, integrity of the individual and meaningful relationships;
- the discussion on the rights violated due to ill health did not explore consequences in terms of freedom, justice and meaningful relationships; and
- the discussion on the impact of health care interventions on rights focused on all elements of the rights lens except for justice.

We clearly need to understand better the rights-health link. Even more, though, we need to practice it. As has been raised extensively in the Indian literature on tuberculosis control, there is a need to develop and use sociological and economic parameters and indicators for assessing the overall impact of tuberculosis control programmes on the disease and society (Nagpaul, 1992).

Of the many issues raised above, the ones left unexamined are perhaps the most important. The critical implications raised by human rights analysis of equality in health have not been discussed. As mentioned in the introduction, an exploration of the issues of equality in health necessitates a consideration of the relationship between the individual and all those who have power to affect his or her health. Related to this is the question of why disease control programmes are often designed within a restrictive biomedical framework, with a narrow and often constraining definition of the problem and its solution. In addition to the programmatic perspectives it provides, human rights analysis has indeed the potential to revolutionise health care provision.

References

Basu, S. (1995) Social assessment study: Perception, attitude, experience of tribal communities vis-á-vis the role of health providers for the acceptability and demand for tuberculosis treatment in tribal areas. Draft report submitted to World Bank.

Bayer, R. and Dupuis, L. (1995) Tuberculosis, public health, and civil liberties. *Ann. Rev. Publ. Hlth.* **16**, 307–326.

Commonwealth Human Rights Initiative (1991) *Put our World to Rights.* London: Commonwealth Human Rights Initiative.

Evans, D., Head, M. and Speller, V. (1994) *Assuring Quality in Health Promotion: How to Develop Standards of Good Practice.* London: Health Education Authority.

Farmer, P. (1997) Social scientists and the new tuberculosis. *Soc. Sci. Med.* **44**, 347–358.

Johansson, E., Diwan, V. K., Huong, N. D. and Ahlberg, B. M. (1996) Staff and patient attitudes to tuberculosis and compliance with treatment: An exploratory study in a district in Vietnam. *Tubercle Lung Dis.* **77**, 178–83.

Liefooghe, R., Michiels, N., Habib, S., Moran, M. B. and De Muynck, A. (1995) Perceptions and social consequences of tuberculosis: A focus group study of tuberculosis patients in Sialkot, Pakistan. *Soc. Sci. Med.* **41**, 1685–1692.

McKeown, T., Record, R. G. and Turner, R. D. (1975) An interpretation of the decline of mortality in England and Wales during the twentieth century. *Populations Studies* **29**, 391–422.

Nagpaul, D. R. (1967) District tuberculosis programme in concept and outline. *Ind. J. Tuberc.* **14**, p. 186.

Nair, D. M., George, A. and Chacko, K. T. (1997) Tuberculosis in Bombay: New insights from poor urban patients. *Hlth. Pol. Plann.* **12**, 77–85.

Narayan, R. and Srikantaramu, N. (1987) Significance of some social factors in the treatment behaviour of tuberculosis patients. *NTI Newsletter* **23**, p. 76.

Porter, J. D. H. and Ogden, J. (1997) Social inequalities in the emergence of infectious disease. In: Shetty, P., Strickland, S., eds. *Biology and Social Inequality.* Cambridge: Cambridge University Press.

Rangan, S. (1995) User perspective in urban tuberculosis control. In: Chakraborty, A. K., Rangan, S. and Uplekar, M., eds. *Urban Tuberculosis Control: Problems and Prospects.* Bombay: The Foundation for Research in Community Health.

Rubel, A. J. and Garro, L. C. (1992) Social and cultural factors in the successful control of tuberculosis. *Publ. Hlth. Rep.* **107**, 626–636.

Toubia, N. F. (1994) From Health or Human Rights to Health and Human Rights: Where do we go from here? *Hlth. Hum. Rights.* **1**, 136–142.

Twumasi, P. A. (1996) Non-compliance with tuberculosis treatment: The Kumasi experience. *Tropical Doctor* **26**, 43–44.

Uplekar, M. and Rangan, S. (1996) *Tackling TB: The search for solutions.* Bombay: The Foundation for Research in Community Health.

CHAPTER 20

THE OWL AND THE PUSSYCAT WENT TO SEA: MOVING TOWARDS INTERSECTORAL POLICIES TO PREVENT THE UNEQUAL DISTRIBUTION OF TUBERCULOSIS

Carolyn Stephens

Introduction — A History of Butchery, Mercury and Myopia

> Fade far away, dissolve, and quite forget
> What thou among the leaves hast never known,
> The weariness, the fever, and the fret
> Here where men sit and hear each other groan;
> Where palsy shakes a few, sad, last grey hairs,
> *Where youth grows pale, and spectre thin, and dies...*
>
> (Keats, 1820, Ode to a Nightingale)

John Keats was born in London in 1795, the eldest son of a horse stable manager. His mother died of tuberculosis in 1810 and his uncle had died at the age of 14 of the same disease. His younger brother Tom died of tuberculosis in 1818, just a few months before Keats discovered that he too had contracted the disease. By the time Keats' most beautiful poetry was published in 1820, he was desperately ill. In 1821, at the age of 26, he too died of the disease which had wracked his whole family, and which crippled British society of all classes at the time.

> As Brown came into the bedroom with a glass of spirits, Keats was just slipping between the sheets. As he did so he coughed; it was only a slight cough, but Brown immediately heard him say "*That is blood from my mouth*". He was examining a single drop of blood upon the sheet. As Brown came forward, he said, "*Bring me the candle, Brown and let me see this blood*". They both stared at it; then, looking up with a steady calm which Brown would never forget, he said, "*I know the colour of that blood; it is arterial blood. I cannot be deceived in that colour. That drop of blood is my death warrant. I must die*." (Gittings, 1979)

Why start a chapter on intersectoral policy approaches to tuberculosis control with an 18th century British poet, most famous for his role as a Romantic poet writing of the impermanence of life and the importance of beauty and truth? It is not simply because Keats and his family had such intimate and terrible experiences with the disease which still devastates so many poor families in Africa, Asia and Latin America. Before becoming one of the world's most renowned Romantic poets, Keats had trained, in 1811, as an apprentice to a surgeon and had graduated in medicine. Aside from his love of poetry, Keats had already noted (along with all his colleagues) that the surgeon training him was "neat-handed, but rash in the extreme" a "butcher" who made "all the students shudder from apprehension" (Cooper, 1814, cited by Gittings, 1979). In addition, Keats was studying at a time when the treatment for infectious conditions, such as common sexually transmitted diseases, often involved the use of highly toxic substances — such as mercury — of which Keats disapproved. A common remedy for tuberculosis was blood-letting — which he blamed, in part rightly, for his deep fatigue, as he died slowly and painfully.

Keats knew then, both through his studies and his personal experience, the limitations of curative medicine. At this time tuberculosis was 'incurable' and its transmission cut across classes, affecting the wealthy more occasionally than the poor, but nevertheless affecting them. Eighty years later Robert Koch discovered the agent responsible for tuberculosis, but medical science was still unable to alleviate the problem of this disease. In 1989, Randall Packard, writing on tuberculosis as a major disease for the black labouring populations in South Africa, supported authors such as Dubos and McKeown in stating that "declines in tuberculosis were largely independent of medical intervention, particularly prior to the 1950s. It appears instead that (declines were due to) improvements in housing, working conditions, and nutrition in the middle years of the nineteenth century" (Dubos and Dubos, 1954; McKeown, 1979; Packard, 1989).

At the end of the 20th century, health professionals are faced with the indisputable fact that all efforts, both national and international, have failed to contain and control tuberculosis. Perhaps as importantly, all efforts in this age of technical skill and medical excellence seem to have failed signally to support and promote the ways in which tuberculosis can be **prevented**.

This chapter will address the importance of moving 'upstream', from control and treatment of tuberculosis within a biomedical framework, and back once more towards intersectoral policies to **prevent** tuberculosis. It will focus on tuberculosis as a disease of inequality — concentrating on policies to prevent tuberculosis in the growing populations of cities. The chapter will examine the importance of spreading responsibility for devising policies for the prevention of tuberculosis across diverse sectors. It will therefore address the importance of intersectoral collaboration — from rendering epidemiological data on tuberculosis understandable and relevant to other sectors (such as planning, housing, social policy, engineering, law) to developing integrated policy interventions. Finally, these issues will be discussed within a conceptual framework which outlines the disciplinary blocks to intersectoral collaboration and the paradoxical policies needed for removing these blocks.

Why Go 'Upstream'? The Evidence from Inequality and the Myth of 'Re-Emerging' Disease

As other chapters in this book have demonstrated, the epidemiology of tuberculosis is the epidemiology of inequality. Tuberculosis is one of the most widely cited of the 're-emerging' infectious diseases which appear to be concentrating in 'the exploding cities' of the South or the 'underclass' of the North (Stephens, 1996). Many cities are in a 'health crisis' — linked to the increasing concentration of the poor in urban centres (World Health Organization, 1993). Associated with the compromised immune defences brought about by HIV infection, tuberculosis is on the increase and is 're-emerging' in some cities in Europe. In reality, however, for the urban poor in the South, tuberculosis never went away. In the North, debate centres on whether or not tuberculosis, the old disease of 'urban poverty', is returning solely through its link to HIV or also as a symptom of increasing polarisation of social groups, in which the conditions of the relative poor have deteriorated dramatically. In reality, the two are linked: AIDS and HIV are now diseases of relative poverty in the North and South, affecting those forced into hazardous sex trades as well as those relying on unsafe drug use (Porter and Ogden, 1998). Drug use itself is linked to coping strategies in situations of social stress brought on by widespread insecurities in employment — particularly for young people. Increasing levels of homelessness in some northern cities, as well as increasing 'ghetto-isation' of certain social groups seem also to be linked to the re-emergence of urban tuberculosis. Thus, for example, a study of childhood tuberculosis in the Bronx, New York, suggests an increase, between 1970–1990, in residential crowding and childhood tuberculosis (Drucker, 1994). Children living in areas where over 12% of the households were severely overcrowded were six times more likely to develop active tuberculosis than their neighbours. Overcrowding was associated with increased household poverty, greater dependence on public assistance, Hispanic ethnicity, larger household size, and a high proportion of young children. In London, studies of urban health inequalities in 1994 revealed that tuberculosis particularly affected the unemployed and those in rented accommodation. A recent analysis of tuberculosis in London (Wilkinson *et al.*, 1998) shows ten-fold differentials in age- and sex-adjusted hospital admissions for 2,157 wards in London between 1992 and 1995 — associated with deprivation, population density and proportion of black and South Asian residents. The authors conclude that there is a strong concentration of disease in deprived urban areas. South Asian immigrants with a high preva-lence of disease in their countries of origin may arrive already infected or with active disease (see Chapter 13). These people, themselves from low-income nations, move into low-income neighbourhoods with poor conditions, in otherwise affluent London. As Wilkinson and colleagues conclude, "inequalities in London tuberculosis disease rates point to the extreme social contrasts still existing in our society".

The current epidemiological pattern of tuberculosis should be ex-pected — it reflects the history of the disease's rise, fall and rise (Reich-man, 1991). Thus, for example, tuberculosis 're-emerged' this century during the 1940 wartime conditions characterised by malnutrition and physical and mental stress (Packard, 1989). In addition, movements of people under social and economic pressures at that time, disseminated and exacerbated the disease. The poor, carrying their disease from their countries of origin ended in the poor, crowded areas of North American cities. Thus, Packard (1989) cites Griggs' argument that tuberculosis was a disease of poverty, moving with the poor, whose low incomes led them to the worst housing in the cities that they moved to. Thus, Packard writes of "the immigration of Europeans into Boston and New York, and the movement of black people from rural areas to the cities of the American South. . . this 'immigration effect' was no doubt generated as well by the ghetto conditions in which many immigrants lived during their early years of settlement".

The epidemiological data must therefore be put in the context of population movements and macro-economic policy shifts. Movements into cities are a major part of the equation. By the year 2025, three out of five people will live in urban areas, the majority in developing countries where 40–70% of the population live in low-income settlements

(United Nations Centre for Human Settlements, 1996). This movement is also taking place in the context of gross polarisation in wealth and assets between people. This chapter is also written at a time when the United Nations reports that "the share of the poorest 20% of the world's people in global income stands at a miserable 1.1%, down from 1.4% in 1991 and 2.3% in 1960" (United Nations Development Programme, 1998). At the same time, the value of the combined assets of the 447 persons who are billionaires exceeds the combined incomes of the poorest 50% of the world's population — some 1.3 billion people. In the North and South, the 're-emergence' of tuberculosis is thus concurrent with the process of polarisation between social groups, with growing inequalities in conditions and opportunities between people. New terms such as 'social exclusion' are used to define the trap of multiple deprivation which has re-emerged in the North and never disappeared from most of the South (UNDP, 1997). These processes combined lead to increasing evidence of the 'ghetto-isation' of the urban poor into overcrowded, poorly serviced and ill-ventilated housing in all parts of the world.

Through the creation of the new conditions for exposure to disease, the current 're-emergence' of tuberculosis is linked to other processes of economic and social 're-emergence' — movements of people particularly the poor, from their land into cities, and from poor Southern nations to low-income urban areas of the North. Figure 1 shows the relative risks of tuberculosis in four contemporary urban centres, demonstrating the strong gradient in relative risks between people living in conditions of multiple deprivation, including crowded housing, economic poverty, poor nutrition and limited access to clean water and adequate sanitation. The figure shows the unequal burden of tuberculosis between groups in all centres, but the scale of the problem is most severe in the city with the most unequal distribution of multiple resources — Cape Town.

A final point must be made about the epidemiology of tuberculosis — it reflects the epidemiology of other illnesses of multiple deprivation. Most historical and modern epidemiological evidence points to the complex links of tuberculosis with poverty and inequality. The multiple deprivation experienced by the world's majority is linked to multiple disease outcomes — many of these outcomes then exacerbate risks of others. Thus, diarrhoeal diseases, linked to faecally contaminated water, food and soil, exacerbate nutritional deficiencies. Families in poverty, already compromised nutritionally by their

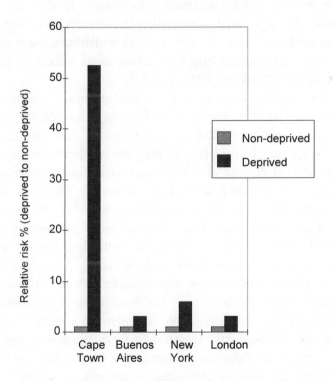

Fig. 1.   The unequal burden of tuberculosis. Relative risks for the urban poor.*

*Cape Town (Yach and Harrison, 1995) death rates; Buenos Aires (Bianco, 1984) death rates; New York (Drucker *et al.*, 1995) case rates; London (Landon, 1994) case rates.

inability to purchase nutritious food, are then put further at risk by their
sanitary conditions. Shift-sleeping in crowded conditions and working
in hazardous cramped workplaces predisposes to other common infectious and chronic diseases in both children and adults. Thus, as Packard
points out for South Africa, synergism between health outcomes mul-
tiplies the risk of disease, implicating all aspects of deprivation in the
causality of any one outcome. In this context "the health cost of inadequate sanitation was not limited to diarrhoea-related deaths. Parasitic diseases have an adverse effect on nutritional levels, particularly on
protein absorption and are a significant co-factor in the production of
tuberculosis. An additional synergistic relationship may have been set
up by increased crowding and the ways in which measles transmission
increased, with its catalyst effect to tuberculosis infections in measles
affected children" (Packard, 1989, p. 142).

In the face of this policy context, a fundamental challenge is posed
to the public health community — and perhaps for nothing more than
for the control and prevention of tuberculosis. Can the majority of
tuberculosis specialists continue to stay so far downstream — in the
field of biomedical control and treatment of a disease with such well-
known links with the multiple risks of poverty? In terms of 'public'
health strategy, the current policies seem to be incapable of addressing
the issue of secondary control, let alone primary prevention. But why
is this so? This cannot be driven by biomedical arrogance, generated
by the success of sophisticated medical technology. It could indeed be
argued that the feverish debate over tuberculosis control measures at
the present time reflects the dismay and frustration of the community of
tuberculosis workers at being unable to reach the poor with affordable,
effective health services and treatments for a disease so synonymous
with urban poverty. Tuberculosis remains a critical disease in need of
complex 'upstream' policies addressing issues such as housing, nutrition,
and labour conditions and opportunities.

How can the public health community develop better strategies to
prevent tuberculosis — strategies which will complement and reinforce
the policies for control and treatment? The next section will consider

the field of intersectoral action and address the issue of how to enhance the collaborative relationship between health specialists and other professionals.

Facilitating Interdisciplinary Understanding and Intersectoral Action

At the end of the 20th century, there are strong calls for more interdisciplinary research processes and intersectoral and multisectoral intervention strategies. These calls have been made for some time — the original primary health strategies were focused on intersectoral action and in 1986 the World Health Organization (WHO) promoted once more the idea of intersectoral policy; and this has been the focus of more recent initiatives such as Healthy Cities and Local Agenda 21 (Dooris, 1997).

Interdisciplinary research will not only enhance the capacity of public health professionals to understand the relationships between environment, development and health, but will also guide towards better multi- and intersectoral collaboration and policy making. Yet, in attempting to move forward, few seem to appreciate fully how firmly history has embedded the largely Western models of scientific thought which developed in Europe during the 16th and 17th century. The impacts of these systems of thought are still felt internationally and they are evident in all spheres of research and policy. They are clearly evident in the continued academic emphasis on single-discipline specialisation within training processes and in institutional administrative structures which mirror disciplinary boundaries. Within universities, departments are often organised by discipline and training continues to emphasise that excellence in understanding and skills is achieved through specialisation in one discipline. Political institutions mirror this: ministries and departments within national and local governments are also organised around sectoral boundaries. Finally, at the international level, even the United Nations organisations are grouped thematically in a way which reflects, in part, disciplinary boundaries.

It is clear that economic, social and health problems do not respect disciplinary boundaries — just as many environmental hazards do not respect the national boundaries humans have set up to organise their social and political systems. This is recognised by an increasing number of professionals who work in interdisciplinary teams and on intersectoral projects. But creating the framework for moving across sectors is not easy. By the time those working in the fields of environment, development and health realise the need to develop interdisciplinary research processes or intersectoral projects, which rely on collaboration and communication, they are already well-trained in their independent languages, conceptual approaches and skills. Ironically, those living in the period when our current systems first evolved recognised that the scientific advances they were making might lead eventually to the reductionism we see today. Thus, 250 years ago, a European writer, Jonathan Swift, predicted that the scientific methods developed at the time would not create *wisdom* in decision making for human development. In *Voyage to Laputa* in *Gulliver's Travels*, written in 1726, Swift warned that wise decisions stem from a recognition and appreciation of life's complexity. He argued, just as many in the research and policy making community do again today, that the "whole is more than the sum of the parts". He also warned against the false dichotomy of research and policy making. His Laputan island, floating high above reality in the sky, was an early image of 'ivory tower' research — Swift believed that research conducted in isolation of the policy process would lead to myopic tendencies in human understanding.

At the end of the 20th century the early concerns of Swift are shared by workers in many disciplines. The debate related to interdisciplinary research and intersectoral action reflects wider discussion in much western scientific thought and expresses a concern which has developed in many fields. There are increasing calls for scientists to collaborate more fully across disciplines, and also calls to reform the bases of individual sciences in order that they may become better guides for wise human action in the face of complex global crises which threaten human society as a whole. But, as Box 2 suggests, the problem of interdisciplinary dialogue and collaboration is as entrenched as 17th century humanists thought they might become.

> *"We make ourselves into Blues and Greens and Reds. And then we are surprised when the Blues speak a different language to the Reds and to the Greens. It is as if I am speaking Ukrainian while you are speaking Urdu. The language we use defines our perspective on problems and our identification of solutions"*
>
> **What language are you speaking?** Mike Cohen (Senior Environmental Adviser, World Bank — speaking to students of the London School of Hygiene and Tropical Medicine 1997).

Creating better interdisciplinary communication and greater intersectoral dialogue can facilitate both interdisciplinary research processes and intersectoral actions. There have, in recent years, been some advance in the development of interdisciplinary communication and it is now clear that such communication should start of the stage of conceptualisation of the 'problem' (Briggs *et al.*, 1996, Stephens, 1997). This requires that different disciplines recognise and respect the fact that they start from very different points in conceptual terms. This is difficult when specific disciplinary approaches traditionally claim precedence in conceptual understanding and setting of priorities. For example, for some, a biomedical scientific discipline such as epidemiology is the basic means to guide priority setting on public health and medicine. More recently, however, epidemiologists themselves have expressed concerns about the inherent reductionism of the discipline suggesting, as Steve Wing does, that *"the field should adopt a less reductionist approach... our dominant epidemiology begins with the assumption that things work separately and independently, that exposure can be separated from the practices which produce them. An epidemiology oriented towards massive and equitable public health improvement requires reconstructing the connections between disease agents and their contexts"* (Wing, 1994).

This does not necessarily mean that epidemiologists should abandon the skills of rigorous critical biomedical analysis of human health, but it opens two new strands of scientific possibility. First, it allows epidemiologists to move, as physicists have already done, towards development of epidemiological methods to address the complex, synergistic interactions of multiple exposures and health impacts — moving the discipline towards 'post-normal' science (Funtowitz and Ravetz, 1994). Secondly, adopting a less reductionist approach allows health professionals to make their work more accessible to those in other disciplines. This, in turn, allows for a stronger collaborative coalition of professional action to prevent as well as treat and control illness. This is perhaps the most productive and practical reason for health professionals to look for ways to develop less reductionist approaches.

This raises an important question, particularly for tuberculosis specialists. Perhaps there is no disease in the world that would benefit more from these collaborations than tuberculosis — finally persuading the specialists out of their corner and into cooperation with diverse professionals in the field of disease **prevention**. Yet improved scientific understanding and interdisciplinary development of policy relies on collaboration from the outset of priority setting between disciplines as diverse as mathematics, physics, epidemiology, engineering, environmental science, as well as the political, social and economic sciences. Such collaboration moves us forward from list-driven, downstream, myopic understanding, but it requires careful appreciation of the conceptual contribution of each discipline, as well as negotiation of roles in ways which show respect for each discipline.

There is progress in this area at a number of levels. For example, in response to the needs for conceptual advances, an ambitious framework has been developed by the Office of Global and Integrated Environmental Health of the WHO in collaboration with the United Nations Environment Programme and the United Nations Development Programme. This is known as the DPSEEA (Driving forces; Pressures; State; Exposures; Effects; Actions) framework (Briggs et al., 1996).

This framework builds on the environmental information systems of 'pressure-state-response' used to structure reporting on the state of development and environmental conditions internationally. The framework was developed initially by the Organisation for Economic Co-operation and Development, following an idea of the Canadian Government and it advances the debate on intersectoral collaboration in two ways. First, it organises concepts and disciplines to include those working at the level of chemists and pharmacologists developing new treatment regimes for disease to the level of political scientists working on the 'driving forces', the most fundamental processes in the development and environment system. Second, and perhaps as importantly, it reveals the attempts of health professionals within the UN system to negotiate and compromise on a joint framework, rather than each sectoral agency developing competing frameworks, and mismatched policies.

Thus, *Driving Forces* are the processes responsible for the pressures on the environment in which people live. Most profoundly, driving forces are the economic and political processes which guide national and international development. Driving forces of economic and political development generate the patterns of development which dictate the distribution of resources and people and which lead to *Pressures* on the environment. Pressures occur in the process of resource extraction, processing and distribution to consumption and waste release. The pressures on the environment lead to changes in the *State* of the environment. These changes can be far-reaching and complex, altering the existence and severity of natural hazards; creating new man-made hazards; and affecting resource availability. In the course of these changes in the state of conditions which humans experience, *Exposures* to hazards occur. *Exposure* refers to the direct juxtaposition of people and environmental conditions. Exposure is not an automatic consequence of the existence of a hazard since it requires that people are present at both the place and at the time that a hazard occurs. Exposure to environmental hazards in turn leads to health effects. These vary depending on the type of hazard to which people have been exposed and the level of exposure. The number of people involved and their personal susceptibility

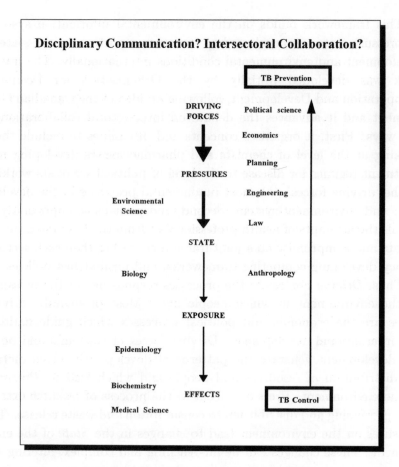

Fig. 2. Some areas in which interdisciplinary communication and intersectoral collaboration are required.

to ill health is also important. Figure 2 shows how the DPSEEA framework can be linked to the disciplinary focus of each professional.

Actions, or policies to address environmental health impacts, are the final element of the DPSEEA framework. In practice, these actions could occur at any stage of the framework.

How would such a framework assist in the development of the prevention of the inequitable distribution of tuberculosis? For a start, it helps to clarify conceptually where each discipline works and where each could contribute. Figure 2 shows that different disciplines focus their attention at very different stages of the DPSEEA framework. It is, for example, at the intersection of exposure, health effect and susceptibility that epidemiologists tend to work. This keeps the discipline downstream unless epidemiologists are prepared to begin dialogues with those in other disciplines who work at other levels of the framework. Equally, planners and engineers will start with an understanding of *Pressures* in the environment and the effect of these pressures on the *State* of the environment. Their work leads them to act at the level of changing conditions in the environment affecting, for example, water supplies, sanitation and the planning of housing. Lawyers will change the regulatory system, thereby affecting the pressures and conditions which people experience. Political scientists may start from the *Driving Forces* which influence development decisions and economic policy. Anthropologists may come to this framework at the point of *State* of the environment and the interface of the environmental social and economic conditions with communities and individuals. The conceptual advances take the debate to the point where each profession is able to recognise its strength and place in the overall understanding. When this is taken to reality, tuberculosis specialists can begin to see that they should be collaborating with planners, lawyers and engineers as well as with anthropologists. The final section of this chapter will discuss this briefly.

Moving Upstream — Beyond the Conceptual Advance

The direct international actions to alleviate the health burden of tuberculosis are focused currently at the level of biomedical control and treatment. Yet, at the level of driving forces, current political and economic forces tend to oppose any attempts at downstream control of this disease by exacerbating urban poverty and creating conditions of social exclusion (United Nations Centre for Human Settlements, 1996; Stephens, 1997). Going to the other end of the chain, shifts in the system of health care delivery will operate at the stage of dealing with the health effects of tuberculosis — but as political pressure pushes the system towards privatisation of services, the tuberculosis public health community struggles to keep the services affordable and accessible to the poor (see Chapter 18).

Against these pressures, there is a strong movement of many professionals towards collaborative understanding of poverty, health and development. This extends from the recent work in the field of law aimed at developing the notion of 'environmental justice', to the re-awakening of the role of public and environmental health as a discipline which had its roots in the 19th century movements of social justice. This last section discusses briefly the convergence of professionals from very different sectors around the key risk factors for tuberculosis — urban poverty, access to services, and crowded conditions in poorly ventilated housing.

Public health professionals have long recognised the importance of good nutrition, housing and work conditions as preventive factors against tuberculosis. In the UK, the 1998 'Green Paper' on Public Health once again emphasised the role of housing in ill health, and the fundamental role of inequality and poverty in perpetuating the conditions for ill health. But the role of lawyers and planners, or more accurately the legislature and planning, in tuberculosis prevention has only recently regained recognition by health professionals. Yet, as shown in Box 3, the important role of these professionals in the prevention of tuberculosis is exemplified by the recent pressure from lawyers and planners to improve living conditions for low-income urban people through adopting a 'rights' approach to access to resources and pushing reforms of legislation which creates barriers to poor people's access to land and housing (SOAS, 1996). For example, the 'Habitat Agenda' emerging from the 1996 UN Summit on Human Settlements highlighted rights to housing as a key issue internationally. The agenda, developed by planners and urban specialists, calls for a commitment by all governments to guarantees of security of tenure as a key policy issue for urban centres internationally, the settings in which most people will live by

---

The Driving Forces for Urban TB — planning, legislature and policy

- **Insecurity of Home, Land and Person** — where the poor have no access to secure homes;

- **Misuse of Planning Mechanisms**: regional plans discriminating against the poor and forcing ethnic and economic segregation;

- **Abuse of Law**: laws which protect landlords not poor tentants;

- **Privatised Service Provision**: where landlords are given the responsibility to provide services (not enforced).

The Consequences: Urban Poverty and the conditions for multiple disease

- Multiple occupancy, renting squatters vulnerable to forced evictions if they complain, living in crowded ill-serviced housing and settlements.

The Way Forward

"Institutionalise the legislative, planning and housing rights that will break the grip of the "institutionalised insecure housing and living conditions experienced by up to 50% of people in cities".

Source: Kothari, M. (1997). Fighting Forced Evictions in The Habitat II Land Initiative Access to Land and Security of Tenure.

2025. Security of tenure may seem far from the field of tuberculosis control but it is a key link in a chain of cause and effect, liberating people from crowded, ill-ventilated informal settlements where they pay high rents and have no control over their facilities, and the legislative systems which favour 'slum landlords' and penalise the renting poor. This issue was pushed high on the 'Habitat Agenda' through a collaboration between lawyers working on environmental justice and housing planners keen to develop ways to protect the housing rights of poor urban citizens. This policy links with the prevention of tuberculosis through its promotion of conditions for healthier domestic living. It is linked to the declarations of the Beijing Summit on Women in 1995 which declared that: "men and women shall have full and equal access to economic resources, including the right to inheritance and ownership of land and property" (Beijing Platform for Action, paragraph 63 in Quist, 1997). This is not all simply rhetoric of UN conferences: as highlighted in Box 4, the new government in South Africa has placed access to land and housing high on its agenda.

South Africa's New constitution

Rights to housing (Article 26):

1. Everyone has the right to adequate housing.

2. The state must take reasonable legislative and other measures within its achievable resources, to achieve the progressive achievement of that right.

3. No one may be evicted from their home or have it demolished, without an order of court made after considering all the relevant circumstances.

4. No legislation may permit arbitrary evictions.

Source : SOAS (1996)

Complementing this pressure from lawyers and planners, the public health community has highlighted 'healthy housing' as a key strategy within the Healthy Cities movement internationally (Dooris, 1997). In the UK, the 1998 'Green Paper' on public health highlights housing as a key part of the UK strategy 'Towards a Healthier Nation' (Department of Health, HM Government, 1998).

Conclusions: The Owl and the Pussycat leave Laputa?

When public health professionals combine with lawyers and planners to provide information, advocacy and technical support for rights to housing, strong pressure is created across a professional and public coalition in favour of the rights of the poor. This pressure can be brought to bear on governments and private agencies to ensure that barriers to healthy living conditions are removed. This coalition is not a panacea, and nor is it simple to achieve. Professionals are still trained to specialise and think territorially. As the Association of Public Health commented on the UK Green Paper: "the themes are still constructed in a biomedical model". This need not be a problem if other disciplines understand and can use this model, but if it alienates them, it is not helpful. As Dooris comments in his review of the Healthy City and Agenda 21 models: "is there an added value in frameworks which cover the same ground — health for all, strategic planning and local initiatives — or should competing frameworks be merged?" The answer lies perhaps in each discipline developing its strength, but reaching out with respect to other disciplines — as many philosophers of science, such as Midgely and Lubenchek have argued for a while.

This chapter emphasises, then, some common themes:

- Shared conceptual and professional humility.
- Shared and complementary information systems.
- Shared and reinforced understanding.
- Coalitions of advocacy across professions.
- Coordinated 'joined up' policies across sectors.
- Patience and an awareness of history.

It would be naïve to suggest that tuberculosis specialists will feel comfortable collaborating with lawyers and planners until they begin to value such collaborations and until public health professionals are taught how to share concepts, information and plans. But it may be good to end on the challenge of the injustice of the distribution of tuberculosis in South Africa. Thus, it may be asked, when the territorial barriers are down, whether tuberculosis specialists would advocate effective treatment of tuberculosis as a solution to South Africa's most unjust disease, or whether they would prefer to put their epidemiology to the support of the legislative demands for access to adequate living conditions for all.

References

Bianco, M. (1983) *Health and its Care in Greater Buenos Aires.* UNICEF/WHO meeting on health care in urban areas. Geneva: World Health Organization.

Briggs, D., *et al.* (1996) *Linkage Methods for Environment and Health Analysis. General Guidelines. A Report of the Health and Environment Analysis for Decision-Making (HEADLAMP) Project.* Geneva: World Health Organization.

De Cock, K. M., *et al.* (1995) Tropical medicine for the 21st century *Br. Med. J.* **311**, 860–862.

Department of Health, HM Government. (1998) *Towards a Healthier Nation.* London: HM Stationery Office.

Dooris, M. (1997) Health and Local Agenda 21: Integrating strategies in local government to achieve action. In: *Sustainable Development Background Paper for UK National Roundtable of Local Governments.* Bristol: The Create Centre.

Drucker, E., Alcabes, P., Bosworth, W. and Sckell, B. (1994) Childhood tuberculosis in the Bronx, New York. *Lancet.* **343**, p. 8911.

Dubos, R. and Dubos, J. (1953) *The White Plague.* Boston: Little, Brown and Company.

Funtowicz, S. O. and Ravetz, J. R. (1992) Three types of risk assessment and the emergence of post normal science. In: Krimsky, S. and Goldng, D., eds., *Social Theories of Risk*, pp. 251–275.

Gittings, R. (1979) *John Keats.* London: Penguin Books, 552pp.

Keats, J. (1988) Ode to a nightingale 1820. In: Barnard, J., ed. *John Keats: Selected Poems.* London: Penguin Books, pp. 169–171.

Landon, M. (1994) *Intra-Urban Health Differentials in London.* London: London School of Hygiene and Tropical Medicine, pp. 1–33.

McKeown, T. (1979) *The Role of Medicine. Dream, Mirage or Nemesis?* Oxford: Blackwell, pp. 1–190.

Packard, R. M. (1989) *White Plague, Black Labour. Tuberculosis and the Political Economy of Health and Disease in South Africa.* South Africa: University of Natal Press.

Porter, J. D. H. and Ogden, J. A. (1998) Social inequalities in the re-emergence of infectious diseases. In: Strickland, S. S. and Shetty, P., eds. *Human Biology and Social Inequality.* Cambridge: Cambridge University Press, pp. 96–114.

Quist, E. (1997) Promoting women's equal access to land. In: *UN Centre for Human Settlements, 1997 Habitat Debate. United Nations*: The Habitat II Land Initiative, Vol. 3, No. 2.

Reichman, L. B. (1991) The U-shaped curve of concern. *Am. Rev. Resp. Dis.* **144**, 741–742.

SOAS (School of Oriental and African Studies). (1996) *Claiming our Future Environmental Justice Workshop*. London: SOAS Law Department.

Stephens, C. (1996) Review article: Healthy cities or unhealthy islands? The health and social implications of urban inequalities. *Environment and Urbanization* **8**, 9–30.

Stephens, C. (1997) *Environment, Health and Development: Negotiating with Complexity in Priority-Setting Processes*. Geneva: World Health Organization.

Swift, J. (1726) Voyage to the Island of Laputa. In: *Gulliver's Travels*. London: Penguin Books, 1984.

UNDP (United Nations Development Programme) (1997) *Human Development Report 1997*. Oxford: Oxford University Press.

United Nations Centre for Human Settlements (HABITAT) (1996) *An Urbanizing World. Global Report on Human Settlements 1996*. Oxford: Oxford University Press.

Wilkinson, P. *et al.* (1998) *Wide socio-economic variation in tuberculosis in London and the South East*. Abstracts of the 1st world congress on Health and Urban Environment, July 1998, p. 329.

Wing, S. (1994) Limits of epidemiology. *Medicine and Global Survival* **1**, 74–86.

White, K. L. (1991) *Healing the Schism. Epidemiology, Medicine and the Public's Health*. New York: Springer-Verlag.

World Health Organization (1993) *The Urban Health Crisis: Strategies for Health for All in the Face of Rapid Urbanization*. Geneva: World Health Organization.

Yach, D. and Harrison, D. (1996) *Inequalities in Health Determinants and Status in South Africa*. Pretoria: South African Medical Research Council.

CHAPTER 21

EDUCATIONAL APPROACHES IN TUBERCULOSIS CONTROL: BUILDING ON THE 'SOCIAL' PARADIGM

Thelma Narayan and Ravi Narayan

Introduction

From the orthodox biomedical perspective, tuberculosis is a 'chronic mycobacterial infection' requiring early diagnosis by sputum microscopy and culture; radiological investigation; and chemotherapy, consisting of prompt, regular and extended treatment by a combination of anti-tuberculosis drugs. This perspective generates a restricted view of the challenges of educational approaches in tuberculosis control as it focuses primarily on motivating patients to take regular treatment and not to become 'defaulters'.

There is an urgent need to broaden the understanding of the disease by applying a socio-epidemiological perspective, which focuses on the larger socio-economic-political-cultural context in which the disease spreads and thrives in the community. This paradigm shift in understanding would lead to a recognition of a multi-disciplinary and multi-dimensional educational response that should become a major part of the control effort. The most significant aspect of this proposed change would be the contextualisation of tuberculosis control efforts to the important policy imperatives of equity and social justice — helping initiatives to reach those who are not reached by our present educational or health care efforts.

In this chapter this broader understanding is explored and a framework for a multi-pronged educational initiative that addresses these imperatives is evolved.

Recognising and Evolving the 'Social' Paradigm

The Medico Friend Circle is a national network of doctors and health workers in India concerned that health care and medical education in the country should become more relevant to the needs of the poor and the marginalised. In 1985, it organised an interactive dialogue on 'Tuberculosis and Society' which brought together 110 doctors, social workers, health and development activists, and many others concerned about

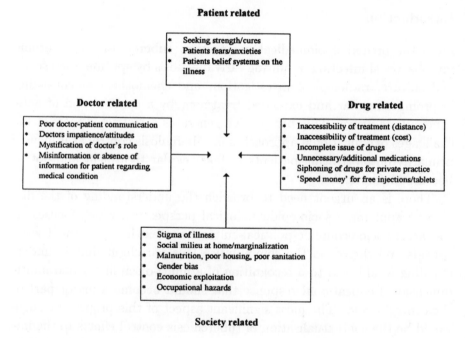

Fig. 1.   The Social Paradigm — Some Significant Social Factors.
Source: Sadgopal (1983) and Medico Friend Circle (1985).

Table 1. Responding to the Social Paradigm — Some Suggestions.*

System Development

- Increasing health budget and reducing urban bias.
- Increasing accountability and responsiveness in the health care delivery system.
- Training paramedicals and community-based health workers to enhance accessibility.
- Reorienting medical/nursing education towards the social paradigm.

Community Involvement

- Interactive, culturally sensitive health education efforts.
- Tackling stigma of disease among health professionals, community and patients.
- Enhancing community participation at all levels.
- Tuberculosis control linked to grassroots peoples' movements.

Seeking New Partnership

- Involvement of Trade Unions and the 'Womens movement'.
- Involvement of local healers and practitioners of all systems of medicine.
- Involvement/orientation of community leaders, politicians, policy makers.
- Introducing 'Tuberculosis Control' in High School Science syllabus.

Tackling the Determinants of the Disease

- Intersectoral action to improve nutrition, housing, sanitation, working environment and wages.
- Minimum Wages Act and Right to Work.
- Land Reform.

---

*Source: Sadgopal (1983) and Medico Friend Circle (1985).

the tuberculosis problem in India. While the discussions explored the challenges of case-finding, case-holding and the alternative 'regimens of chemotherapy' there was also an identification of a large number of significant social/societal factors and issues of concern, from the field experience of the participants, that constituted a 'social paradigm' (Medico Friend Circle, 1985).

Figure 1 lists some of the factors that appear to play a key part in the patient's experience of the disease and the response of various types of health care providers to the disease (Sadagopal, 1993; Medico Friend Circle, 1995). Table 1 lists a series of ideas and initiatives that were suggested during the group discussions as ways and means of addressing the social factors and issues of concern listed in Figure 1 (Medico Friend Circle, 1985).

It was evident at this meeting that if the factors responsible for the occurrence, spread and maintenance of the disease were social and societal, then the responses needed to be social/societal as well. This shift of emphasis would not only change the framework of tuberculosis control but would lead to a broader framework of educational effort to support action towards control.

Table 2.   Tuberculosis and Society — Levels of Analysis and Solution.*

Levels of Analysis of Tuberculosis	Causal Understanding	Solutions/Control Strategies
Surface phenomenon (medical and public health problem)	Infectious disease/germ theory	BCG, case-finding and domiciliary chemotherapy
Immediate cause	Undernutrition/low resistance, poor housing, low income/poor purchasing capacity	Development and welfare-income generation/ housing
Underlying cause (symptom of inequitable relations)	Poverty/deprivation, unequal access to resources	Land reforms, social movements towards a more egalitarian society
Basic cause (international problem)	Contradictions and inequalities in socio-economic and political systems at international, national and local levels	More just international relations, trade relations, etc.

*Source: Narayan (1998).

More recently, a comprehensive review has once again stressed that the level and depth of analysis of the problem of tuberculosis and its causative factors influence the construction of the solution. Table 2 indicates different levels of analysis and different solutions and control strategies, highlighting once again the shift from a 'biomedical' to a 'social' paradigm (Narayan, 1998).

Widening the Educational Framework: Reaching All

The orthodox biomedical paradigm usually results in an educational effort that has a two-pronged focus: on the patient and on the health team. Health education efforts are directed at the patients to make them more informed and aware of all aspects of the disease and its treatment and the basic rules to prevent spreading the infection to others in the family or the community.

Instruction in all aspects of tuberculosis, including epidemiology, clinical, laboratory, therapeutic, preventive and public health aspects, has been an important part of medical and nursing education as well as a component of the curriculum of paramedical workers and health auxiliaries for many years.

The biomedical paradigm also stresses the technological component of tuberculosis control — BCG vaccine, sputum microscopy, radiological diagnosis, and varying regimens of chemotherapy. It focuses on individual patients, stresses only physical aspects of the illness, highlights mainly the role of the health care provider — doctor or nurse — and considers the role of the patient as a passive beneficiary of a top-down providing system who must be prevented, through health education, from becoming a 'defaulter'. Finally, the biomedical paradigm also stresses the challenges of research in molecular biology or pharmacotherapeutics.

The new 'social paradigm' discussed in the previous section and increasingly recognised in the last decade (CHC, 1989; Qadeer, 1995; Nikhil, 1995; Uplekar and Rangan, 1996; Narayan T, 1997; Narayan R,

1997; Chaturvedi, 1997) requires a totally different framework of education that is both multi-dimensional and multi-pronged in its orientation. While neglecting neither the patient nor the health care provider, the focus of such education goes beyond to a larger section of society and a broader range of groups in the community so that tuberculosis control efforts get the support, encouragement and involvement of many people. These include:

The patients' family. This is particularly important because tuberculosis has psycho-social dimensions that need family support for their amelioration. Care providers are therefore an important focus group.

The people of the community in which the patient lives. These include community leaders — both formal and informal, school teachers, non-governmental organisations, women's groups, other community-based organisations and educational institutions (Kaul, 1996).

Occupational groups. Those in which the patient works and, particularly, the occupational groups in which the risk of tuberculosis is higher.

Health care providers. This focuses beyond education of doctors nurses and paramedical personnel to a host of other formal and informal health care providers including practitioners of alternate systems of medicine, traditional birth attendants and other types of local folk healers, private practitioners and health teams, and technicians of the large number of private laboratories and health institutions.

Marginalised social groups. The 'social paradigm' should also lead to a special educational effort focused towards high risk groups and marginalised groups in society, including residents of urban slums, those who are HIV positive and those with AIDS, the homeless, destitute and pavement dwellers, ragpickers and street children, addicts — both drug users and alcoholics — and refugees, including those displaced by war, ethnic conflicts and development projects.

Policy makers. Most significantly, however, the recognition of the 'social paradigm' leads us to focus educational/awareness building efforts towards those within society who make decisions, those who are involved in policy planning and implementation, as well as those who support the programme initiatives. These include political leaders at all levels — particularly elected representatives at state, district and municipal corporation levels, government bureaucrats and technocrats, the pharmaceutical industry, and civic society. Finally, all those groups who are contributors to the 'watch dog' role of civic society also need to be addressed through educational efforts: these include the media, consumer groups/organisations/associations and non-governmental organisations.

Content of Educational Approaches: From 'Biomedicine' to 'Socio-epidemiology'

The recognition of the 'social paradigm' will necessitate a different framework of tuberculosis education and so the focus and content will have to experience a paradigm shift. The focus will move from individual tuberculosis patients, increasingly to focus on a community of potential sufferers. It will move beyond the physical dimension and explore the psycho-social-economic-cultural and political dimensions of tuberculosis including relationship to poverty, the problem of stigma and marginalisation, and the 'social burden' of the disease. It will move beyond vaccine/drug distribution to include components that enhance awareness, motivation and empowerment of patients through counselling. The focus will therefore be on educational and social processes and other enabling and autonomy-building skills, and will emphasise the supportive role of family members, other care providers, community leaders and grassroots and community-based health workers. It will also emphasise a change of role of the patient from a passive beneficiary of treatment to an active participant of the control strategy whose autonomy and sense of responsibility is to be respected and enhanced.

Clearly, such a framework of education must emphasise the key contributions from behavioural science and a qualitative approach to research, including both action and participatory research, and must encourage attempts to understand attitudes, belief systems, knowledge levels and practice options at the community level. This would also encourage an increasing shift from the orthodox 'clinical' and 'molecular biology' fixation of tuberculosis researchers to a more broad-based sphere of interest.

Table 3.   The Paradigm Shift.*

Parameter	Biomedical Approach		Social/Community Approach
Focus	Individual	→	Community
Dimensions	Physical (tuberculosis pathology)	→	Psycho-social, economic, cultural, political and ecological (stigma, poverty, social burden)
Technology	Drugs/vaccines	→	Education and social processes
Type of service	Providing/Dependence creating	→	Enabling/Empowering Autonomy building
Patient	Passive beneficiary	→	Active participant
Research	Molecular biology	→	Socio-epidemiology
	Pharmaco-therapeutics	→	Behavioural sciences

*Adapted from CHC (1989).

Table 3 summarises this shift so that the broadening of the framework and content is clearer. It is important here to emphasise that a case is being made not for a biomedical versus a community/social model of public health dialectic, but for the broadening of the orthodox biomedical approach by the inclusion of a social/community/societal dimension (CHC, 1989). This will make the tuberculosis control initiative more holistic, more responsive, more relevant and definitely more effective in the complex environment and societal reality in which tuberculosis thrives and continues to be a major public health problem today.

An important feature of this recognition of the social paradigm in tuberculosis is the consequent need to give socio-economic-political-cultural determinants an important role in policy review and programme planning.

Many determinants of tuberculosis have been known for some time (Narayan, 1997):

(1) Tuberculosis is related to industrialisation, which resulted in a process of urbanisation with overcrowded, unhygienic living conditions for the working class in the new industrial and mining towns. These were further complicated by low wages and longer hours of work. Research has indicated that, in the USA and Africa, there was an increase in the prevalence of tuberculosis at a time of industrial and urban growth.

(2) Population growth, migration, colonialism and war-initiated epidemic waves of tuberculosis in different regions of the world.

(3) The incidence of tuberculosis often increases in times of war and during ethnic conflicts and among refugees. In India, tuberculosis was a big problem among post-partition refugees.

(4) Disrupted social conditions, malnutrition, poor housing and physical and emotional stress are predisposing factors. In India, it is not surprising that the incidence of tuberculosis is relatively high among Tibetan refugees in the resettlement colonies.

(5) Housing is a key factor, especially small, overcrowded tenements in shanty towns and urban slums.

(6) Poor sanitation and unregulated growth of hazardous industries further compound the problem.

(7) Smoking, pollution and rapid industrialisation driven by an economic imperative which sacrifices safety procedures and compromises regulatory mechanisms are all contributory factors.

(8) Finally, there is growing evidence that new economic trends that promote 'globalisation', liberalisation and privatisation — increasingly have an adverse effect on the health of the poor by making health care more and more inaccessible (Chaulet, 1998). In Africa and the Philippines, the documented ill effects include a higher incidence of tuberculosis. State-run health services

experienced cut-backs in expenditure which particularly affects services for the poor.

While these factors are all very significant, it is equally significant that most of the literature, pamphlets and reports from the World Health Organization (WHO), the Government of India and non- governmental organisations ignore these dimensions (National Tuberculosis Institute, 1994; Government of India, 1995; World Health Organization, 1995a, 1995b; World Health Organization/UNAIDS, 1996; Voluntary Health Association of India, 1994, 1996; Chakraborthy and Choudhury, 1997). Hence the narrow biomedical perspective continues.

Educational Approaches — What Do We Seek to Achieve?

While all educational approaches at all levels, and for all the target groups mentioned earlier, must emphasise these broader factors in addition to the biomedical ones, the objectives of education will shift from enhancing case-detection, case-management, and tuberculosis treatment *per se* to a host of initiatives that would address the determinants and deeper causes of the illnesses. Tuberculosis treatment and control will become part of a wider social movement that seeks to address poverty, illiteracy, poor environment, marginalisation, unplanned urbanisation and industrialisation, poor housing and to increase access to, and options of, health care for the poor.

In 1981, the Indian Council of Social Science Research and the Indian Council of Medical Research in their Health for All Strategy in India, outlined a prescription for Health for All, which included such a broad concept of health action (ICSSR/ICMR 1981). They emphasised the need for a mass movement to reduce poverty and inequality and to spread education, to organise the poor and underprivileged to fight for their basic rights, and to move away from the counterproductive consumerist Western model of health care and replace it by an alternative based in the community.

More recently, echoes of this broader action are seen even in the writings of orthodox epidemiologists who stress that medicine and politics should not be kept apart. The late Professor Rose wrote, in what was perhaps his final work after decades of extensive epidemiological research, that "Medicine has indeed delivered effective answers to some health problems and it has found the means to lessen the symptoms of many others. But by and large, we remain with the necessity to do something about the incidence of disease, and that means a new partnership between the health services and all those whose decisions influence the determinants of incidence. The primary determinants of disease are mainly economic and social and therefore its remedies must also be economic and social. Medicine and politics cannot, and should not, be kept apart" (Rose, 1992).

The objective of a comprehensive educational initiative — comprehensive both in target groups and in content — is to facilitate a more comprehensive anti-tuberculosis programme that would locate programmatic action in a mosaic of multi-dimensional and multi-sectoral action impacting on all aspects of the problem. Such a programme would include an increase in health budgets — including funding for tuberculosis control, poverty alleviation programmes focused on marginalised peoples, housing and planned urbanisation programmes, occupational safety focused on high-risk individuals and high-risk occupations, personal and social support to affected people and their families — particularly those from the marginalised sections and initiatives to address social and economic inequality and injustice.

Such a broad based, social/societal-oriented model of a health programme for tuberculosis would then strike at the roots of the problem and not fritter away resources in superficial biomedical reductionist strategies that have a limited impact on the disease.

It is rather unfortunate that, in more recent times, the WHO and other international funding agencies have failed to establish their programmes for tuberculosis on a broad base and have advocated ideas such as DOTS that are at best 'reductionist' and at worst totally inadequate for the treatment of the complex social pathology of tuberculosis in society. This continued 'technomanagerialism' at the cost of a comprehensive, integrated social strategy is particularly disappointing and, as usual, the poorest among the tuberculosis patients will bear the consequences of this public health reductionism (Banerji, 1996, 1997).

Educational Initiatives — Moving from Content to Process

In the earlier sections of this chapter, the 'who', the 'what' and the 'why' of educational initiatives in tuberculosis control in the context of the 'social paradigm' have been explored. In this section, the 'when' and 'where' of some aspects of such an educational response are explored. Broadly, these are described under the headings of basic and continuous health professional education and patient/community education.

Health Care — Professional Education

There is urgent need to enhance and strengthen the framework of tuberculosis education for medical practitioners and nurses. To make an impact on professional education, there is need to focus both on 'basic education' and continuing education.

Basic Education

There a is need to make tuberculosis education comprehensive, integrated, multi-systemic, multi-disciplinary, problem-based and sociologically and epidemiologically orientated. Doctors and nurses must be sensitised to the wider socio-economic and cultural factors in the disease causation and encouraged to see the patients as active participants and not as passive beneficiaries of the control strategy.

Increasing patient awareness and understanding of the disease process is a challenge in doctor-patient communication and, rather than 'victim blaming' and considering the patient as a 'potential defaulter', an attempt must be to enable and empower the patient to adhere to treatment and other procedures.

Skills in listening, motivation and supportive counselling need to be enhanced and humane attitudes and behaviour towards patients, which are primarily non-stigmatising, must be emphasised. Education in pathology and therapeutics must be balanced by instruction in ethics and the social sciences. This is particularly important because the availability of effective chemotherapy has often tended to emphasise the curative aspects of the disease control strategies while disregarding the caring aspects. Tuberculosis is a very stressful disease and, although the clinical manifestations are irksome and often very discomforting, the patient suffers more than just physical illness. It is very important that the curing aspect of disease control strategies becomes more effective, but it is equally important that the caring aspects of the strategies are enhanced.

It is also important to ensure that training moves from didactics and a focus on minutiae to a more interactive, bedside and community-based education that emphasises the practical aspects of the disease and enhances skills in patient care and counselling. Where necessary case studies may replace case demonstrations. But the training must always be rooted in the human problem.

While stressing the component of tuberculosis in medical and nursing education will enhance the leadership of the tuberculosis control team, it is equally important to impart proper knowledge, skills and attitudes in tuberculosis treatment to all grades of health care workers — multi-purpose and community-based — who are often the peripheral health workers. They are most in touch with those who suffer from tuberculosis. An initiative at this level will strengthen first-line/first-level care and will ensure that the patient, who according to most socio-epidemiological surveys is already 'knocking at the health service door' (Narayan, 1998), will be given a supportive and relevant response by adequately sensitive and skilled health workers.

Continuing Education

While the focus on basic professional education will ensure that health professionals of the future will be better informed, better skilled, and better orientated to the socio-epidemiological challenges of tuberculosis control strategies, an urgent need today is to reach the present generation of health care providers with relevant, meaningful, authentic and practical information and updates on tuberculosis to enhance their involvement in, and contribution to, the fight against this disease. For it to be effective, this must be sponsored by professional associations or colleges and the National Health Programmes.

Much of the ongoing education on tuberculosis in many developing countries is presently done by the pharmaceutical industry. The focus and content of education is often orientated towards the promotion of specific prescriptions or remedies over others that are available in the market; to enhancing brand choice and subtly promoting the 'me-too' drugs that have additional, and usually unnecessary, components such as cosmetic embellishments or they may contain irrational combinations of drugs. In addition, they are often inadequately evaluated. Depending on the skills and vigilance of drug controlling agencies and the level and extent of legislation in each country, this 'drug' education is often supported by the subtle misinformation in which indicators for treatment are enhanced and side effects and contraindications are played down, thereby enhancing profits and sales, often at the cost of patient safety. It is not at all surprising that the Report on Health for All Strategy of ICMR/ICSSR (1981) exhorts us that "eternal vigilance is required to ensure that the health care system does not get medicalised, that the doctor-drug producer axis does not exploit the people, and that the 'abundance' of drugs does not become a vested interest in ill health".

In the area of anti-tuberculosis drugs, however, sometimes other forms of irrationality creep into the situation. If such drugs are included in the essential drug list and the prices are controlled, then the mark-up allowed on them is often reduced, leading to a decreased incentive for drug manufacturers to produce them. Shortages of anti-tuberculosis drugs have not been uncommon in the past.

Another challenge in current continuing medical education (CME) is to ensure the emphasis on the use of standardised regimes for treatment which have often been evolved at the national level by expert committees who have considered clinical and epidemiological factors in the situation analysis and have looked at other relevant factors including the availability and cost of drugs and the logistics of their supply and distribution.

A number of very effective drug regimens for tuberculosis have been evolved on the basis of extensive and good clinical and field trials. Unfortunately, private practitioners and even hospital-based clinicians in most countries tend to evolve their own very individualistic, and often irrational, regimes based on what they consider to be 'clinical experience'. Costly and therapeutically unsound regimens, supported by a host of complementary and supplementary medications that are invariably unnecessary, ineffective and irrational are all part of regular practice. At best, these are merely symptomatic and play on the psychology of the patient. A good CME programme in tuberculosis should not only emphasise rational and therapeutically sound regimens but also discourage the use of all types of irrational and unnecessary complementary medication and always stress the social context as well.

Patient/Community Education

Education of the patients, their relatives and those caring for them within the family is an important challenge in tuberculosis control.

While making the patients aware of all aspects of the disease, its prevention and cure, the challenge is to do so by means and orientation that primarily enhance their autonomy, provide informed choices and options for treatment, and enable and empower them to abandon superstition and stigmatising concepts and to take responsibility for their own health. Motivation and supportive counselling must be built into the whole educational effort so that the patients build up confidence in 'cure' in an environment of 'care'. The effort must also emphasise 'care' after 'cure'.

Such effective education is best achieved by culturally sensitive, interactive, low-cost approaches including puppetry, street theatre, folk methods, role play or even flipcharts and flashcards, and planned games whereby the patients learn in small groups, at their own pace, supported by other adult learners in an environment of collective trust and sharing. Whether clinic or community-based, the process of health education is as important as its content (Kaul, 1996).

Case Study: Health Education for Tuberculosis in Urmul Trust (a non-governmental organisation in Rajasthan)

Health education is working on three fronts (Kaul, 1996):

(1) Street theatre and puppet shows in the villages highlight the symptoms of the disease and the need to identify it as early as possible. It also gets the message across that irregular treatment is not only detrimental to the patients but also to people around them so that they must chip in to ensure that the patients take the full course of treatment without a break.

(2) The importance of the regimen and its regularity and duration and what to do in case of side effects are explained to the patients and their relatives in groups. All this is done with the help of television, puppet shows or playlets on the day of the tuberculosis camp held on a fixed day of the month.

(3) The doctor spends at least 15 minutes with each new patient and at least 5 minutes with each old one.

In addition, every few months, some cured patients are assembled to talk to the newer patients. The camp-like atmosphere on a single day of the month encourages the patients to share experiences.

In a country such as India and in most other parts of the developing world, the large majority of the people are illiterate or semi-literate and 'adult learning' techniques need to be used, moving away from the didactic approaches of orthodox education.

Recent studies and experiments done by a group of non-governmental organisations in India have demonstrated that even visual aids used in pamphlets, posters, flipcharts and flannel graphs need to be culturally sensitive and geared to the perceptions of illiterate adults which are rather different from those of urban literate adults. While an understanding of 'magnification' and 'depth perspective' by those who have had some school education including an exposure to scientific concepts and experimentation and demonstration may be taken for granted, these are not comprehended in the same way by adults without a basic school education.

Health education materials must therefore be developed locally and must relate sensitively to local socio-cultural realities. Decentralised health education efforts are therefore a very important component of any health programme strategy.

The centralised production of DOTS-related educational materials and the attempts to distribute so-called standardised, top-down guidelines on contents and messages are the very antithesis of current understanding of adult education for health and are another example of the overemphasis of the 'global' approach in what is essentially a local approach or strategy.

Much health educational material including that currently available for tuberculosis is still rather urban in orientation, context and visual content. A concerted effort needs to be made to ensure that material more relevant to rural and indigenous populations is evolved so that the process of learning and motivation is greatly enhanced.

There is, nowadays, a tendency to get on the 'electronic bandwagon' and videos, slides, cassette sets and even computer software programmes are being promoted. While they have their uses in situations where there is electricity and where people are habituated to such adjuncts to learning and recreation, they are not as widely relevant or as effective as they are often perceived to be. To an illiterate audience, they are often more a source of entertainment than an effective tool for learning and, of course, the absence of continuous electricity in a large number of urban towns and in most rural and tribal areas in many developing countries limits their use and effectiveness. Even in this era of space and cyber technology, traditional and time-tested folk methods and interactive approaches still have great relevance and their importance must not be underestimated or inadvertently played down.

Conclusion: Towards an Alternative Strategy

In these reflections on educational approaches to tuberculosis control, an attempt has been made to highlight the following:

- Tuberculosis control initiatives need to move from the ortho-dox biomedical approach to a more social/community-oriented approach.
- This shift of emphasis will depend upon a creative educational initiative that helps to broaden the understanding of the prob-lem and locate it in the wider social paradigm.
- The focus of education must expand beyond patients and health providers to a wide range of other involved persons including the patients' families, the people in the community where the dis-ease occurs, occupational groups, health care providers includ-ing those in the private and alternative sectors, marginalised social groups, policy makers and society at large.
- The educational process must be primarily enabling and em-powering and must transform the role of the patients from pas-sive beneficiaries to active participants in the programme.
- Treatment and control of tuberculosis must form part of the wider social movement that seeks to address poverty, illiteracy and poor environment, marginalised peoples and unplanned ur-banisation and to increase access to, and options for, health care for the poor. Such a broad-based model would then strike at

the roots of the problem and not fritter away valuable resources in implementing superficial, biomedical, reductionist strategies.

- Health care professionals must be sensitised to the wider socio-economic and cultural factors in the causation of disease and are encouraged to see the patients as active participants in the control strategy rather than passive beneficiaries.

- Skills in listening, motivation and supportive counselling must be enhanced and humane, primarily non-stigmatising, attitudes and behaviour towards patients must be emphasised.

- An initiative at this level will strengthen primary health care and ensure that the tuberculosis patient will be given a supportive and relevant response by sensitive and skilled health workers.

- A good continuing medical education programme in tuberculosis should not only emphasise rational, epidemiologically sound treatment regimens, but also de-emphasise all sorts of irrational and unnecessary complementary medication, as well as stressing the social context.

- Culturally sensitive, interactive, low-cost educational approaches, such as puppetry, street theatre, folk methods, role play or even flipcharts, flashcards and planned games, that enable the patients to learn in small groups, at their own pace and with the support of other adult learners in an environment of collective trust and sharing, must be promoted.

- Health education materials must be locally developed and be both sensitive and relevant to local socio-cultural realities. Decentralised health education efforts are therefore a very important component of any health programme strategy.

- All this will lead to the tuberculosis control initiative becoming more holistic, more responsive, more relevant and definitely more effective in the complex environment and societal reality in which tuberculosis thrives and continues to be a major public health problem today.

The continuing problem of tuberculosis has been accepted all over the world as a major public health issue of our times. Much is planned and much is being done. The sustained success of our efforts will, however, be determined by the extent to which we understand and respond to the challenge of the 'social paradigm' and the creative nature of our supportive educational response. The way forward is a paradigm shift from 'Directly Observed Therapy, Short Course' (DOTS) to 'Community Orientated Tuberculosis Service' (COTS).

Are we ready for this paradigm shift?

References

Banerji, D. (1996) *Serious Implications of the Proposed Revised National Tuberculosis Control Programme for India*. Voluntary Health Association of India /Nucleus for Health Policies and Programmes. New Delhi: Voluntary Health Association of India, pp. 1–100.

Banerji, D. (1997) Voice for the Voiceless — The Revised National Tuberculosis Control Programme: A negligent approach. *Health for the Millions* 23(March-April), pp. 30–32. (Published by Voluntary Health Association of India, New Delhi.)

Chakraborthy, A. K. and Choudhury, S. (1997) *National Tuberculosis Programme: Stopping the Killer*. Bangalore: Action Aid.

CHC (Community Health Cell) (1989) Community health in India. *Health Action* 2, 5–25. (Published by Health Action For All Trust, Secunderbad).

Chaturvedi, G. (1996) Tuberculosis Programme in India: Some social issues. In: Chaturvedi, G. *et al.*, eds. *Tuberculosis Control in India — Developing Role of NGOs*. (Theme in Development series, No. 4). Bangalore: Action Aid, pp. 96–102.

Chaulet, P. (1998) After health sector reform, whither lung health? *Int. J. Tuberc. Lung Dis.* 2, 349–359.

Government of India, (1995) *Revised National Tuberculosis Control Programme with World Bank Assistance*. New Delhi: Government of India.

ICSSR/ICMR (Indian Council of Social Science Research/Indian Council of medical Research) (1981) *Health for All: An Alternative Strategy*. Pune: Indian Institute of Education.

Kaul, S. (1996) Tuberculosis Control under an NGO in Western Rajasthan. In: Chaturvedi, G., *et al.* eds. *Tuberculosis Control in India — Developing Role of NGOs*. (Themes in Development Series No. 4). Bangalore: Action Aid, pp. 37–44.

Medico Friend Circle. (1985) Tuberculosis and society. *Medico Friend Circle Bulletin* No. 111 (March), pp. 1–6 (Published by Medico Friend Circle, Bangalore).

Narayan, R. (1977) Editorial: Resurgence of malaria. *Nat. Med. J. India* 10, 157–158.

Narayan, T. (1997) *Tuberculosis: Persistent Killer*. Chennai, India: The Hindu Survey of Environment, pp. 71–75.

Narayan, T. (1998) *A Study of Policy Process and Implementation of the National Tuberculosis Control Programme in India*. Doctoral Thesis, London School of Hygiene and Tropical Medicine.

National Tuberculosis Institute, (1994) Facts and figures on tuberculosis and the National Tuberculosis Programme. Bangalore: National Tuberculosis Institute, Government of India.

Nikhil, S. N. (1995) Socio-cultural dimensions of tuberculosis. *Health For the Millions* 21 (January–February), pp. 43–46 (Published by Voluntary Health Association of India, New Delhi).

Qadeer, I. (1995) National Tuberculosis Control Programme — A social perspective. *Health For the Millions* 21 (January–February), pp. 10–13 (Published by Voluntary Health Association of India, New Delhi).

Rose, G. (1992) *The Strategy of Preventive Medicine*. Oxford: Oxford Medical Publications, pp. 1–138.

Sadagopal, M. (1983) Health care versus the struggle for life. *Medico Friend Circle Bulletin*. No. 93 (September), pp. 1–5, and No. 94 (October), pp. 2–5 (Published by Medico Friend Circle, Bangalore).

Uplekar, M. and Rangan, S. (1996) *Tackling Tuberculosis: The Search for Solutions*. Bombay: The Foundation for Research in Community Health.

Voluntary Health Association of India (1994) *A Report on the National Consultation on Tuberculosis*. New Delhi: Voluntary Health Association of India.

Voluntary Health Association of India (1996) *Tuberculosis: A Critical Public Health Challenge* (ANUBHAV Series). New Delhi: Voluntary Health Association of India, pp. 1–28.

World Health Organization (1995a) *Stop Tuberculosis at the Source: WHO Report on the Tuberculosis Epidemic*. Geneva: World Health Organization.

World Health Organization (1995b) *Tuberculosis Fact Sheet No. 93*. Geneva: World Health Organization.

World Health Organization/UNAIDS (1996) *Tuberculosis in the Era of HIV*. Geneva: World Health Organization.